SPORTS INJURIES

Lars Peterson is Associate Professor of Orthopedic Surgery at the University of Gothenburg and works from the Eastern Hospital, Gothenburg, Sweden. He is Chairman of the Swedish Society of Sports Medicine, and a member of both the Sports Research Council and the Medical Committee of the International Association of Football.

Per Renström is also Associate Professor of Orthopedic Surgery at the University of Gothenburg and works from Sahlgren's Hospital, Gothenburg, Sweden. He is Vice-Chairman of the Swedish Society of Sports Medicine, and a member of the Scientific Committee of the International Federation of University Sport (FISU).

Both authors are active athletes, with special interests in ice hockey, soccer, cross-country skiing and tennis. They have both held positions in American universities as Visiting Professors and have lectured world-wide on their research work.

SPORTS INJURIES

Their prevention and treatment

Lars Peterson, MD, PhD

Associate Professor, Department of Orthopedic Surgery,
Eastern Hospital, Gothenburg,
Sweden

and

Per Renström, MD, PhD

Associate Professor, Department of Orthopedic Surgery,
Sahlgren's Hospital, Gothenburg,
Sweden

North American editor:
William A Grana, MD
Associate Professor, Division of Sports Medicine,
Department of Orthopedic Surgery,
University of Oklahoma School of Medicine,
Oklahoma City, Oklahoma

Foreword by Robert J Johnson, MD
Professor of Orthopedic Surgery,
Head of the Division of Sports Medicine,
University of Vermont College of Medicine,
Burlington, Vermont

YEAR BOOK MEDICAL
PUBLISHERS INC
CHICAGO

© Lars Peterson/Per Renström 1983
Originally published in Sweden in cooperation with the Swedish
Sports Federation and Folksam Insurance Company

© Martin Dunitz Ltd
English Language edition 1986

Published 1986 by Year Book Medical Publishers Inc
35 East Wacker Drive, Chicago, Ill. 60601

First published in the United Kingdom in 1986
by Martin Dunitz Ltd, London

Library of Congress Cataloging in Publication Data

Peterson, Lars.
  Sports injuries

  Translation of: Skador inom idrotten.
  Bibliography: p. 463
  Includes index.
  1. Sports – Accidents and injuries. I. Renström, Per.
II. Title. (DNLM: 1. Athletic Injuries. QT 260 P485s)
RD97.P4813   1986   617'.1027   84–25658
ISBN 0–8151–6678–8

Phototypeset in Ehrhardt by Input Typesetting Ltd, London
Printed and bound in Singapore
by Kyodo Shing Loong Printing Industries Pte. Ltd.

Contents

General Principles of Sports Injuries 18

Acute Treatment of Athletes at the scene of the injury 64

The Biomechanics of Sports Injuries 71 (*Olle Bunketorp*)

Preventive Measures 86

5

Methods of Treatment 150

6

Sports Injuries by Specific Area 174

Foreword

Robert J. Johnson, M.D.
Professor of Orthopedic Surgery, Head of Division of Sports Medicine, University of Vermont College of Medicine, Burlington, Vermont
The work that follows should be of specific interest, and is strongly recommended, to coaches, trainers, physical therapists, school nurses, physicians, athletes, and all others interested in the varied problems of sports medicine. The thrust of the book is to provide, in an organized manner, the general principles of care for most injuries and conditions that afflict athletes. It provides, in a clear fashion, the major treatment options available to the physician as well as the athlete and allied health personnel. Specific valuable advice is provided concerning the diagnosis of both common and unusual conditions. Much emphasis is placed on the rehabilitation of athletes following injury and, of equal importance, the means of preventing injury.

The authors are well-known authorities on many facets of sports medicine in Scandinavia, and are well respected worldwide by their colleagues. Dr Peterson is presently Associate Professor of Orthopedic Surgery, as well as a boarded General Surgeon at the University of Gothenburg's Eastern Hospital. He is currently President of the Swedish Sports Medicine Society, and a member of the International Soccer Federation's (FIFA) medical committee. He is a member of the Swedish Sports Research Council, as well as other national and international sports medicine organizations. Dr Renström is an Associate Professor of Orthopedic Surgery at the University of Gothenburg's Sahlgren's Hospital. He is Vice-President of the Swedish Sports Medicine Society, and is a member of the International University Sports Federation's scientific committee. Both Dr Peterson and Dr Renström have published numerous articles and scientific papers on sports medicine subjects. They also pursue vigorous and athletic endeavors themselves and have cared for numerous sports teams, both regionally and internationally.

This unusually well-illustrated text was originally published in Swedish in 1977, and was extensively revised in 1983, and again in 1986 for this translated edition. It has previously been published in Russian, Danish, Finnish, Dutch and German. In addition to this English translation, it is presently being translated into French and Japanese. To date, over 100,000 copies have been printed, attesting to its popular appeal in the various countries. This work has been utilized as a text in the education of physical therapists, trainers and nurses. I believe that Dr Renström and Dr Peterson are to be congratulated heartily for their efforts in providing the sports medicine world with a text of this quality, and I know that readers will find it enjoyable and informative.

INTRODUCTION

Sports injuries occur as a result of physical activities carried out either for general recreational purposes or with more professional goals in mind. They may be caused by accidents or by overuse, and they do not necessarily differ from injuries sustained in non-sporting activities.

Most sports injuries are minor and would not prevent the average athlete from continuing his daily work, but as many people become more seriously committed to sporting activities, continuing daily work is no longer the only consideration. The injury must be treated effectively so that leisure activity can also be resumed at the earliest opportunity.

Those athletes who participate at championship level require not only correct diagnosis of their injuries but also early treatment with complete healing so that they can continue to produce good performances with as short an absence as possible from their sporting activity. Even the more casual enthusiast, upon whom demands are not so great, may suffer both physically and psychologically as a result of minor injuries and may be prevented from pursuing the sport which usually contributes significantly to his sense of well-being and to the quality of his life.

Progress in diagnosis and treatment is rapid in the field of sports medicine, and to keep this book abreast of recent developments we have revised it extensively since it was first written. Our thanks are due to the many people who have contributed their expertise towards this new edition which we hope will satisfy a need in the world of sport and be of use to athletes, their trainers and their medical advisers.

In a complex subject such as sports medicine, good illustrations are of greatest importance. Illustrations in the first edition of this book were prepared by Tommy Bolic Eriksson who fulfilled our intentions skillfully and with great imagination. These illustrations are retained in this book and have been coloured by Tommy Berglund who has also produced a large number of excellent additional coloured illustrations. Tommy Berglund has shown his great ability to understand and illustrate our ideas.

Our friend, Ole Roos, who is the photographer at the Sahlgren's Hospital in Göteborg, has given us his support and professional help at all times of the day with the photographs in the book. His professional skills are gratefully acknowledged.

A basic knowledge of biomechanics is necessary in order to understand the mechanism behind injuries. Our friend and colleague, Dr Olle Bunketorp, has written the chapter on biomechanics and for this we are very grateful.

Careful and planned rehabilitation is essential after an injury. We therefore considered a detailed description of rehabilitative training to be of importance in this book. Eva Faxén, RPT, who is working with us at the Skåtas Sports Medicine Clinic and at the hospitals, has put much work, ideas and energy into the rehabilitation chapter and we are extremely grateful to her for her work. Valuable advice has also been given by Roland Thomée, RPT.

In managing the original Swedish edition, Editor Kerstin M. Stålbrand made an invaluable contribution with her excellent scrutinizing of the language and for her numerous and intelligent comments.

The second edition, which has been widely extended with the inclusion of coloured photographs, would not have been published in this way without the imagination, risk-taking and whole-hearted support from Ebbe Carlsson, former head of Tidens Förlag Publishing House in Sweden.

For work on this English edition, we want to thank Dr Kate Hope, Great Britain for her valuable contributions to editorial details and for her suggestions on the realistic treatment of sports injuries in Great Britain. We grately appreciate her beautiful language.

We would also like to thank Editor Sally Jones for her continuous support, careful scrutinizing of every detail, and for her patience with all our comments and delays.

Our colleague and friend, Dr Mark Pitman in New York, has read the manuscript and given many valuable suggestions. Mark has also been kind enough to write a section on throwing injuries, making particular reference to baseball injuries which are more of a problem in the United States than in Scandinavia. We are grateful to Mark for his support.

We would also like to thank Professor Robert J. Johnson, Burlington, Vermont for his support and for his kind foreword to the American edition.

Professor Moira O'Brien, Dublin, Ireland has carefully read the whole manuscript. She has given many valuable comments based on her long experience in sports medicine and for this we are very grateful.

We would like to thank the Swedish Sports Federation and Folksam Insurance Company for their help in the production of this book.

Many other friends and colleagues have given their views on parts of the manuscript and we want to thank Professor Bengt Saltin, Dr Ann-Sofie Saltin, Professor Nils Svedmyr, Associate Professor Tore Mellstrand, Associate Professor Bengt Eriksson, Professor Bertil Stener, Professor Ian Goldie, Dr Ake Andien-Sandberg, Bengt Sevelius – Managing Director of the Swedish Sports Federation and Nils Stjernfeldt, Arne Brundell, Yngve Tillborg and Tore Brodd for their assistance and constructive criticism.

We are happy that this book has caught the interest of so many people. The contents of this book may sometimes be controversial. A book like this contains a large number of facts which are based and coloured by our own philosophy and by our personal experiences.

Göteborg in February, 1986

Lars Peterson   Per Renström

SPORTS AND INJURIES

'If we could give every individual the right amount of nourishment and exercise, not too little and not too much, we would have found the safest way to health.' Hippocrates 460—377 BC

Despite Hippocrates' statement made almost twenty-five centuries ago, it is only recently that sport has been widely accepted as an integral part of keeping fit. Enthusiasts rightly encourage participation in sport as one aspect of leading a healthy life, but it should be remembered that 'fitness' is not the same as 'good health' and that physical activity can only contribute to fitness when undertaken on a regular basis and supported by good dietary habits.

Sport — the essence of keeping fit
Even in the absence of scientific proof, few people doubt the beneficial effects of sport on their fitness and sense of well-being. They see physical effects in the strengthening of muscles, improved mobility and balance, increased stamina and better weight control; and at the same time it extends their recreational and social lives. In medical terms there are strong indications that regular physical activity contributes towards preventing cardiovascular disease and delaying the onset of those degenerative disorders which are an inevitable part of ageing.

Awareness of the potential benefits of exercise, together with a changing social and economic climate, has meant that most of us now have a considerable amount of leisure time at our disposal, and has led to an explosion in the numbers of people participating in sports on a regular basis. Simultaneously there has been a change in attitudes in competitive sport which has meant greater pressure upon individuals to produce ever more spectacular results. Both developments have involved increased pressure on medical services. Fortunately, there has not been a marked increase in the incidence of injuries caused by accidents, perhaps because basic training and equipment have improved. The incidence of injuries caused by overuse, however, has increased as more people have started jogging and taking part in events such as marathons which were once regarded as being suitable only for experienced athletes. Many overuse injuries can and should be prevented by a wider knowledge of preventive measures and their application.

Although this book deals with the injuries which are one of sport's drawbacks, it is worthwhile remembering that, overall, the advantages gained from sporting activity both by the individual and by society as a whole, far outweigh the disadvantages. Add to this the fact that many athletes are young and active individuals, and it becomes clear that increased resources in sports medicine for prevention, treatment and rehabilitation make sound economic sense.

Physical activity is of value to all the tissues of the body, providing it is performed correctly.

IMPORTANT FACTORS IN RELATION TO SPORTS INJURIES

For every sport, a number of factors of varying degrees of importance must be considered in relation to injury.

1. The athlete's qualifications

— *Age* affects the strength and resilience of the tissues. Muscular strength begins to decline at the relatively early age of thirty to forty years, while elasticity in tendons and ligaments decreases from the age of thirty and the strength of bone after the age of fifty.

Inactivity accelerates the natural degeneration of muscles, tendons, ligaments, articular surfaces and bone structure, while activity tends to delay it. Physical achievement reaches its peak between the ages of twenty and forty, unlike intellectual ability which is at its best between thirty and sixty years of age.

— *Personal characteristics* such as temperament and maturity may affect the athlete's tendency to take or to avoid risks.

— *Experience* is important. Beginners often suffer more injuries than experienced athletes.

— *Level of training* is significant since injuries occur more often at the beginning of the season and towards the end of matches and are caused by inadequate basic physical fitness. Too much training, on the other hand, may cause injuries as a result of overuse.

— *Technique* is of the greatest importance to anyone taking part in such sports as high jump, javelin throwing and tennis. Faulty technique can contribute to overuse syndromes and cause traumatic injuries, for example, in Alpine skiing.

— *An insufficient warm-up period* may contribute to muscle and tendon injuries.

— *Intensive competition and training programmes* which do not allow a sufficient recovery period after maximum effort increase the risk of injury.

— *Health problems* (for example, infections and flu-like illnesses) increase the risk of complications such as inflammation of cardiac muscle. No athlete should participate in training or competition until his temperature has returned to normal after an illness.

— *A balanced and nutritious diet*, including adequate fluids, is a prerequisite for sporting activities.

— *General measures*, including sufficient rest and sleep, and avoiding alcohol, reduce the risk of injury.

2. Sports equipment and facilities

— *Equipment* used in any sport may be inadequate, poorly designed and/or defective.
— *Protective clothing* can be faulty, insufficient or even discarded.
— *Sports facilities* are not always suitable for the activities for which they are used.
— *Lighting* of the sports area may affect the judgement of distances, the perception of colours and the athlete's visual acuity.
— *Unsuitable weather conditions* increase the risk of injury.

3. Characteristics of sports

Different sports make different demands on the athlete. Competitive sport perhaps involves an increased risk of injury, but some people have a positive need to participate at this level and gain great satisfaction from doing so. Top athletes are often held up as examples to the young who are encouraged to attend sports grounds and running tracks as a result. Also, top level sport arouses great public interest and plays an important part in the everyday life of many people, so is not to be discouraged.

Regardless of the level at which it is played, each sport is unique in terms of the demands it places on participants and its special characteristics which can cause both overuse and traumatic injuries.

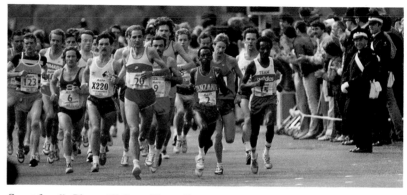

Sport for all. *Photo: All-Sport/Trevor Jones.*

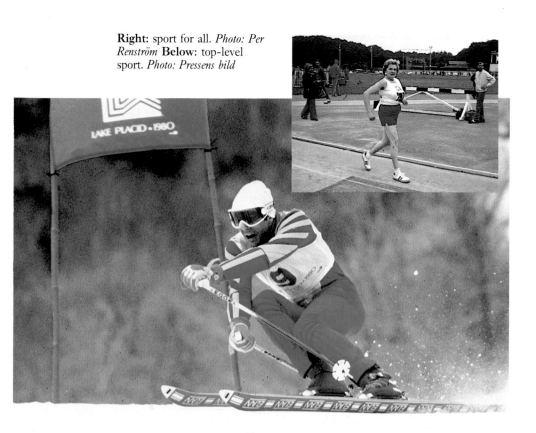

Right: sport for all. *Photo: Per Renström* **Below:** top-level sport. *Photo: Pressens bild*

SPORTS MEDICINE — A DEFINITION

Sports medicine encompasses the following elements: preparation and training, prevention of injuries and illness, diagnosis and treatment of injuries and illness, and rehabilitation and return to active participation in sport. This definition relates to the athlete, the sport, sporting equipment and diagnostic instrumentation.

Preparation and training

Preparation and training includes instruction in training methods, technique, dietary requirements, the negative effects of drugs and alcohol, and psychological preparation for competition.

Training methods

A good, general conditioning achieved through, for example interval and endurance training programmes, is the basis of all sporting activities, though there are many other factors involved in creating a good athlete.

Strength training includes isometric exercise and different types of dynamic training. A good example of an effective dynamic strength training

15

method which has been developed in recent years is isokinetic strength training in which muscles are made to work against accomodating resistance. Increased flexibility can be achieved by stretching exercises — a modern form of mobility training which has proved to be very effective in preventing injuries to muscles, tendons and joints. General conditioning, strength and flexibility exercises are essential for all sport-specific training and aim to improve skill in each sport.

Technique

Technique is improving constantly in most sports. As sport becomes more demanding, correct techniques are crucial if inadvertent overuse injury is to be avoided.

Diet

Physiologists have described how important it is for the athlete to follow a balanced diet before and after training sessions and competitions and to compensate for fluid loss during and after exercise. It is surprising how many athletes are unaware of these facts. It is important to maintain a well-balanced diet before, during and after practice and competition.

Drugs and alcohol

Taking drugs to improve performance is nothing short of cheating and can increase the risk of injury. All forms of drug-taking in connection with sport are to be deplored.

Alcohol has deleterious effects upon performance for up to 48 hours after consumption, which again increases the risk of injury and tends to cancel out the beneficial effects of training. Sport and alcohol should not be combined.

Tobacco, too, has a detrimental effect on performance in addition to its other harmful side-effects.

Psychological preparation

Performance is in many ways dependent upon psychological preparation, and a well-balanced and motivated athlete will usually perform well even though psychological effects may be difficult to evaluate scientifically.

Prevention of injury and illness

The prevention of illness and injury in sport depends, at least in part, on appropriate clothing (including protective clothing), equipment, rules, facilities and health controls.

Clothing

In many sports, shoes or boots are the most important items of clothing. They should be designed to meet the demands made on the foot by each particular sport; today's market offers plenty of choice for all types of sporting activity. Joggers, for example, require shoes which give adequate support and a sole thick enough to provide shock absorption on hard running surfaces, whereas those involved in court games such as squash require shoes which provide them with a closer contact with the court surface. In Alpine skiing, the design of boots, bindings and skis has improved significantly to decrease the incidence of injury, but has resulted in a changed injury panorama.

Protective clothing	Specialized protective clothing has been developed for many sports such as fencing, ice hockey, cricket, baseball, American football and riding. Pioneers in sports medicine have made efforts not only to ensure that such protective clothing (equipment) achieves the required standards but also to ensure that it is used.
Equipment and rules	Equipment used in sport can itself cause injury, particularly if it is used incorrectly. Both equipment and the rules of the game should be amended if they are in any way likely to contribute towards causing injury.
Sports facilities	At one time only technology and economics were considered when sports facilities were built — medical expertise was not consulted. Now times are changing and the authorities have realized, for instance, that surfaces and turfs should be designed and constructed to take account of the demands to be made upon them by different sporting activities.
Routine medical examinations	Routine medical examinations can never entirely eliminate the possibility of latent cardiovascular disease, but they can be useful in revealing hidden infections and areas weakened by old injuries. They are probably most useful when they are carried out on a selective basis according to the particular sport in question. Examinations before competition and at the beginning of the season are important because they highlight the athlete's risk areas and help the trainer to design specific training programmes. In most sports, an evaluation of the musculo-skeletal system is of special value.

Diagnosis and treatment of injury and illness

Serious acute injuries are generally treated adequately in hospital and it is the sub-acute and chronic injuries which present more of a problem to the coach or trainer in sport. Meniscal and overuse injuries, including inflammation of periosteum, tendons and bursae, are often difficult to diagnose and treat and are not always well understood.

Rehabilitation and return to sporting activities

Injuries heal at varying paces depending on their severity and location. If rehabilitation is to be complete, it is essential that whoever is treating the injury should have a thorough knowledge of the healing process in different tissues and should also be thoroughly familiar with the demands of the sport concerned. Then the various elements of the rehabilitation programme can be introduced appropriately to ensure a successful return to active sport.

General Principles of Sports Injuries

INJURIES DUE TO TRAUMA

Skeletal injuries (fractures)

Skeletal injuries are relatively common in sport, especially in contact sports such as soccer, rugby, American football, team handball, field and ice hockey, and in individual sports such as Alpine and crosscountry skiing, gymnastics and riding.

A fracture should be considered a potentially serious injury since not only is the skeleton injured but also the soft tissues in the immediate surrounding area, that is, tendons, ligaments, muscles, nerves, blood vessels and skin. Fractures may occur as a result of direct trauma, for

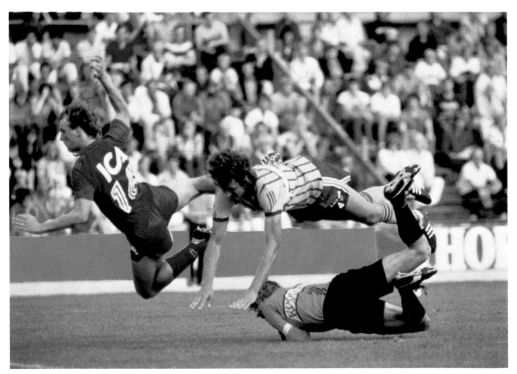

Situation picture giving warning of possible injury. *Photo: Bernt Claeson/Pressens bild*

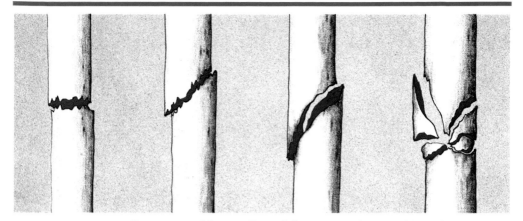

Different types of fracture **From left:** transverse fracture, oblique fracture, spiral fracture and comminuted fracture.

example an impact to the leg, or indirect trauma, as when the foot is trapped causing the athlete to fall awkwardly and break his leg.

Types of injury Skeletal fractures may be classified as transverse, oblique, spiral or comminuted (see diagram above). When the fractured ends of the bone pierce the skin the injury is known as an *open* or *compound fracture*. When the skin remains undamaged it is a *closed* or *simple fracture*. With compound fractures there is a great risk of infection in the bone, and special treatment is required. If the fracture involves an adjacent articular joint surface it is called an *articular surface fracture*. An *avulsion fracture* means that a bone attached to a muscle or ligament has been torn away.

The different types of fracture displacement are: angulation, rotation and shortening. The aim of any treatment should be to return the fractured ends as precisely as possible into their correct position, that is, to reduce displacement and return the bone to its normal alignment by manipulation.
For fractures in children and adolescents see page 409.

Location The sport being played at the time of injury may well determine the site of a fracture. Fractures of the lower leg predominate amongst soccer players, whilst fractures of the forearm are common in gymnasts and fractures of the clavicle in riders.

Associated soft tissue injuries The soft tissues around a fracture are often damaged at the same time, by sharp fragments of bone (see diagram on page 20), and the more violent the impact the greater the risk of extensive soft tissue injury. Such injuries can increase haemorrhage and delay healing and may, in fact, cause more problems than the fracture itself.
It is rare for major blood vessels and nerves to be damaged when a fracture occurs, but this may be a complication of fractures of the humerus just above the elbow and fractures of the wrist.

Symptoms and diagnosis The following features suggest that a fracture has occurred:
— Swelling and progressive bruising in the injured area as a result of damage to the soft tissues and small blood vessels.

19

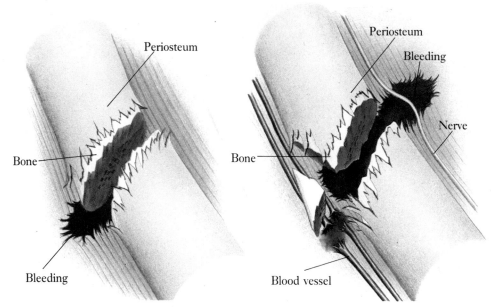

Fracture with bleeding and rupture of the periosteum.

Fracture with bleeding and rupture of the periosteum, also affecting nerves and blood vessels.

— Tenderness and pain around the site of injury caused by both movement and loading of the limb.
— Deformity and abnormal mobility of the fractured bone.

In certain circumstances, fractures may cause few or none of these signs and symptoms. This can be true of fractures of the neck of the femur or of the humerus when the fractured surfaces of the bone are driven into each other, becoming firmly impacted and giving the fracture stability.

Treatment

When a fracture is suspected, the *athlete* or *trainer* should:
— cover an open injury with a clean bandage or cloth;
— immobilize the limb by splinting;
— elevate the injured limb;
— arrange transport to hospital for treatment and possibly X-ray examination as soon as possible. There will be many situations when no aids, such as bandages or splints, are available, in which case improvisation is necessary. Clean handkerchiefs, belts, straps, items of clothing and sporting equipment can all be used. Elegance is not important, but effective immobilization is essential if pain and further injury are to be prevented. It is usual for an injured upper limb to be supported by strapping it to the body, and for an injured leg to be strapped to the other leg. Immobilization should include the joints on either side of the fracture.

It is the *doctor's* function to correct any significant displacement as soon as possible in order to control bleeding, reduce pain and improve blood supply.
— In cases of fracture without displacement, the injured part is immobilized and supported by the application of a plaster cast. Ambulatory

treatment and early protected motion can be important in many fractures and may allow an early return to training and competiton. This can be achieved by use of fracture bracing, orthotics and, in some cases, by external fixation (that is, using a frame system).

— In cases of fracture with displacement, the fractured ends are re-aligned by manipulation (reduced) either without surgery (a *closed* procedure), or with surgery (an *open* procedure). In the latter case, internal fixation of the fracture is achieved by the use of cerclage (steel wire), screws, rods, pins or nails. Internal fixation usually also requires the application of a plaster cast, which can be removed after a comparatively short time. Some cases of internal fixation allow early immobilization without a plaster cast.

After-care Active muscular exercises such as flexing and lifting (see pages 419–462)

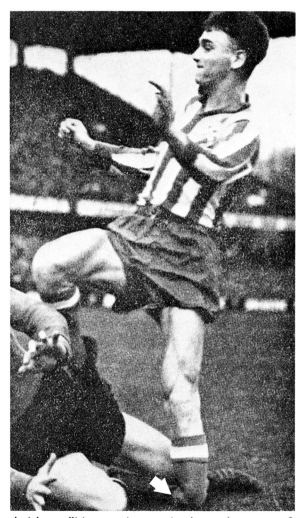

A violent collision may, in exceptional cases, have very unfortunate consequences. In this case the impact was so violent that both the ankle bones were broken (see arrow). The player, however, recovered completely and could play football again one year after the accident.

must involve all parts of the body not enclosed in plaster to maintain general cardiovascular fitness and avoid muscle atrophy. Muscles inside the plaster casts can be exercised isometrically. Sometimes the cast allows joint motion — a so-called cast brace — and then dynamic exercises can be included.

The length of time spent in plaster varies from case to case according to the location of the fracture, its severity and the rate of progression through the healing process. A fracture of the wrist, for example, may be immobilized for 4–6 weeks, whereas a fracture of the lower leg is likely to be in plaster for at least 3 months. Once the plaster is removed, at least an equal period of time needs to be spent undergoing rehabilitation.

Joint ligament injuries

A joint is formed by cartilaginous articular surfaces covering the ends of adjoining bones. Not all joints are identical in structure, but, in general, one articular surface is convex (the ball) and the other concave (the socket), the two fitting together to a varying degree in different joints. In the hip, for example, the ball is almost entirely surrounded by the socket, while the 'sockets' of the knee and finger joints are very shallow.

The opposing ends of the bones are joined by a capsule of connective tissue which surrounds the joint. The joint capsule is lined by a membrane which secretes synovial fluid, and, at points where the strain imposed on the joint is greatest, is strengthened and protected by bands of connective tissue (ligaments) which also limit abnormal movement. The entire joint is surrounded by muscles and tendons.

The stability of a joint is influenced by both active and passive factors. Active stability is maintained by muscle activity, which is under the control of the individual, while passive stability is maintained mainly by the ligaments. Without adequate passive stability a joint is unable to function normally.

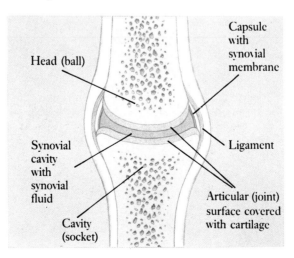

Head (ball)

Capsule with synovial membrane

Synovial cavity with synovial fluid

Ligament

Cavity (socket)

Articular (joint) surface covered with cartilage

Example of the structure of a joint.

Types of ligament injury A ligamentous injury occurs when a joint is forced beyond its normal range of movement. A ligament tear may affect any number of ligament fibres, from a few to the entire ligament.

1. A *partial* tear by definition involves only part of the ligament fibres and does not affect joint stability.
   a)   Part of the ligament may be torn, while the rest is undamaged (see diagram 1a below).
   b) & c) Part of the ligament attachment may have been torn away from its insertion, with or without a fragment of bone (see diagrams 1b and 1c below).

2. A *complete* tear involves most, or all, of the ligament fibres, and the affected joint is unstable.
   a) The ligament may be totally torn and the ends separated from each other (see diagram 2a below).
   b) The entire ligament attachment may have become detached from the bone (see diagram 2b below).

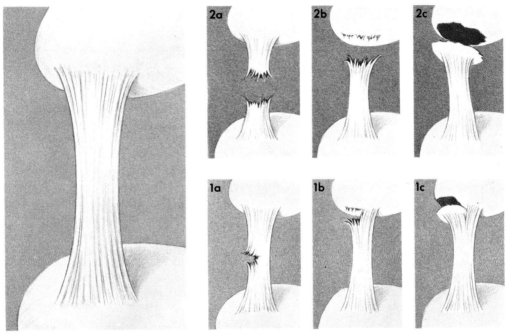

Examples of different types of partial and total ligament ruptures. See the section 'Types of injury' opposite.

   c) The fragment of bone to which the ligament is attached may have been torn away from the rest of the bone (see diagram 2c above).

A partial tear corresponds to a grade I tear (disruption of a few fibres) and a minor grade II tear (disruption of less than half the fibres). In both cases, the joint is stable. A complete tear corresponds to a major grade II tear (disruption of more than 50 per cent of the fibres) and a grade III tear (disruption of all the fibres). In both cases the joint is unstable.

A disruption of the fibres of the ligament is often accompanied by bleeding which spreads into surrounding tissues and is frequently seen as bruising.

Injury to a ligament within the joint or to the joint capsule may cause haemorrhage into the joint space. Injuries to the ligaments can also be accompanied by damage to the articular cartilage surfaces.

Location	Joint and ligament injuries are common in sport and occur most frequently in the ankle, knee, elbow, wrist and shoulder.
Symptoms and diagnosis	The following symptoms suggest that a ligament injury has occurred: — Bleeding causing bruising, swelling and tenderness around the affected joint. — Bleeding causing a haemarthrosis. — Pain when the limb is moved or loaded. — Instability of the joint depending upon the extent of injury. (compare partial and complete tear).

In all cases of ligament injury, the joint should be tested for stability.

Treatment	In cases of acute ligament injury, the *athlete* or *trainer* should: — apply cooling (for example, an ice pack) to the joint; — support the joint by elastic bandaging; — encourage rest and unloading of the injured area; — elevate the limb according to the guidelines on page 68. The *doctor's* function is to: — determine the stability of the joint by stability testing. Especially with a knee joint injury, proceed to arthroscopy (see page 294), and if the pain is severe, perform stability testing under anaesthetic; — if the joint is stable, provide early mobilization exercises or apply a supportive adhesive strapping, tape or cast for a short period of a few days to some weeks, depending upon the type, the seriousness and the location of the injury; — if the joint is *unstable*, decide whether the treatment should be non-operative with early protected motion exercises; *or* application of supportive adhesive strapping, tape, brace or cast, followed by a cast brace for a period for 3–6 weeks depending upon the type, seriousness and location of the injury; *or* decide on surgical treatment of the unstable joint.
Rehabilita-tion	Active muscular exercise and mobility training is of the greatest importance during the rehabilitation phase and should be carried out with co-operation between the athlete, trainer, coach, doctor and physiotherapist. The healing of a ligament after an injury can take a long time (usually more than 6 weeks). During the healing process, the ligament should be protected to some extent and strapping, taping (see page 158) and bracing (see page 122) are of value at this stage. Early motion exercises for the joint as a whole are desirable but they might create a dilemma for the doctor applying treatment. They must not affect the healing of the injured ligament.

Dislocations

Types of injury	As described above, all joints are surrounded by a joint capsule and ligaments. For a dislocation to occur, at least part of the capsule and its

ligaments must be torn; therefore any dislocation involves injuries to these structures and sometimes to the articular cartilage. Rehabilitation will depend upon how quickly these damaged tissues heal.

Total dislocation (luxation) of a joint indicates that the opposing articular surfaces have become separated and are no longer in contact with each other. *Partial* dislocation (subluxation) of a joint indicates that the articular surfaces remain in partial contact with each other but are no longer correctly aligned. Again, there may be capsule, ligament and cartilage injuries.

Location

Total dislocations most frequently affect the shoulder, elbow, finger joints and patella, while partial dislocations usually affect the knee, ankle and acromioclavicular joint.

Treatment

When a dislocation occurs or is suspected, the *athlete* or *trainer* should:
— treat the affected joint with cooling and rest;
— arrange immediate transport to a doctor.

The *doctor's* function is to reduce the joint, that is, to manipulate the articular surfaces of the bones back to their normal positions performed with the patient under anaesthetic. This is usually done after a preliminary X-ray to ensure that no fractures are present.

Further treatment is aimed at restoring the stability and function of the joint. Depending upon the degree of instability present, the doctor will suggest the most suitable treatment for the joint involved. This can include early mobilization with strength training or immobilization for a varying period of time (1–6 weeks) and, thereafter, exercises or surgical treatment. Injuries may recur in the shoulder joint and the patella; young athletes are particularly susceptible especially after inadequate treatment and/or rehabilitation. Dislocations may be complicated by damage to nerves and blood vessels.

> In the absence of a fracture or dislocation, all injuries which cause swelling in and/or around joints and all sprains associated with bleeding, swelling and tenderness should be treated as ligament injuries.

Muscle injuries – strains

Muscle injuries are amongst the commonest, most misunderstood and inadequately treated conditions in sports medicine. Their significance is often underestimated because most patients can continue their daily activities soon after injury. According to some studies, muscle injuries account for 10–30 per cent of all injuries in sport. Furthermore, it has been found that 30 per cent of all soccer injuries are muscle injuries.

Muscles can be damaged both by direct trauma (impact) and by indirect trauma (overloading). The resulting injuries can be divided into ruptures and haematomas.

Ruptures can be total or partial and may be subdivided into distraction and compression ruptures.

Haematomas may be either inter- or intramuscular and there are major differences between the treatment and prognosis of the two types.

Muscle injuries are usually benign but often annoying for the athlete because inadequate treatment can cause long absences from sporting activity. Some knowledge of the normal structure and function of muscles is necessary in order to understand how injuries may best be prevented and treated.

Muscle structure

The human body possesses more than 300 clearly defined muscles comprising about 40 per cent of the total body weight.

Each muscle has an upper origin (head) and a lower insertion, with the

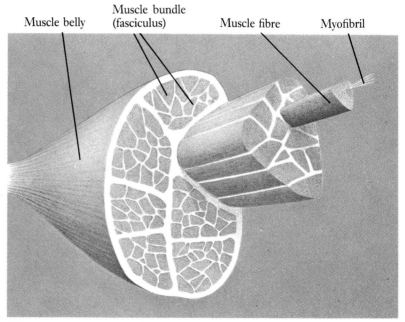

Muscle belly   Muscle bundle (fasciculus)   Muscle fibre   Myofibril

Schematic representation of the structure of a muscle.

bulky part between them (known as the belly) forming the actively contracting portion. The muscle often has a tendon by which it is attached to the skeleton (at the so-called muscle–tendon junction). A skeletal muscle is composed of thousands of long, narrow muscle cells or fibres containing contractile elements and is surrounded by a membrane or sheath. The muscle fibres are bound together in bundles (fasciculi) which, in turn, combine to form the muscle belly. In some muscles, the belly is divided into several parts. Each belly has its own origin or head, a muscle with two heads being known as a biceps, three heads a triceps, and four heads a quadriceps.

There are two types of muscle fibre — *slow* (type I or red) and *fast* (type II or white). Slow fibres obtain their energy from oxygen via the

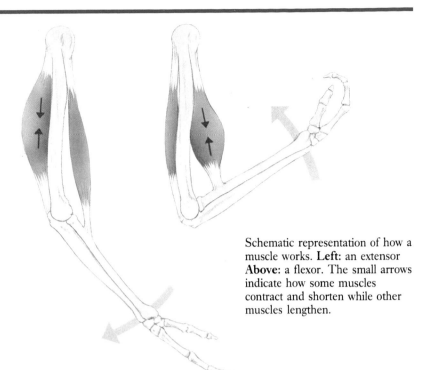

Schematic representation of how a muscle works. **Left:** an extensor **Above:** a flexor. The small arrows indicate how some muscles contract and shorten while other muscles lengthen.

blood stream, while fast fibres obtain theirs from glucose which is stored in muscular glycogen and converted into energy without the use of oxygen (anaerobically). Slow fibres, in comparison to fast fibres, are smaller in size, have a lower anaerobic glycolytic capacity and a slower speed of contraction; they are supplied with a greater network of small blood vessels (capillaries), fewer nerves and have a lower level of endurance. The slow fibres respond very well to dynamic exercise while the fast fibres respond better to static exercise especially of high intensity. The fast fibres are subdivided into types IIa and IIb. The former are characterized by great strength lasting over a long period, and the latter by similar strength over a short period. When a muscle is contracted, the different fibres are activated sequentially — type I, followed by type IIa and finally type IIb.

There are considerable variations in the composition of individual muscles. The most usual combination is that of equal numbers of fast and slow fibres, but in an athlete who participates in endurance sports (for example, marathon running) there will be a preponderance of slow fibres while in a sprinter there will be more fast fibres. A knowledge of fibre distribution in muscles is important when training for specific sports.

Muscle tissue is invested with an extensive network of small blood vessels (the capillaries) averaging about 3,000 per sq mm on cross section. When the muscle is at rest, 95 per cent of the capillaries are closed, but when physical activity is undertaken they open progressively to ensure an ample blood flow to the working tissue.

Training results in the following effects on muscle:
— muscle enzymes (protein catalysts) increase;
— the number of units (mitochondria) in which energy conversion takes place increases;

— storage of fuel for the production of energy increases;
— the capillary network increases;
— muscular volume increases (hypertrophy).

This combination of effects increases muscle strength, stability, stamina and a capacity for rapid contraction. Various types of muscle training are described on page 89.

Types of injury to the muscle–tendon complex

Muscles and tendons function together as units. In principle, injuries can affect the muscle origin, the muscle belly, the point at which muscle and tendon merge (the muscle–tendon junction), the tendon itself, and the insertion of the tendon into bone and periosteum (see diagram below).

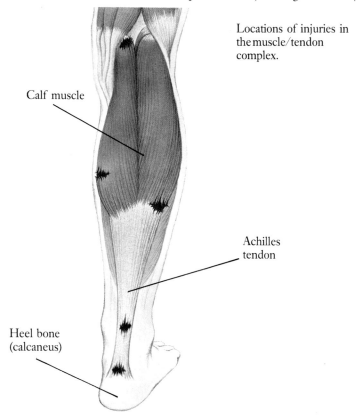

Locations of injuries in the muscle/tendon complex.

Calf muscle

Achilles tendon

Heel bone (calcaneus)

Muscle ruptures

A muscle fibre is a highly specialized unit which responds rapidly and adapts quickly to change. Damaged muscle can heal quickly, with fibres reformed in about 3 weeks. When injury occurs, however, there is almost inevitably some degree of bleeding and this can affect the healing process mechanically by reducing contact between the ruptured ends of the muscle fibres. If bleeding can be controlled, healing is more likely to be quick and complete.

Sporting activities can cause a number of different types of muscle rupture.

1. *Distraction* ruptures. These are caused by overstretching or overload, and are often located in the superficial parts of muscles or at their insertions and origins. These ruptures occur as a result of the intrinsic force an athlete can generate in his own muscles.
2. *Compression* ruptures. These occur as a result of direct impact (trauma). The muscle is pressed against the underlying bone, for example when a player's knee hits another's thigh during a soccer game, and heavy bleeding deep within the muscle may result.

A distinction should be made between *total* ruptures, when all the muscle fibres are torn, and *partial* ruptures which involve only some fibres.

Factors which contribute to muscle ruptures

A number of factors are important in contributing towards the occurrence of muscle ruptures:

— the muscle may have been poorly prepared because of inadequate training or lack of warm-up;
— the muscle may have been weakened by previous injury followed by faulty rehabilitation;
— the muscle may previously have been extensively injured with resultant scar tissue formation. (Scar tissue is less elastic than muscle and, therefore, more liable to recurrent injury);
— a muscle which is overstrained or fatigued is injured more easily;
— tense muscles which do not allow a full range of joint movement may be injured in sports demanding flexibility;
— muscles subjected to prolonged exposure to cold are less contractile than normal.

In sports demanding maximum muscular work extended over a period of 0.5–4 minutes, for example, weight training, Alpine skiing or 200m free-style swimming, the formation of lactic acid within muscle cells is one of the factors which limits performance. The cell environment is disturbed to such an extent that its usual chemical processes are disordered resulting in impaired co-ordination and an increased risk of injury.

Distraction ruptures

Distraction ruptures frequently occur in sports that require explosive muscular effort over a short period of time, for example in baseball, sprinting, jumping, American football and soccer. When the demand made upon a muscle exceeds its innate strength, rupture may occur; for example, in overload during eccentric muscle contractions. Other examples in sport include sudden stopping, deceleration (eccentric work), rapid acceleration (concentric work) or a dangerous combination of deceleration and acceleration when turning, cutting, jumping and so on.

Distraction ruptures often occur in muscles that move two joints, for example, the hamstring muscles which flex the knee and extend the hip joint. These muscles cannot perform the two functions at the same time during running so they are strictly governed by a sensitive neuromuscular system. Failure of this system will potentiate injuries. Other examples of muscles susceptible to distraction ruptures are the quadriceps muscle in the front of the thigh, the gastrocnemius muscle in the calf and the biceps muscle in the upper arm.

The symptoms of a muscle rupture depend on its severity. Ruptures are classified as partial or total. Another form of rupture classification describes different degrees of strains; so first and second degree strains are partial ruptures and third degree strains are total ruptures or disruptions.

Partial ruptures A *first degree or mild strain* describes an overstretching of the muscle with a rupture of less than 5 per cent of the muscle fibres. There is no great loss of strength or restriction of movement. Active movement or passive stretching will, however, cause pain around the area of damage and there will be some discomfort. It should be remembered that a small rupture or mild strain can be just as distressing to the athlete as a more serious injury.

A second degree or moderate strain involves a more significant but less than total tear to the muscle. The pain will be aggravated by any attempt to contract the muscle.

A total rupture (or *third degree/severe strain*) involves total disruption of the muscle.

Symptoms and diagnosis The following features suggest that a distraction rupture has occurred.
— A sharp or stabbing pain is felt at the moment of injury and reproduced by contracting the muscle concerned. Usually, there is little pain if the muscle is rested.
— In a partial rupture, the resulting pain can inhibit muscle contraction. In total ruptures, the muscles are unable to contract for mechanical reasons.
— In partial ruptures it is sometimes possible to feel a defect in part of the muscle on examination. In a totally ruptured muscle the defect can be felt across the entire muscle belly. The muscle may 'bunch up' and form a lump resembling a tumour.
— There is often localized tenderness and swelling over the damaged area.
— After about 24 hours, bruising and discoloration may be seen, often below the site of injury; these are signs of bleeding within the damaged muscle. Muscle spasm may occur.

Clinical examination by local inspection and palpation is initially carried out to analyse the degree of trauma. The most effective diagnostic test is often a test of function, with or without resistance.

Healing When a muscle is overstretched, the muscle fibres and blood vessels will tear. The torn ends will retract from the injured area leaving it filled with blood. Initially there will be inflammation and thereafter resorption of the bleeding. The repair of a muscle injury involves two 'competitive' events: *Formation of new muscle fibres* (regeneration) and the simultaneous *production of scar tissue* (granulation tissue).

Skeletal muscle possesses a high capacity to regenerate but the new muscle fibres will be shorter and incorporate inelastic scar tissue. If the scar covers a large area, function will be impaired because contraction is restricted. Areas of different elasticity may be formed in the muscle which increase the risk of recurrence of rupture. It is therefore important to follow a muscle injury with a long-lasting rehabilitation programme.

Compression ruptures

When direct impact is the cause of injury, deep rupture and bleeding can occur as the contracted muscle is compressed against the underlying bone. Compression ruptures can also occur in superficial muscles, in which case the symptoms are similar to those caused by distraction ruptures (see above).

Muscular haematoma

During physical activity there is a substantial redistribution of blood flow. In the muscles, it increases from about $1\frac{1}{2}$ pt (0.8 1)/min (15 per cent

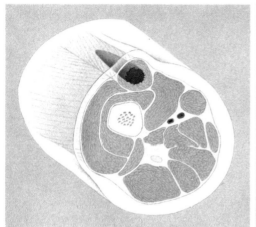

Example of a superficial intramuscular haematoma.

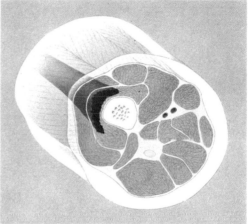

Example of a deep intramuscular haematoma.

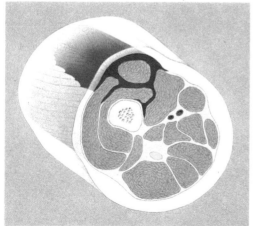

Example of an intermuscular haematoma.

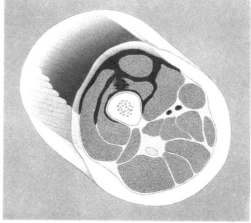

Example of a deep intramuscular haematoma with an intermuscular spread.

31

of cardiac output) at rest to 32 pt (18 1)/min (72 per cent of cardiac output) during strenuous effort. It follows that the blood supply to the muscles during sporting activity is enormous; the extent of bleeding when the muscle is damaged is directly proportional to muscle blood flow and inversely proportional to muscle tension at the time of injury. The effect of an injury depends upon its location and extent rather than upon its cause, and in the following paragraphs no distinction will be made between compression and distraction ruptures. Treatment, healing and rehabilitation will also vary according to the type, location and extent of haemorrhage and ruptured tissue.

1. Intramuscular haematoma

Bleeding within a muscle may be caused by rupture or impact. It begins within the muscle sheath (fascia), and causes an increase in intramuscular pressure which counteracts any tendency to further bleeding by compressing the blood vessels. The resultant swelling persists beyond the first 48 hours and is accompanied by tenderness, pain and impaired mobility. Swelling may increase as the bleeding draws fluid from the surrounding tissue (osmosis), and muscle function may be completely absent. If the muscle sheath is damaged, blood may spread into the space between the muscles (see below) or out into the surrounding tissues. Intramuscular haematoma may create an acute compartment syndrome (see page 321) due to increased intracompartmental pressure.

2. Intermuscular haematoma

Bleeding may occur between muscles when a muscle sheath (fascia) and its adjacent blood vessels are damaged. After an initial increase, causing the bleeding to spread, the pressure falls quickly. Typically, bruising and swelling, caused by a collection of blood, occur at some distance from the damaged area 24–48 hours after the injury due to gravity. Because there is no sustained increase in pressure, the swelling is temporary and muscle function returns rapidly. Provided immediate treatment is available, recovery can be expected to be speedy and complete.

Treatment of muscle rupture and haematoma

The *athlete* or *trainer* should stop or control muscle bleeding irrespective of its cause, by use of the following measures:
— encouraging rest;
— cooling the affected area;
— bandaging the injured part;
— elevating the limb;
— relieving load on the limb. If the injury affects the leg, crutches should be used until a definite diagnosis has been made. When an arm is involved, splinting may help during the acute phase.
The body's defence against bleeding (coagulation or clotting) comes into action as soon as the injury occurs and continues to function for several hours. The repair mechanism, however, is unstable during the first 24–36

hours, so that further bleeding may occur as a result of another impact, vigorous muscular contraction or unprotected weightbearing. *Massage, which is, in effect, repeated minor trauma, should not be used within 48–72 hours of a muscular injury.*

Whenever there is any suspicion of a major muscle rupture or significant bleeding, a doctor should be consulted as soon as possible.

The *doctor's* action will depend upon the extent of the injury. If it is severe, admission to hospital for observation is usual as the bleeding and swelling may increase, impairing the blood supply and raising the intramuscular pressure; this can be dangerous if left unmonitored. If the bleeding is not extensive, or if there is any uncertainty about the nature or extent of the injury, 48–72 hours' rest may be prescribed. Precise diagnosis can be difficult in the acute phase and for the first 2–3 days an injury should be considered as potentially serious.

Constant re-examination of the injured area is necessary in order to distinguish between intermuscular and intramuscular bleeding. Decreasing swelling and rapid recovery of function would suggest the former, and persistent or increasing swelling with poor function the latter.

After 48–72 hours the following questions should be answered:
1. Has the swelling resolved? If not, intramuscular haematoma is probably present.
2. Has the bleeding spread and caused bruising at some distance from the injury? If not, haematoma is probably intramuscular.
3. Has the contractile ability of the injured muscle returned or improved? If not, the injury probably involves intramuscular haematoma.
4. Is the haematoma a symptom of a total or partial muscle rupture?

It is important that an accurate diagnosis is made, because premature exercise of a muscle affected by extensive intramuscular haematoma or a complete rupture can cause complications in the form of further bleeding and sometimes increased scar tissue formation. This in turn is likely to lead to a more protracted healing process and possibly even permanent disability.

Treatment beyond the first 72 hours depends upon the diagnosis which has been made.

Treatment after 72 hours
After initial acute treatment, minor partial ruptures, intermuscular haematomas and minor intramuscular haematomas should be managed by the following measures:
— support with an elastic bandage;
— apply heat locally. Contrast treatment using heat and cold may sometimes be of value;
— active muscle exercises which adhere to specific principles and are carried out in the following order:
  1. Static exercises without load (see pages 91–2).
  2. Static exercises with light load.
  3. Limited dynamic muscle training with exercises within the active range of movement to the pain threshold (see pages 92–3).
  4. Dynamic exercises with increasing load.

5. Stretching exercises to improve range of movement. It is important not to neglect exercising the muscles which act in the opposite direction (antagonists) to the one which has been injured (see pages 96–7).
6. Co-ordination (proprioceptive) training (see page 97).
7. Gradually increasing activity and load on the injured muscle. If a lower limb is affected, it may be advisable to precede running by cycling and swimming.
8. Sport-specific training (see page 97).

If the symptoms caused by the injured muscle fail to improve, it is important to reconsider intramuscular haematoma and tissue damage. In order to elucidate the situation, the doctor may take one or more of the following steps:
— carry out a further local examination;
— measure intramuscular (intracompartmental) pressure;
— puncture and aspirate the injured area with a wide-bore needle if fluctuation is present;
— request soft tissue X-rays without, and sometimes with, a contrast medium;
— carry out an ultrasound examination;
— undertake surgery.

When the diagnosis is established, the *doctor* has a number of treatment methods at his disposal:
— an elastic support bandage and a programme of muscle exercises as outlined above;
— anti-inflammatory medication;
— surgery should be considered in cases of extensive bleeding especially when it is intramuscular and involves complete or partial rupture affecting more than half the muscle belly. It is particularly important when the damaged muscle is unique in the function it performs or is without agonists (muscles with similar function) for example, pectoralis major. The aim of surgery is to remove any intervening blood clots and repair the torn muscle fibres by suturing them together. This procedure ensures the least possible scar formation; this is important for full recovery as scar tissue is less elastic than muscle tissue and therefore at greater risk of further injury (see diagram on page 35). A period of immobilization in a plaster cast is usually necessary after muscle surgery.

Rehabilitation

Rehabilitation after surgery is planned by discussions between the athlete and his doctor, taking into consideration the location and severity of the injury. Studies have shown that when rehabilitation is started early, healing is more rapid, with restoration of circulation and improvement in strength. The athlete can begin static muscle exercises (see page 91) with the doctor's agreement, soon after the surgery, and later progress to dynamic strength and flexibility training.

Return to sporting activity

A muscle injury can be considered completely healed when there is no pain or tenderness on full contraction of the muscle. Once complete muscle function, full flexibility in adjacent joints and a normal pattern of movement are regained, a full training programme can be resumed.

The time taken for a muscle rupture to heal varies between 3 and 16 weeks depending upon the location and extent of the injury. In cases of intramuscular haematoma, in which tissue damage is often a feature, the healing time is usually between 2 and 8 weeks, whereas sporting activity can often be resumed only 1 or 2 weeks after an intermuscular haematoma.

Conditioning exercises and gradually progressive muscle exercise against resistance should take priority over explosive training exercises when sporting activity is resumed.

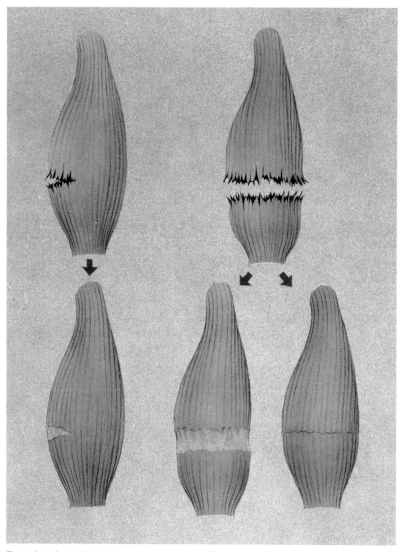

Partial and total muscle ruptures and healing results. **Top left:** partial muscle rupture. **Top right:** total muscle rupture. **Lower left:** healed partial muscle rupture which has not been operated on. **Above middle:** scar tissue of healed total muscle rupture which has not been operated on. **Lower right:** healing of total muscle rupture which has been operated on; the haematoma is removed and the torn muscle ends are sutured together.

Complications of muscle injury

1. **Scar tissue formation**

   Muscle fibres which have been overloaded with resultant bleeding and rupture become less contractile. The space between ruptured muscle fibres fills with blood which clots and is gradually converted into connective tissue. This in turn is gradually converted into scar tissue. This healing process leaves the muscle with areas of varying elasticity, and further injury (rupture or haematoma) may then occur if the muscle is exercised too hard too soon. If scar tissue causes persistent problems it may be necessary to remove it surgically.

2. **Heterotopic bone formation (Myositis ossificans, 'Charley-horse')**

   Direct impact causes intramuscular and/or intermuscular bleeding. If immediate treatment is inadequate, deep located intramuscular haematoma may gradually become calcified and ossified. Ossification continues as long as healing is disrupted by repeated impact or contraction. This will result in areas of varying strength and elasticity in the affected muscle, with a correspondingly increased risk of further injury. Ossification is a lengthy inflammatory process for which doctors hesitate to recommend active treatment for a long period of time. If muscle function and flexibility are significantly impaired for more than 6–10 weeks and X-rays reveal signs of ossification, then, in our experience, surgical removal of the ossification should be considered.

3. **Muscle ruptures may mimic tumours**

   Complete muscle ruptures can sometimes be misinterpreted and diagnosed as tumours during their later stages. When the area involved is examined, a mass is found and this appears to increase gradually in size. A thorough clinical examination is essential if the correct diagnosis is to be made.

   The following sequence of events is typical. The adductor longus muscle is located on the inner (medial) side of the thigh and its function is to draw the leg inwards (adduction). As shown in the diagram on page 38, it has its origin in the pubic bone and is inserted into the femur. Partial rupture usually affects its origin and total rupture its insertion. The latter may occur completely painlessly, and without causing any major problems. Gradually, however, an enlarging lump in the thigh becomes more noticeable. It may be mistaken for a tumour, but in fact is caused by an increase in muscle bulk. The original muscle, having shortened following rupture, is forced to work over a shorter distance, and therefore harder than previously, when a new insertion is formed by scar tissue (see diagram page 38).

   The diagnosis of 'old total rupture of adductor longus' is not difficult to make in this case, providing examination takes place with the muscle in both the relaxed and contracted states (see diagram page 38).

Tendon injuries

A muscle is usually attached to bone by a tendon through which the effects of muscle contraction are conveyed. The muscle produces force only when contracting and this has a stretching effect on the tendon. Tendons are very strong and have a tensile strength of 50–100 Newton/mm^2. They withstand tensile forces well, but resist shearing forces less effectively and provide little resistance to compressive forces. A tendon consists mainly of collagen, which provides great mechanical strength, and elastin, which provides elasticity.

In the normal resting state, a tendon has a wavy configuration, but if it is strained by more than 4 per cent, the wavy pattern disappears and the collagen fibres are subjected to stress. At 4–8 per cent strain, the cross-links joining the collagen molecules together will start to break as the fibres slide past one another. At 8–10 per cent strain, the tendon will begin to fail and the weakest fibres will rupture.

Tendons are most vulnerable to injury when:
1. Tension is applied quickly and sustained without adequate warm-up.
2. Tension is applied obliquely.
3. The tendon is tensed before the trauma.
4. The attached muscle is maximally innervated and contracted.
5. The muscle group is stretched by external forces.
6. The tendon is weak in comparison to the muscle.

All these factors can apply to athletes of all ages.

Types of injury

Injuries to tendons can be divided into ruptures (strain) and inflammations. By the age of thirty, the tendons begin to lose their elasticity with increasing degenerative changes, but the process can be delayed by regular exercise. Inflammation in tendons can result in decreased strength and a susceptibility to rupture even under normal load. Therefore, measures to prevent tendon rupture in athletes are essential.

Injuries to tendons are often located in areas of poor circulation. Achilles tendon injuries, for example, may be located 1–2 in (2–5 cm) proximal to the tendon's attachment to the calcaneus where there is a decreased vascularity. Injury to the supraspinatus tendon may be located $\frac{1}{2}$–1 in (1–2 cm) from its attachment to the humerus, where blood supply is also poor.

Achilles tendon injuries can be classified in different ways. From a clinical point of view, it is practical to differentiate between rupture and overuse syndromes because of differences in treatment and prognosis. Ruptures can be divided into total (3rd degree strain) and partial (1st and 2nd degree strain) ruptures, and overuse syndromes into tendinitis, peritendinitis, (tenosynovitis and tenovaginitis), tenoperiostitis and bursitis associated with tendinitis due to partial ruptures (tendinosus).

Total tendon rupture (3rd degree strain)

Total tendon rupture often occurs in a degenerated tendon and is especially common in older athletes who return to sport after some years' absence from training. Similar ruptures afflict badminton players in particular, but also tennis, team handball, basketball, rugby, American football and soccer players, long-jumpers, high-jumpers and runners.

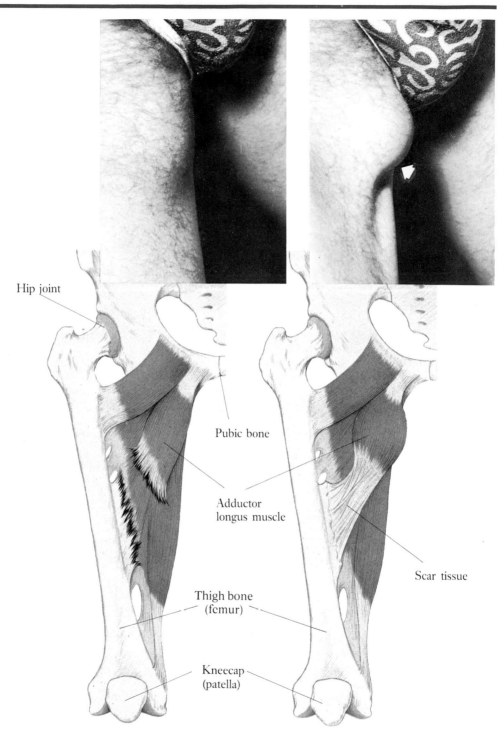

Hip joint

Pubic bone

Adductor
longus muscle

Scar tissue

Thigh bone
(femur)

Kneecap
(patella)

Example of a total rupture in the attachment of the muscle that draws the leg inwards (the adductor longus muscle). **Top left:** the muscle in a relaxed state. **Top right:** the muscle in a contracted state. **Lower left:** rupture in the attachment of the muscle to the thigh bone (femur). **Lower right:** healing with scar tissue.

Symptoms and diagnosis	Total tendon rupture may become apparent as follows: — The athlete may be aware of a sudden 'snap' followed by intense pain when the injury occurs. — The injured athlete is unable to perform those movements for which integrity of the affected tendon and its attached muscle is required. — A defect, associated with pronounced tenderness, may be felt in the tendon. — Swelling and bruising, indicating bleeding, occur soon after the injury. — A thorough clinical examination will confirm the diagnosis.
Location	The tendons most frequently affected by complete rupture are the Achilles tendon, supraspinatus tendon, biceps tendon, quadriceps and patellar tendon.
Treatment	The *athlete* or *trainer* should give immediate treatment according to the guidelines given on page 65. The *doctor* has a choice of treatment methods depending on the injury location: 1. Surgery, especially when young athletes are injured, followed by immobilization in a plaster cast for 4–6 weeks; 2. Immobilization alone, in a plaster cast; 3. Early mobilization with exercises.

Partial tendon rupture (1st and 2nd degree strain)

In this type of rupture, the tendon is only partly torn. Depending on the extent of the injury, the affected athlete may not always be aware that a rupture has occurred, but believes the tendon to be overused and inflamed. Partial ruptures can be divided into acute and chronic injuries.

Symptoms and diagnosis of acute partial tendon rupture	Acute partial tendon rupture may become apparent as follows: — A history of a sudden onset of pain often in combination with a specific event or movement. — Pain occurs in the injured area on further activity and when movements in adjacent joints are made against resistance. — A localized distinct tenderness in the injured area. — Swelling, and sometimes a haematoma, may occur. — A small, tender defect can be felt in the tendon soon after the injury.
Symptoms and diagnosis of chronic partial tendon rupture	Chronic partial tendon rupture may become apparent as follows: — A history of sudden pain is common but often no trauma can be remembered. — As illustrated by the pain cycle (see page 41), pain may be experienced during the warm-up but may then disappear only to reappear with greater intensity later. — Pain may be elicited in the injured area by moving the adjacent joints against resistance. — A localized distinct tenderness may be present. — Some swelling may be seen.

39

Location	The tendon most frequently affected by both acute and chronic partial rupture is the Achilles tendon but the injury may also occur in the patellar tendon, rotator cuff tendons and the adductor longus tendon.

Treatment of acute injuries

The *athlete* or *trainer* should give immediate treatment to a partial tendon rupture as follows:
— treat with ice, compression bandage, rest, and elevation. Sometimes crutches can be of value;
— consult a doctor to confirm the diagnosis and thereafter decide upon further treatment.

The *doctor* may:
— apply a plaster cast or other supportive bandage especially during the acute phase;
— prescribe an exercise programme of gradually increasing intensity;
— prescribe anti-inflammatory medication.

If a partial tendon rupture is inappropriately treated, inflammatory tissue will form in the injured area and heal only with difficulty. If the healing is prolonged, chronic inflammation may result, giving the same symptoms as those which occur in chronic tendinitis. It is, therefore, essential that these injuries are treated correctly from the start. When neglected they can be amongst the most difficult of all sports injuries to treat.

Treatment of chronic injuries

The *athlete* or *trainer* should:
— try an exercise programme including a combination of stretching and eccentric exercises (see page 92);
— use a supportive bandage, tape or brace to unload the injured area;
— use a heat retainer.

The *doctor* may:
— prescribe anti-inflammatory medication;
— carry out surgery if the symptoms are prolonged and incapacitating.

Even small partial ruptures should be treated with great concern and respect otherwise they will heal with scar and granulation tissue. These can cause further problems and lead to a chronic condition which is often very difficult to treat.

OVERUSE SYNDROMES

Overuse syndromes are particularly difficult to diagnose and treat. These injuries are becoming increasingly common as participation in sport in general and the intensity and duration of training increase.

Despite documentation on overuse injuries as early as 1855, little research has been carried out and today's knowledge is based mainly on practical, clinical experience.

Overuse injuries are generally caused by overload or repeated microscopic injuries to the musculo-skeletal system. Tissues can withstand great loads but there is a critical limit to this capacity, which varies greatly between individuals.

There are many intrinsic and extrinsic factors which make tissues susceptible to injury:

Intrinsic – such as malalignment of the leg, muscle imbalance and other anatomical factors.

Extrinsic – such as training errors, faulty technique, incorrect equipment and surfaces, poor conditions.

The actual frequency of injury due to overuse is unknown as such cases rarely require examination by a doctor/physician; but some researchers

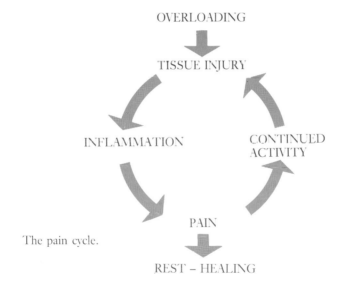

OVERLOADING

TISSUE INJURY

INFLAMMATION

CONTINUED ACTIVITY

PAIN

The pain cycle.

REST – HEALING

suggest that between 25–50 per cent of athletes visiting sports medicine clinics have sustained an overuse injury. In one study, 15 per cent of these were female. The age of occurrence of overuse injury also varies: they are most common in top level athletes between the ages of twenty and twenty-nine, but in non-competitive athletes between the ages of thirty and forty-nine. In adults, overuse injuries are more prevalent after 2 years of regular daily training. With reference to the type of sport involved, 80 per cent of overuse injuries occurred in endurance sports, such as long distance running, or individual one man sports that require skilled technique and repetitive movements, such as tennis, gymnastics, weight-lifting; 80 per cent of these injuries occurred at the lower extremities of the body, most frequently at the knee (28 per cent) and the ankle, foot and heel (21 per cent).

Inflammation

Inflammation represents the body's response to tissue injury caused by pressure, friction, repeated load or overload and external trauma. Trauma is associated with some degree of bleeding, which in turn causes swelling and increased pressure. Both extrinsic and intrinsic factors (see above) contribute to the inflammatory reaction in tendons, tendon and muscle attachments, bursae and the periosteum. Common combinations of frequency and loading causing overuse injuries when applied, are:

normal load at high frequency;
heavy load at normal frequency;
heavy load at high frequency.

Inflammation, sometimes accompanied by pus formation, also occurs in response to bacterial infections. It both confines and combats such infections as well as stimulating healing.

Whatever the nature of the underlying cause, the inflammatory response leads to impaired and painful mobility of the affected part and so enforces rest. If it affects gliding surfaces, such as those of tendons and their sheaths, crepitus or 'creaking' might develop. If inflammation goes unchecked, scar tissue will develop and, for this reason, early intensive treatment is recommended.

The single most important step in the management of inflammation is the removal or reversal of its cause and, in addition, reduction of swelling to relieve pain, improve mobility and encourage healing.

Symptoms typical of inflammation include the following:

— Swelling caused by accumulation of fluid.
— Redness caused by increased blood flow.
— Local rise of temperature, caused by increased blood flow around the injured area.
— Tenderness on touching the affected area.
— Impaired function of the affected part because of swelling and tenderness.

Inflammation often begins insidiously and, initially, pain and stiffness may decrease or even disappear after warm-up. Usually, however, the pain returns and intensifies during continued activity and unless a rest break is taken, there is a great danger of entering the 'pain cycle' (see diagram on page 41). Unless the cycle is interrupted, chronic pain results and can be extremely difficult to treat.

Pain should be interpreted as a warning sign of tissue injury and should lead to a rest from activity.

Inflammation of muscle-tendon attachments to bone (tenoperiostitis)

Attachment of a muscle to bone involves a gradual transition from muscle-tendon to cartilage and from mineralized cartilage to bone. Bone-tendon junctions are poorly supplied with blood because the fibrocartilage creates a 'barrier'; this may explain why these injuries often take a long time to heal and often become chronic.

Inflammation of the muscle-tendon attachment is caused by repeated strain on the attachment and periosteum. The resultant minor ruptures and bleeding cause irritation and inflammation. Growing individuals rarely suffer from tenoperiostitis because their tendons and muscles are relatively stronger than bone. Instead, they sustain inflammation and fragmentation of bone, for example Osgood-Schlatter's disease in the knee and calcaneal apophysitis.

Location

Tenoperiostitis occurs most frequently in the elbow area ('tennis elbow' and 'golfer's elbow'), in the groin at the attachment of the adductor longus muscle, in the knee at the proximal and distal attachments of the patellar tendon, in the Achilles tendon insertion into the calcaneus, and in the attachment of the plantar fascia into the calcaneus (plantar fasciitis).

Symptoms and diagnosis

Tenoperiostitis is characterized by development of the following:
— Pain at the attachment site of a muscle or tendon to bone.
— Slight swelling and some degree of impaired function.
— A distinct, localized tenderness to pressure over the affected attachment.
— An increase in pain at the site of attachment when the muscle group concerned is contracted.

Treatment

When tenoperiostitis develops the *athlete* or *trainer* should:
— restrict the activity which triggers the pain; sometimes crutches can be beneficial;
— cool the injury with ice packs in the acute phase to reduce pain and swelling;
— give support with strapping or taping;
— apply local heat and use a heat retainer after the acute phase.

The *doctor* may use one or more of the following treatment methods:
— anti-inflammatory medication;
— prescribe an exercise programme according to the principles on page 90.
— local steroid injections at a later stage combined with rest for 1–2 weeks;
— surgery in patients with prolonged pain and chronic conditions.

Prevention

The following measures will help to reduce the likelihood of tenoperiostitis developing:

— correct training techniques;
— equipment appropriate for the sport concerned (new equipment, especially footwear, should be 'worn in');
— clothing and equipment suitable for the athlete concerned;
— good basic training, and specialized training aimed specifically at vulnerable areas.

Muscle inflammation (myositis)

Myositis is rare and mainly affects the muscles of the thigh, back, shoulder and calf.

Symptoms and diagnosis

The following indications may suggest a diagnosis of myositis:
— Pain in the affected muscle group on exertion.
— Symptoms increase as effort becomes more intensive and repetitive.
— Tender, firm areas may be felt on examination of the muscle.
— Muscle cramp may occur.

Treatment

When myositis occurs, the *athlete* or *trainer* should:
— rest the muscle in question or reduce training;
— apply local heat and use a heat retainer.

Inflammation of the tendon (tendinitis) and its sheath (peritendinitis, tenovaginitis)

An inflammatory reaction in a tendon and its sheath may be initiated by repetitive one-sided movements or by persistent mechanical irritation. The condition frequently becomes chronic and difficult to treat.

Location

The Achilles tendon is most frequently affected by tendinitis, along with the tendon of the long head of the biceps, the supraspinatus tendon and the extensor tendons of the wrist and ankle.

Symptoms and diagnosis

Tendinitis and peritendinitis cause the following signs and symptoms:
— In the acute phase, pain and occasionally crepitus felt in the affected tendon during and after exercise. In chronic conditions, initial pain will often disappear during warm-up (pain cycle see page 41).
— Impaired function.
— Soft tissue X-rays show swelling and sometimes calcification of the affected tissues.

Treatment

When tendinitis/peritendinitis develops the *athlete* or *trainer* should:
— cool the injured area during the acute phase;
— rest the affected part actively until the pain resolves;
— apply local heat and use a heat retainer;
— consult a doctor if the problem persists despite these measures.

The *doctor* has at his disposal the following treatment methods:
— an exercise programme which should start as soon as healing permits. In the initial phase, isometric exercises, without load, should be carried out; thereafter, dynamic exercises can begin and should include eccentric exercises, combined with careful stretching. At no time should these exercises exceed the pain threshold;
— supportive strapping and taping;
— anti-inflammatory medication;
— high voltage galvanic stimulation;
— ultrasound or short-wave therapy;
— surgery.

> Not many sports injuries are as difficult to treat as tendinitis and the athlete should rest the affected part as soon as the symptoms appear. Failure to do this can result in chronic tendinitis which will put an end to any future sporting activity.

Prevention

Bearing in mind the potential seriousness of tendinitis, preventive measures, as set out below, should be encouraged:
— thorough warm-up before activity and cool down afterwards;
— varied training with avoidance of repetitive, one-sided movements;
— gradual adaptation to new conditions, for example change of playing surface;
— equipment adjusted according to the environment;
— good basic training to delay the onset of degenerative tissue changes; good general conditioning.

Inflammation of the periosteum (periostitis)

Periostitis of the lower leg is a common condition in athletes, especially those who change from one playing surface to another in spring and autumn and those who change their techniques or equipment. Any athlete who trains intensively on a hard surface may be affected, as may runners who run on tip-toe or with their feet turned outwards and those who use spiked shoes. Poor metatarsal arches and increased pronation (see page 355) may contribute to the problem. The cause of this pain syndrome is still under debate. Some suggest traction periostitis may cause microfractures in underlying bone. Compare compartment syndrome (see page 321) and medial tibial stress syndrome (see page 326).

Symptoms and diagnosis

Periostitis should be suspected if:
— Pain is felt on the inside of the shin on activity; as load increases, the pain becomes more intense.
— Local tenderness and swelling can be felt along the inner (medial) anterior edge of the shin.

Treatment

When periostitis develops, the *athlete* or *trainer* should:
— encourage rest. Physical fitness can be maintained by cycling without ankle movement;

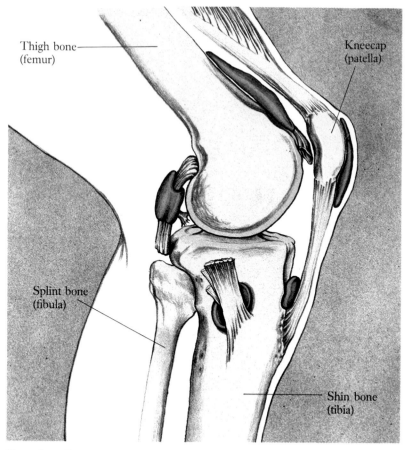

Thigh bone (femur)

Kneecap (patella)

Splint bone (fibula)

Shin bone (tibia)

Examples of bursae around the kneecap.

— apply local heat and use a heat retainer;
— consult a doctor if the problem persists.

The *doctor* may use the following methods of treatment:
— anti-inflammatory medication;
— adhesive strapping or tape;
— local applications which increase blood flow, for example, heparin paste;
— local steroid injections;
— surgery.

Symptoms similar to those of periostitis which persist despite treatment may indicate the presence of a stress fracture (see page 324), which may be revealed by an X-ray or bone scan.

Prevention Periostitis can be prevented by:
— gradual adjustment to changes of surface and intensity of training;
— use of appropriate equipment, particularly footwear;
— adaptation of technique to the surface used.

Injuries affecting bursae

Bursae are small fluid-filled sacs whose function is to reduce friction and distribute stress. They may be found between a bone and a tendon, between two tendons, or between a bone or tendon and the overlying skin. There are a number of permanent bursae around the hips, knees, feet, shoulders and elbows, and some of these are linked with the adjacent joints. The bursa in the posterior aspect of the knee (popliteal, Baker's or semimembranosa-gastrocnemius cyst), for example, is connected with the knee joint, while that located beneath the iliopsoas muscle may be connected with the hip. Acquired bursae are found in areas which are subject to repeated stress, friction or pressure such as those over protruding bones.

The conditions which affect bursae are inflammatory (bursitis) or caused by impact with subsequent bleeding (haemobursa).

Inflammation of a bursa (bursitis)

Bursitis may be classified as frictional, chemical or septic according to its cause. It can occur in isolation or as part of a generalized inflammatory or infectious disease such as rheumatoid arthritis or tuberculosis.

1. Frictional bursitis

This condition occurs when a tendon, the Achilles tendon for example, moves repeatedly over a bursa. The mechanical irritation stimulates inflammation which in turn causes fluid to be secreted into the bursa with resultant swelling and tenderness. Fluctuation of the fluid can often be felt when the bursa is examined, and, if the inflammation is intense and particularly when it is superficial, the overlying skin is red and hot.

Location
Frictional bursitis occurs in athletes who carry out repetitive movements for example, tennis players, runners training on one side of the road. It frequently affects bursae in the shoulder, elbow, hip and knee and around the heel.

Treatment
The *athlete* or *trainer* should:
— encourage rest until the pain has resolved completely;
— cool the injured area with an ice pack;
— apply a bandage to compress the bursa;
— relieve any external pressure on the bursa (for example, by applying a piece of plastic foam with the centre cut out);
— apply local heat and use a heat retainer after the first 24 hours;
— consult a doctor if the swelling is extensive or the pain severe and persistent.

The *doctor* may:
— aspirate the fluid from the bursa, sometimes in combination with compression;
— prescribe rest;
— inject steroids locally;
— remove the bursa by surgery. Removal of the underlying bone may sometimes be necessary if it has been a factor in causing the bursitis;

47

— request a contrast X-ray of the bursa (bursography) if there is doubt about the diagnosis. Perform bursoscopy (inspection of the bursa using an arthroscope).

2. Chemical bursitis

Chemical bursitis is caused by substances formed as a result of inflammatory or degenerative conditions of tendons and should be treated by a doctor at an early stage. The signs and symptoms will resemble those described above. The doctor may initially drain the bursa and inject it with steroids, but if the symptoms persist, surgical excision will become necessary.

Chemical bursitis is generally diagnosed in athletes of thirty or over who have been involved in racket or throwing sports for a number of years. It frequently affects the bursa overlying the supraspinatus tendon in the shoulder and may be associated with calcium deposits from the tendon draining into the bursa (calcific bursitis). In some cases, the bursitis can be secondary and initiate so-called pseudogout.

3. Septic bursitis

Septic bursitis is caused by bacteria entering a bursa either from the bloodstream or from the outside environment through damaged skin, for example where abrasions or blisters have occurred. Superficial bursae, around the elbows and knees, are most frequently affected, and athletes, and soccer players, who are likely to suffer dirty abrasions are most vulnerable. Septic bursitis may rarely occur after aspiration.

Symptoms and diagnosis

Septic bursitis is suggested by:
— Pronounced pain and tenderness.
— Marked swelling and redness of the affected area.
— Considerable impairment of function.
— Underlying changes in bone, revealed by X-ray, after protracted infection.

When mechanical irritation is the cause, symptoms include:
— Swelling.
— Local increase in temperature.
— Redness.
— Tenderness.
— Pain on attempted movement.

Treatment

When septic bursitis is suspected the *athlete* or *trainer* should:
— rest and relieve pressure on the affected area;
— keep damaged skin clean by washing with soap and water;
— consult a doctor as early as possible.

The *doctor* may:
— treat the underlying cause when bloodstream infection is present;
— prescribe antibiotics;
— drain the infected bursa;
— possibly apply compression and support for a few days;
— resort to surgery if the infection fails to resolve.

48

Bleeding into a bursa (haemobursa)

The usual cause of bleeding into a bursa is a direct impact such as a fall (see diagram on page 311). It may also be caused indirectly by tendon rupture or by bleeding within a joint to which the bursa is connected. Blood within the bursa causes chemical irritation and, if severe enough, may clot and cause adhesion of connective tissue and loose bodies (calcifications). Once this has occurred, chronic inflammation is likely to ensue.

Location

Haemobursae occur frequently in players whose sports require them to make repeated contact with a hard surface or object, for example team handball and volleyball players. Apart from those of the hands, bursae around the knee, greater trochanter of the femur, the elbow and above the supraspinatus tendon may be affected.

Symptoms and diagnosis

In cases of acute injury, a haemobursa is suggested by the following signs and symptoms:
— Swelling of the bursa as it fills with blood.
— Extreme tenderness.
— Pain and impaired function of the part in question.
— Sometimes redness and damage to the skin.

Treatment

When a haemobursa occurs, the *athlete* or *trainer* should:
— cool the area in order to control bleeding;
— apply a compression bandage;
— rest the affected part.

The *doctor* may:
— drain the bursa by aspiration;
— apply a compression bandage and possibly a plaster splint.

Diseases of joints

The articular surfaces of joints are covered with cartilage which has no blood supply and, therefore, does not heal well when injured. Cartilage functions to reduce friction between bones. The nutrients required by the cartilage are supplied by the synovial fluid which is secreted by the membrane lining the joint capsule and which also serves to reduce friction during joint movements.

Osteoarthritis ('Worn joints')

The term osteoarthritis applies particularly to the degeneration and excessive wear of articular cartilages, although gradual changes in underlying bone tissue also occur. The condition is one which develops and advances with increasing age. It may be either 'primary' or 'secondary'.

Primary osteoarthritis, the cause of which is unknown, occurs most frequently in women and diabetics; it is uncommon in Orientals. Obesity is probably of no significance as far as onset of the disease is concerned, but it does accelerate the degenerative process once it has begun.

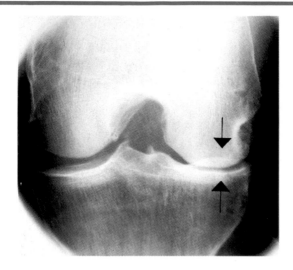

Knee joint under load. The inner side of the knee joint (see arrows) shows changes associated with osteoarthritis.

Secondary osteoarthritis may follow either injury or joint disease. Fractures of articular surfaces, ligament injuries and dislocations are all possible causes, as are infections and rheumatoid arthritis. Persistent inappropriate loading of joints, for example, in joggers who run on a camber, can also result in osteoarthritis, as can running on a hard surface.

Pathological changes

Whether osteoarthritis is primary or secondary, the changes which occur in the joints are similar. Initially the articular cartilage softens. Subsequently the surface becomes uneven, the cartilage 'frays' and develops cracks which may extend down to the bone beneath. Ultimately the cartilage is worn away to reveal the bone which then has to serve as the load-bearing surface of the joint. Simultaneously the bone hardens (sclerosis) and areas of low density (cysts) begin to form. New cartilage cells which are laid down around the worn cartilage become ossified, and bony projections (osteophytes) are formed as a result of thickening of the joint capsule. The changes are seen most frequently in the hip and knee joints, but less frequently in the ankle, and are all clearly visible on X-ray examination carried out with the joint under load.

Symptoms and diagnosis

The following features suggest a diagnosis of osteoarthritis:
— *Pain*. Some pain is usually, though not invariably, present. Even when it is absent during normal daily activities, it can often be precipitated by increasing the load on the affected joint. Initially pain develops gradually, and in athletes it may disappear during warm-up only to return once training or competition is over. Pain at rest occurs when osteoarthritis has reached an advanced stage and at this point sleep may be disturbed.
— *Joint abnormalities*. A variety of changes may be found around an osteoarthritic joint on straightforward clinical examination. They include swelling, impaired range of movement, muscle atrophy, tenderness, crepitus, local increased temperature, and instability and/or abnormal joint movements resulting from ligament laxity.
— *Morning stiffness*. Stiffness typically occurs after a period of inactivity, and a limp may also be present.

— X-ray changes. These include narrowing of the joint space, cysts, osteophytes and sclerosis. There may also be evidence of increased production of synovial fluid.

Treatment

The changes of osteoarthritis cannot be reversed, but a variety of approaches may be adopted to relieve symptoms and to delay further degeneration:
— the load on the affected joint should be reduced. It may be necessary to discontinue weight-bearing sporting activity if, for example, a hip or knee is affected in which case physical fitness can be maintained by cycling or swimming;
— active mobility and muscle-strengthening exercises should be carried out under the direction of a physiotherapist (and possibly in a pool). **Passive exercises, that is those which involve no effort on the part of the patient whose joints are manipulated for him, should be avoided;**
— ultrasound, short-wave therapy and hot packs can have a beneficial psychological effect, and a heat retainer may be used;
— a walking-stick, used on the healthy side, can be of value when one hip or knee is affected;
— bandages of various sorts may be used to relieve the load on joints;
— anti-inflammatory and pain-relieving medication may be prescribed;
— surgery may be necessary when the degenerative changes are severe.

Osteoarthritis and sport

Athletes who suffer from osteoarthritis should take the advice of their doctors with regard to continuing their sporting activities. Each case has to be considered on its merits. In the early stages there is usually no reason to cease participation in sport, though there may well need to be a change in the type of exercise. Cycling and swimming may be recommended rather than running in order to eliminate or at least reduce load on an affected joint. Active mobility and muscle-strengthening exercises should be encouraged in order to prevent or delay deterioration. Once a damaged hip or knee has been replaced surgically by a prosthetic joint, sporting activity should only be resumed after consultation with the doctor in charge.

Rheumatoid arthritis

Rheumatoid arthritis, which is classified as one of the auto-immune diseases though its precise cause is not known, is a chronic inflammatory condition which affects joints, tendons, tendon sheaths (fascia), muscles and bursae as well as other tissues throughout the body. It is three times commoner in women than in men and usually begins between the ages of twenty and thirty or forty-five and fifty-five years.

Pathological changes

The first stage in rheumatoid arthritis is inflammation of the synovial membrane (synovitis) associated with the deposition of protein (fibrin). As a result of the inflammation, fluid is secreted into the joint, causing swelling. The inflammatory tissue grows towards the centre of the joint space and coats the articular surfaces and the surrounding ligaments and tendons. At the same time, the articular cartilage is destroyed systematically from its surface inwards to the underlying bone and cysts form in the adjacent bone. As the inflammatory tissue begins to be replaced by scar tissue, the joint capsule becomes thickened and can consequently impede the mobility of the joint.

Symptoms and diagnosis

The following features suggest a diagnosis of rheumatoid arthritis:
— Pain and swelling of joints.
— Joint stiffness which is particularly pronounced in the mornings.
— Joint deformities, muscular atrophy and tendon abnormalities.
— Periods of relapse and remission in the course of the condition.

For practical purposes, rheumatoid arthritis is considered to be present if three or four of the following criteria are fulfilled:
1. Morning stiffness.
2. Pain and tenderness in at least one joint.
3. Soft tissue swelling or excessive fluid in at least one joint.
4. When 2. or 3. is present, swelling in at least one other joint.
5. Symmetrical joint swelling.
6. Nodules on tendons at sites typical of rheumatoid arthritis.
7. X-ray changes typical of rheumatoid arthritis.
8. Blood tests showing changes typical of rheumatoid arthritis.

Treatment

As with osteoarthritis, there is no cure for rheumatoid arthritis. However, its manifestations and progress can be controlled and symptoms relieved by:
— physiotherapy and maintenance of general physical fitness;
— anti-inflammatory medication;
— immunosuppressant medication;
— local treatment with steroids or gold, for example;
— surgery, in severe cases.

Rheumatoid arthritis and sport

Rheumatoid arthritis does not have to exclude sport. Those physical activities which are known to have a beneficial effect should be encouraged. Above all, athletes with arthritis should indulge in active exercises, that is those requiring muscular effort.

Other diseases of the joints

Osteochondritis dissecans and Bechterew's disease See pages 301/347 and 257.

Joint infections

Infection may reach a joint either via the bloodstream (from the urinary tract, respiratory tract, sinuses, mouth and so on), directly through an open wound or following a surgical procedure. Medical advice is essential if a joint infection is suspected.

Gout

Gout is caused by accumulation of uric acid crystals in joints, and 95 per cent of the victims are middle-aged men. The first metatarsophalangeal joint (at the base of the big toe) is most frequently affected and during an acute attack, which usually lasts for between 2 and 7 days, becomes red, hot, swollen and exquisitely painful. Chronic gout may affect more than one joint, in which case it may mimic other generalized joint diseases.

Medical examination and advice is recommended for the athlete with gout for which treatment may include anti-inflammatory and other medicines, dietary modifications and rest.

Stress fractures of the skeleton

Stress fractures (also called fatigue or insufficiency fractures) occur most frequently as a result of repeated loading of the skeleton over a long period of time and are probably preceded by periostitis.

Causes

Stress fractures can appear after the application of a normal load at high frequency (for example long distance running), of a heavy load at normal frequency (for example, repeatedly running a 100m race carrying a second person) or a heavy load at high frequency (for example, intensive weight training). The latter is the most dangerous as it is not only likely to cause stress fractures but also overloads other tissues.

There are two theories about the origin of stress fractures. The *fatigue theory* states that during repeated protracted effort, such as running, the muscles pass their peak of endurance and are no longer able to support the skeleton during impact applied as the foot strikes the ground. The load is therefore transferred directly to the skeleton. Its tolerance is eventually exceeded and a fracture occurs, for example, when repeatedly bending a paper clip.

The *overload theory* is based on the fact that certain muscle groups contract in such a way that they cause the bones to which they are attached to bend. The contraction of the calf muscles, for example, causes the tibia to bend forward like a drawn bow. After repeated contractions the innate strength of the tibia is exceeded and it breaks.

Stress fractures occur in healthy individuals at all ages from seven years upwards. They follow normal activity and affect healthy bones which have not been subjected to impact. The inadequately trained are more likely than others to suffer these fractures, and they should be suspected in any athlete who complains of bone pain and particularly of pains in the legs during exercise.

Location

About 20–25 per cent of stress fractures occur in the fibula, the tibia and the metatarsal bones. The calcaneus, navicula, femur, humerus, pelvis and vertebrae are affected less frequently.

It is usually the third metatarsal bone which sustains stress fractures. The injury should be suspected if pain has been present for 6–8 weeks or more. It is common in infantrymen in whom it is called a 'march fracture'. In the tibia, it is the upper two-thirds which are most frequently affected, and in the fibula the fracture is usually located 2–3 in (5–7 cms) above the lateral malleolus.

Typically, runners sustain stress fractures of the lower third of the fibula, high-jumpers of the upper third of the fibula and javelin-throwers of the humerus.

Symptoms and diagnosis   The following features suggest a diagnosis of stress fracture:
— Symptoms begin insidiously in 50 per cent of cases, and acutely, without apparent injury, in the remaining 50 per cent.
— In the first week of symptoms pain is felt during training but not at rest. When training is hard the pain increases in intensity and eventually a dull ache persists after exercise.
— Local swelling and tenderness can be felt over the fracture area.
— 40–50 per cent of X-rays show changes initially, but the first indication may be the signs of healing which only occur after 3–4 weeks. This feature emphasizes the importance of repeating X-ray examination if the first X-ray is negative but symptoms persist.
— Radio-isotope scanning may reveal abnormalities when other methods fail to do so.

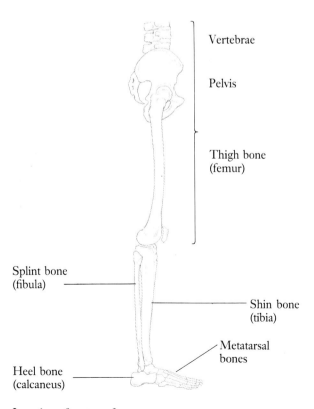

Vertebrae

Pelvis

Thigh bone (femur)

Splint bone (fibula)

Shin bone (tibia)

Metatarsal bones

Heel bone (calcaneus)

Location of a stress fracture.

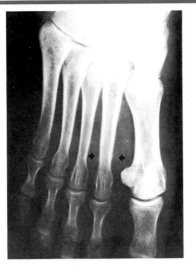 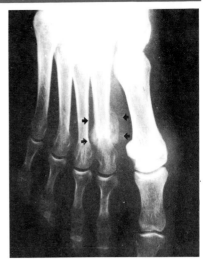

X-ray of the foot showing a stress fracture of the second metatarsal bone at an early stage (see arrows).

X-ray of the same stress fracture six weeks after the first symptom. The ossification around the bone is a sign of healing.

> In cases in which lower leg pain has been diagnosed as periostitis and the symptoms persist, in spite of rest, for more than 2 weeks, stress fracture should be suspected and the limb X-rayed.

Treatment

When a stress fracture occurs, the *athlete* should:
— rest for 4–8 weeks until the pain has resolved and healing can be seen on an X-ray.

The *doctor* may:
— apply a plaster cast for 2–6 weeks if pain is severe or if the fracture is in the tibia;
— prescribe crutches to relieve the injured part;
— check the progress of healing by X-ray examinations.

Prevention

If stress fractures are to be avoided, the athlete should assess his training methods with his coach and doctor, paying particular attention to his footwear and equipment.

MISCELLANEOUS

Open wounds

Open wounds are very common among athletes, particularly those who play contact sports such as soccer, American football, rugby and ice hockey. Riders, orienteerers and cyclists, who are likely to sustain falls on to hard surfaces are also vulnerable.

The way in which a wound is inflicted determines its nature and extent, and the possibilities include cuts, contusions, lacerations, gashes, puncture wounds, and abrasions. Some wounds may only affect the outer layers of skin or they can also damage tendons, muscles, blood vessels and nerves.

The healing of a wound is delayed by the presence of dirt and infection, bleeding, gaps between the wound edges and disturbance of the injured tissue. Treatment aims to eliminate these factors.

Treatment

In order to stop bleeding the *athlete* or *trainer* should:
— **elevate the injured part**. In most cases of limb injury, supporting the limb in a raised position with the injured athlete lying on his back or side is sufficient to stop the bleeding;
— **apply direct pressure**. With one hand on each side of the wound, press the wound edges together while the injured limb is kept elevated, with the help of a third person if necessary. The risk of contamination of the wound is obviously reduced if the wound surfaces themselves are not touched. Should the injured person be alone, he should stop the bleeding by pressing directly on the wound with his hand;
— **apply a pressure bandage** as soon as first-aid supplies have been obtained. The wound edges should be brought into opposition as described above, and, when necessary, a folded pad or clean handkerchief can be bandaged in place to increase the pressure on the area. A tourniquet should never be used and even a pressure bandage must not be kept in position for more than 10–20 minutes. If a pressure bandage has been necessary to stop bleeding, a doctor should be consulted.

Cleaning

Superficial wounds which have been contaminated by dirt must be cleaned carefully within 6 hours, otherwise they will become infected as bacteria begin to multiply and penetrate tissues. It is essential that *all dirt is removed*, especially from abrasions on the face, as retained material can cause disfiguring scars. Heavily contaminated abrasions should be cleaned thoroughly for several minutes with soap and water and a soft nail-brush. They should then be rinsed with plain water, or a saline solution, and covered with a sterile compress, held in place by a bandage. If fluid seeps through the dressing it should be changed daily. If a doctor is consulted he may prescribe medicated dressings to facilitate healing. Small superficial abrasions heal best if well-cleaned and left undisturbed.

Deep wounds include skin, underlying connective tissue and possibly also tendons, muscles, blood vessels and nerves. The wound edges often gape

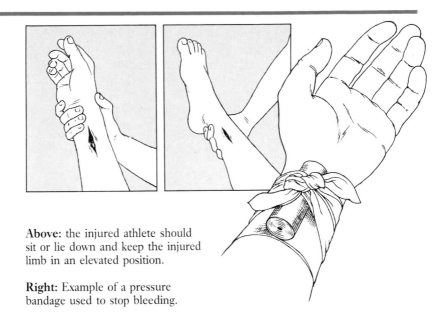

Above: the injured athlete should sit or lie down and keep the injured limb in an elevated position.

Right: Example of a pressure bandage used to stop bleeding.

apart and bleeding can be considerable. Puncture wounds caused by studs or spiked shoes can be treacherous and should always be treated by a doctor. Wounds to the sole of the foot require padding to distribute load when walking.

Deep wounds must be cleansed with extreme care, and, when damage is extensive, it is sometimes necessary for the doctor to excise dead tissue (debridement). A sound rule is that wounds which are not treated within 6 hours should be considered infected.

Some wounds — those which are deep, those which bleed profusely and those whose edges do not lie readily in opposition with each other — need to be stitched by a doctor. Stitching, too, should preferably be done within the first 6 hours of injury.

Infected wounds are characterized by pain, swelling, redness of the skin and local tenderness. Infection can spread from the wound to the lymph glands via the lymph channels (lymphatics). Infection in the leg, for example, spreads to the glands in the groin. When this happens, the lymphatics appear as red streaks in the skin and other symptoms, such as fever and general malaise, commonly occur. The affected lymph glands are swollen and tender. The condition should always be treated by a doctor who will prescribe antibiotics in addition to any other treatment. A period of bed rest may be necessary during the acute illness.

> Athletes must refrain from training or competition during the course of an infection.

Tetanus

All wounds that occur in an outdoor environment carry with them some risk of tetanus, and it is common practice in many countries for babies to be inoculated routinely against the disease.

Primary tetanus inoculation involves a course of three injections administered over a period of 6 months and confers long-lasting immunity. An incomplete course means incomplete protection and everyone should be encouraged to be aware of his inoculation status and to comply with the instructions he is given by his doctor. It is usual for a booster dose of vaccine to be given at the time of any wound which needs the attention of a doctor and is potentially contaminated.

Blisters

Blisters on the feet are the scourge of athletes, and blisters on the hands can be a problem for cross-country skiers, cricketers, rowers, tennis, badminton and squash players. Once a blister is broken it becomes a painful open wound.

The physically handicapped in wheelchairs are a special group who often have trouble with pressure sores and blisters. These can be difficult to treat because of impaired skin sensitivity and poor circulation.

Treatment

Blisters should be treated in the following way:

— when there is any suggestion of a blister forming, a break from exercise should be taken in order to prevent further irritation. The problem area can then be protected with adhesive plaster, or feet can be 'half soled' with adhesive plaster as shown in the diagram below. Avoid creases in the plaster which would encourage rather than prevent blister formation;

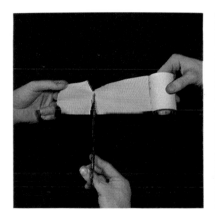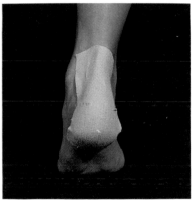

Blisters can be prevented by 'half soling' with adhesive plaster.

— once a blister has formed, its surface should be retained intact as it acts as a barrier against bacteria. Never break a blister deliberately. Large blisters can be punctured at their edges with a sterile needle. The blister can be protected from pressure by means of a piece of plastic foam with its centre cut out;

— if a blister breaks naturally, it is important to clean it carefully with soap and water or antiseptic solution. A sterile non-adherent dressing or, later, a bandage is used to cover the wound.

Preventive measures

Blisters can be prevented by the following measures:

— All equipment should be designed for use in training as well as in competition. Footwear, in particular, should be well worn in.

— Socks should be free from holes, dry, clean and of the right size so that they do not crease. They should be changed frequently.

— Hygiene should be meticulous. The feet should be washed daily and can be rubbed with salicylic acid grease which softens calluses and keeps the skin supple.

— Sensitive skin areas can be protected with adhesive plaster applied firmly and directly to the skin before exercise.

> It cannot be stressed too strongly that blisters *can* be avoided if preventive measures are applied. They may seem trivial but they can necessitate long breaks from training, especially if they become infected.

Friction burns

If an athlete falls during training or competition on a synthetic surface or a synthetically treated floor, he runs the risk of sustaining friction burns. As a rule, the burn affects only the outer layer of skin and in its mildest form causes only superficial redness which needs no treatment, but if contact is hard it may result in an abrasion. If blisters appear in the skin, they should be covered with a clean dressing; if the skin is broken, the wound should be cleansed and dressed as soon as possible by methods already described, in order to prevent infection.

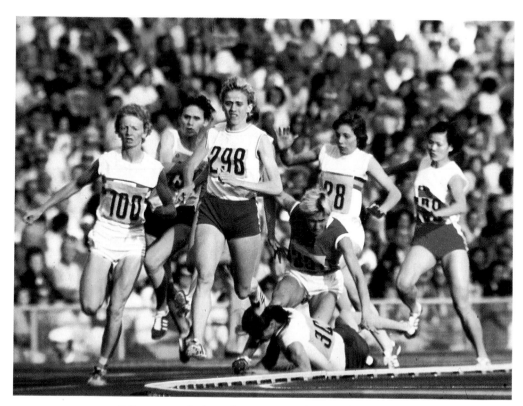

Falls on a synthetic surface can cause frictional burns. *Photo: All-Sport/Don Morley.*

Treatment and prevention	The *athlete* or *trainer* should:

— prevent friction burns by making sure that the correct equipment and clothing for the protection of vulnerable areas is used;

— reduce friction during falls by rubbing exposed parts with greasy ointment;

— treat frictional burns by cleaning the wound carefully with soap and water and dressing with medicated compresses held in place with a bandage.

Muscle cramp

Muscle cramp affects most people at some time in their lives. Athletes may suffer cramp in a muscle during or after strenuous exertion such as a soccer match or a long-distance race.

Causes

— During protracted exercise, especially when the weather is very hot, vast amounts of fluid can be lost from the body. This dehydration predisposes to muscle cramp, though the exact connection is not known. Salt deficiency is not the cause; dehydration by sweating actually causes body salt concentration to increase.

— The type of cramp which affects soccer players towards the end of a match is probably caused by changes in the musculature resulting from earlier muscular bleeding, small muscle ruptures or the athlete's general state of health or training.

— The precise causes of muscle cramp are not clear, but any factors which impair the circulation should be considered. These include close-fitting socks, shoes laced too tightly, an accumulation of lactic acid in the muscles, varicose veins, cold weather and infections.

Prevention and treatment

The *athlete* should:

— prevent muscular cramp by good basic training and warm-up exercises, by using the correct equipment and by ensuring that his body has adequate fluid and salt reserves;

— break off his sporting activity when he has acute cramp and contract the muscle which exerts an effect opposite to the one affected with cramp. For example, if cramp in the calf muscle draws the foot downwards, the foot should be raised carefully, with the knee bent, until it is at right angles to the leg (see photograph on page 62). The movement should not be forced and the affected muscle should be massaged.

If an athlete suffers persistent cramp despite preventive measures, he would be wise to seek a medical examination in order to exclude any specific problems.

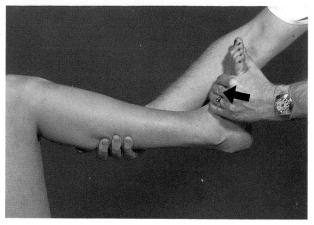

To cure cramp in the calf muscle responsible for drawing the foot downwards, raise the root at right angles to the leg with the knee bent and massage the muscle.

Muscle soreness after training

Soreness, with pain, tenderness, and sometimes swelling of the muscles, can appear a few hours after strenuous training. The pain occurs during both active exercise and passive movements, and the muscles may feel weak. Many athletes experience the problem in late autumn and early spring when they change surfaces and either do not adjust their shoes to the new surface or start training too energetically. The symptoms appear mainly during the kind of exercise in which muscles lengthen and contract simultaneously (eccentric contraction or negative work).

In untrained individuals who are suddenly subjected to strenuous exertion, muscle changes in the form of 'ruptures' of the so-called Z-discs have been seen within 2–7 days. These ruptures have been connected with stiffness after training, and disappear after the musculature has been allowed to rest. The Z-discs contain no sensory bodies and, therefore, do not in themselves cause any pain. When they are ruptured, however, simultaneous ruptures appear in the muscle capillaries and these, combined with altered pressure conditions and impaired blood flow, lead to swelling which in its turn can cause stiffness and pain. The condition is not dangerous and usually disappears after a few days.

Preventive measures and treatment

The following measures help to minimize the problem:
— The training programme should be adjusted according to the level of training achieved and the surface used. Appropriate equipment is important.
— If a minor degree of soreness is felt, training can be continued but should be modified. The intensity of training should always be increased gradually, especially during the initial stages.
— Gentle movements and warm surroundings help to ease the pain.

Stitch

Runners who have not warmed up properly sometimes feel a sharp pain in the upper part of the abdomen a few minutes after they have started to run. It may be located on the right or the left and is more frequent when sporting activity is undertaken immediately after a meal. The pain may be made worse by deep expiration and relieved by deep inspiration.

The real causes of stitch are essentially unknown though some studies indicate that a purely mechanical effect may trigger it. The connective tissue which anchors the abdominal organs bears a much greater load just after a meal and physical activity at this time could cause strain and minor internal bleeding. Other possible causes are lack of a sufficient supply of oxygen to the diaphragm or pain arising from the internal abdominal organs, such as the spleen and the liver, as the blood flow is redistributed.

Treatment

The *athlete* should:
— avoid training and competition for a few hours after main meals;
— run bent forward or stop so that the stitch has time to disappear before the training is resumed;
— squeeze a hard object, for example a stone, in the hands. Most athletes feel that this makes the stitch pains subside, but the mechanism of this phenomenon is unknown.

Acute Treatment of Athletes at the scene of the injury

Treatment of soft tissue injuries

This group of injuries includes:
— muscle and tendon damage (haematoma and/or rupture);
— joint and ligament damage (dislocations and/or ruptures);
— soft tissue injuries associated with fractures.

Acute soft tissue injuries

When muscles, tendons or ligaments are damaged, blood vessels in the area are also torn. As a result bleeding occurs and spreads rapidly into adjacent tissues. The bleeding causes swelling which in turn results in increased pressure on surrounding tissues, which become tense and tender. The increased pressure causes pain in sensitive tissues, and the

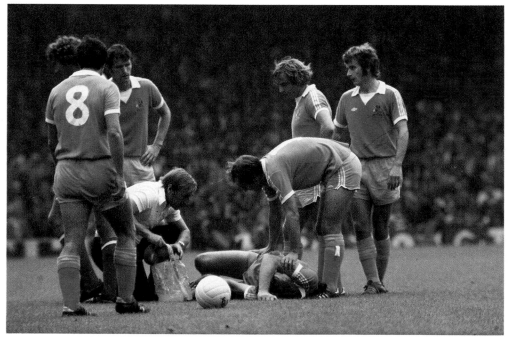

Emergency treatment of injury. *Photo: All-Sport/Don Morley.*

combination of bleeding, swelling and increased pressure can adversely affect the healing process.

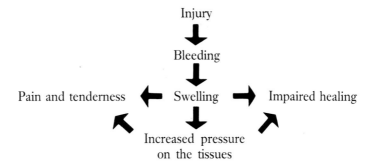

If this cycle of events can be interrupted, healing is enhanced so, in cases of soft tissue injury, it is important to inhibit and control bleeding as soon as possible. Treatment should be started *immediately*. If it is carried out correctly, the initial acute treatment of a soft tissue injury can be the most important factor influencing recovery.

Once bleeding has been controlled, some blood remains in the tissues and has to be removed. This function is performed mainly by the lymphatics. A variable amount of scar tissue forms in the area and constitutes a weak spot in the injured muscle, tendon or ligament. If too early or too heavy a load is applied to this scar tissue, injury is liable to recur.

Sports injuries may take so many different forms that it is impossible to create a standard protocol for their management. Certain guidelines for immediate treatment can, however, be drawn up.

Immediate treatment at the scene of injury

Examination
— A preliminary on-the-spot assessment of the extent of injury should be carried out by the injured athlete or by the trainer. If there is any doubt about the situation, a more careful examination should be carried out in a quiet place such as the changing room.
— The injured athlete should be undressed to the extent necessary for a proper examination of the injured area to take place. Tape, strapping, protective pads and so on are removed.
— The course of events should be analyzed. Listen to the injured athlete's description of how the injury occurred and what symptoms are present.
— The injury should be examined in the light of the history. Is there an effusion of blood, swelling, an open wound or any other abnormal sign?

— A simple functional assessment of the injured part should be made. Can the injured athlete carry out normal movements of the part (with or without a load) without pain?
— The area around the injury should be examined. Is there tenderness in soft tissues or bone? Can a defect be felt in any soft tissue?

If there is swelling and tenderness together with pain when movements are made or a load is applied, treatment should be started as follows.

Cryotherapy (Cooling)

When soft tissue injuries occur, the first priority is to attempt to stop the bleeding since this results in swelling, pain and tenderness. The general rule is that the lighter the bleeding, the faster the effusion of blood disappears and the less scar tissue forms in the injured tissue. Therefore, in cases of soft tissue injuries, reduce the extent of the bleeding by rapid cooling, compression bandaging, an elevated position of the injured limb and rest. This enables the haemostatic functions of the body itself to take effect more easily.

Cooling of body tissues brings about:
— *a local pain-relieving effect* which makes the injured athlete feel better and may well encourage him to return to his sporting activity. Here the trainer has a great responsibility to bear. If an injury needs cooling it is often of such severity that further exertion will only delay healing. Common sense should prevail;
— *contraction of the blood vessels* so that blood flow is reduced in the injured area. Less swelling then occurs and healing proceeds more rapidly.

In the presence of signs of extensive soft tissue injury with bleeding or injury to the skeleton, the injured person must not resume his sporting activity until the injury has healed. Nothing is to be gained by endangering future health.

If cooling is to be effective it must penetrate deep into the injured tissue, and a suitable method must therefore be used. Cooling should be applied long enough for it to be effective, and it is generally true to say that the larger the injured muscle or joint, the longer the cooling should continue. An injury to the ankle or knee should be cooled for periods of at least 30 minutes, an injury to a thigh muscle for periods of 45 minutes.

During the first 2–3 hours following an injury the aim is to provide as continuous a period of cooling as possible. The first disposable ice pack should be changed after 30–45 minutes, at that time checking the appearance of the skin under the pack. During the next 3–6 hours cooling can continue for about 30 minutes per hour to achieve pain relief.

Methods of cooling

Disposable ice packs exert their effect for about 40 minutes after the cold has been released by squeezing hard on the pack. This method has the advantage that the cold penetrates deep down into the injured part and the packs are easy to store.

Reusable ice packs contain an easily moulded viscous substance (a gel) which remains effective for 45–60 minutes after it has been chilled. The pack can be used repeatedly and can be moulded to the shape of the injured part. Again the cold penetrates well into the injured part, but a disadvantage of this type of ice pack is that it must be cooled in a refrigerator and kept in a cooling bag until required. It is, however, ideal for repeated cooling in the home.

> Ice packs must never be placed directly on the skin but should be separated from it by one thickness of elastic bandage, a handkerchief or something similar.

Ice or cold water can be used for cooling injuries when ready-made ice packs are not at hand and also when the injuries involve larger areas which cannot easily be covered with packs of the usual size.

Neither cold water nor ice packs should be used directly on open wounds. *A cooling spray* may be used when local pain relief is the only objective. This applies to areas where the skin is in close contact with the skeleton such as the shins, knuckles and ankles. The cold from such a spray penetrates only $\frac{1}{8}$–$\frac{1}{4}$ in (3–4 mm) into the skin and therefore does not affect underlying injured tissue. There may be some contraction of deeper blood vessels triggered by reflex action, but this effect is probably only slight and transitory. Cooling ceases after spraying has stopped, and the blood flow subsequently increases causing an effect entirely opposite to that desired. Apart from this disadvantage, there is also a risk of inducing cold injuries to the skin when a cooling spray is used.

Compression bandage

At the same time as a soft tissue injury is cooled, a compression bandage should be applied. The aim is to provide counterpressure to the bleeding developing within the injured area so that the body's own haemostatic functions take effect more easily. A compression bandage usually comprises elastic bandages applied with some degree of tension and it is convenient to position an ice pack with the aid of an elastic bandage so that cooling and compression effects are achieved simultaneously. The compression bandage should be held in position after cooling has ceased, providing the location and extent of the injury allow it. Later it may be replaced by a supportive bandage or strapping.

Rest

It is generally true to say that an injured athlete should rest for 24–48 hours and that the injured area should not be subjected to loading (see page 151). It follows, therefore, that he should be assisted from the scene of the injury and taken home or to a doctor, as soon as possible.

Elevation

When an injured part is elevated, its blood flow is reduced, and expelled blood is transported away more easily, thus reducing swelling. An injured leg which is elevated should be supported at an angle of more than 45° when the patient is lying supine. Four or five cushions or a stool placed under the leg will achieve this effect (see photograph on page 68). In cases of extensive bleeding and swelling the injured part should be kept elevated for 24–48 hours if possible. Subsequently, it should be elevated whenever the opportunity arises.

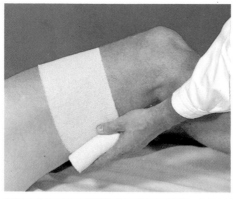

Apply an elastic bandage over the injured area.

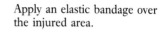

Place ice pack over the injured area.

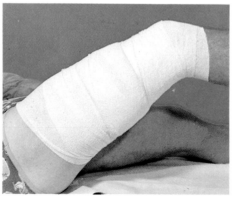

Apply an elastic, compression bandage to hold the ice pack in place. This bandage should cover an area about 8 in (20 cm) above and below the injury.

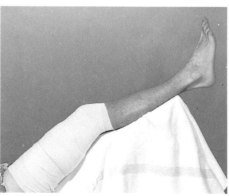

Place the injured leg in an elevated position at an angle of at least 45° to the horizontal.

Heat treatment   If an injury is treated by heat applications in its acute stage the blood vessels expand, and the blood clotting procedure may be disrupted. The amount of fluid in the tissue increases. This leads to increased bleeding in the injured area, increased swelling and higher pressure in the surrounding tissues. The result is severe pain and slower healing than would otherwise be the case.

> Heat treatment should, therefore, not be started until, at the earliest, 48 hours after the injury has occurred. The same applies to massage.

General pain relief   Cooling, compression and rest usually provide relief from pain in soft tissue injuries. Pain-relieving medication should be avoided in the early stages as they can complicate further treatment if continued analysis and medical examination are required.

Equipment   Available equipment should include the trainer's and/or physician's kit. Crutches and stretchers should be available as well as immobilization splints.

Preparation   An emergency plan should be worked out in order to secure adequate acute treatment and transportation. The staff should be well educated and trained.

Summary of treatment in cases of acute injury
Examine the injury.
Apply cooling.
Apply a compression bandage.
Allow the injured person to rest.
If possible, elevate the injured part.
Help the injured person to a doctor if necessary.

Treatment of a soft tissue injury during the first 24–48 hours

When a soft tissue injury does not require medical treatment, but effusion, pain and impaired functioning of the injured part are present, treatment should continue along the following lines:
— *further cooling* if pain relief is the objective;
— *compression bandaging* replaced after a few hours by a support bandage (see page 156);
— *rest* until there are no further symptoms;
— *elevation* of the injured part. If walking is necessary, use crutches to unload the injured area if the lower limbs are involved.

For the treatment of soft tissue injuries after the first 24–48 hours, see the section discussing the injury in question.

A limb which has suffered a soft tissue injury should not be loaded or used until a positive diagnosis has been made. In cases of extensive bleeding, persistent pain and impaired functioning, or when there is uncertainty about the correct treatment method, a doctor should be consulted.

A medical opinion should be sought urgently in any of the following circumstances:

— unconsciousness or persistent headache, nausea, vomiting or dizziness after a head injury (see page 376);
— breathing difficulties after blows to the head (see page 376), neck (see page 385) or chest (see page 386);
— pains in the neck after impact, whether or not they extend to the arms (see page 239);
— abdominal pain (see page 387);
— blood in the urine (see page 388);
— fracture or suspected fracture (see page 18);
— severe joint or ligament injury (see page 22);
— muscle injury (see page 26) or tendon injury (see page 37);
— dislocation (see page 24);
— eye injury (see page 383);
— deep wound with bleeding (see page 56);
— injuries with intense pain;
— any injury in which there is doubt about its severity, diagnosis or treatment.

Injured athletes should seek a medical opinion within 24–48 hours in cases of:

— persistent symptoms arising from injuries to muscle, tendon, joint or ligament;
— severe pain.

It is generally true to say that a doctor should be consulted if there is any uncertainty about the diagnosis, and thus the treatment, of any sports injury.

3 The Biomechanics of Sports Injuries

Biomechanics is the science of the mechanical functioning of the human body, including locomotion, and application of the laws of mechanics helps to explain the mechanisms of injuries caused by accidents and overloading.

Some of the laws of classical mechanics can be used to explain the relationships between the human body and its environment, while other laws relating to the properties of materials describe the stresses to which tissues are subjected.

These laws cannot, of course, be entirely accurate in their prediction when applied to the human body because of individual variations and because of the difficulties encountered in obtaining precise descriptions of the mechanisms of injury. Nevertheless, they provide useful guidelines.

LOAD

Physiological load and adaptability

Man thrives on a certain amount of physical activity which exercises the muscles, skeleton, soft tissues and joints physiologically, that is, within a range in which injuries are rare. The body tissues have the unique ability, not usually possessed by inorganic materials, to adapt to the strain to which they are subjected and to tolerate a progressively increasing load. This adaptability is more evident in the early years than in adult life, but even in the young it is not infallible in preventing injury; the athlete's own ambitions or others' expectations of him may lead him to exceed physiological limits in training or competition.

The capacity for physical adaptation continues to some extent throughout life, and old age alone is not sufficient reason to give up physical exercise even if performance and the level of tolerance of the tissues have decreased.

Overloading and injuries

Body tissue resembles any other material in that it will break when its innate strength is exceeded. The limits of its tolerance depend partly upon its own properties and partly upon the type of load applied. The latter is

71

determined by the magnitude of the forces brought to bear, their points and directions of application and variations in time. The resultant injury may involve tearing or breaking of the tissue concerned, or alternatively, a permanent structural change with consequent functional impairment.

The following explanation includes a number of abstract concepts and mathematical calculations. An understanding of the fundamental ideas is, however, far more important than the ability to make 'detailed' calculations and any reader who finds the formulae difficult should not spend too much time over them.

FORCE AND MOTION

The concept of 'force' is difficult to explain, though most people have some idea of what is meant by the word. The force of gravity, for example, influences us continuously. Even after a short free fall the human body can reach such a speed under the influence of gravity that injury will occur if the fall is brought to an abrupt halt by the environment. Injuries caused by the force of gravity can also occur when no fall is involved, for example in sprains. The relationship between the forces which affect a body and the state of motion or equilibrium of that body can be summarized by the three laws of motion: the law of inertia, the law of acceleration and the law of equal and opposite reaction.

Gravity, inertia and uniform motion

A body has a certain weight which corresponds to its mass, the so-called body weight. The weight is a force which exerts its effect through the body's centre of gravity. If this force were to be unopposed, its tendency would be to move vertically downwards under the influence of gravity. However, if it is counteracted by an equal and opposite force (such as that exerted by the surface on which it lies), it will remain at rest. Similarly, if a body is in motion, it will continue at constant velocity and in the same direction unless outside force is applied.

The force of inertia, that is, the ability of a body to resist a change of motion, is summarized in Newton's First Law and exemplified by centrifugal force:

'Every body continues in its state of rest or uniform motion in a straight line except in so far as it is compelled by forces to change that state'.

The effects of inertia may be felt, for example, when cornering on a bicycle; the bicycle would be inclined to tip outwards if it were not for the weight of the body tipping inwards to counteract the centripetal force.

Translational motion (as described above) is not the only factor which influences the movement of a body through space. Rotational movement around the centre of gravity has to be taken into consideration. Rotational motion also has inherent inertia which is determined by the mass and its distribution around the axis of rotation. Thus, when the mass is close to the axis, the body has less rotational inertia than when it is further away and, by altering the distance of the mass from the axis, the velocity of rotation may be varied. This effect can be seen quite clearly in skating when the velocity of rotation increases as the skater brings his outstretched arms nearer his body during a spin, and also in diving when the diver can stop his rotational motion and prevent a further somersault by straightening out his body before hitting the water.

Force, mass and acceleration

An apple remains hanging from its branch as long as the stalk is attached. The resultant force exerted is zero. If the stalk breaks, the apple falls because the downward force of gravity is no longer counteracted by the lifting force of the branch. During its fall the apple may hit a branch with a certain force so that its direction and velocity are changed. This change of velocity depends on the magnitude of the force and its direction. The velocity of the apple changes both during the free fall and after it hits the branch.

Velocity change per unit of time is called acceleration when the speed increases and deceleration (or retardation) when the speed decreases. Acceleration is directly proportional to force, that is, twice as much force doubles acceleration. Mass and acceleration, on the other hand, are inversely proportional; therefore, the larger the mass, the less acceleration a certain force can achieve.

The relationship between a force and the change in momentum of a body on which it acts is expressed by the equation

$$F = m\,a$$

where F denotes the force in newtons (N), m is the mass in kilograms and a is the acceleration in metres per second^2 (m/s^2). This is summarized as *Newton's Second Law*:

'*Rate of change of momentum is proportional to the applied force, and takes place in the direction in which the force acts*'.

Rotational motion is affected by similar factors, so that change in the forces which cause the body to rotate will change the rotational velocity.

At one time the unit kilopound (kp) was used to denote the magnitude of a force. One kp corresponds to the force of gravity on a mass of 1 kg. On the earth's surface this force gives a mass of 1 kg an acceleration of 9.81 m/s^2 in free fall, so 1 kp equals 9.81 N. Nowadays the newton (N) is used as the unit of force, being roughly equivalent to that force exerted by a mass of 0.1 kg, or a medium-sized apple.

Action and reaction

Forces develop at the points of contact between a body and its environment. The effect of the body on the environment is an *action force* while the effect of the environment on the body is a *reaction force*. According to Newton's Third Law:

'*For every action there is always an equal and opposite reaction*'.

Every force acting on a body possesses a point of action, magnitude and direction. The effect of the force on the body is determined by all these factors. Thus when a person stands up, walks or runs, in accordance with Newton's Third Law, the force of the foot against the surface is always equal but opposite to the force of the surface against the foot.

Friction

If the contact area between the foot and the surface is smooth, the action and reaction forces during locomotion will be directed almost at right angles to the surface, and a gliding motion can easily result. If, on the other hand, the contact area is rough, some force is necessary to initiate the same effect. This force, the *frictional force*, arises from the properties of the surface and that part of the action/reaction force which is directed at right angles to the contact area and is known as the normal force.

The relationship between the action/reaction force, the normal force and the frictional force is illustrated by the diagram on page 75 in which the foot exerts force A on the surface. The reaction force R exerted against the foot is equal in magnitude to A but operates in the opposite direction. R can be divided into two components, N and F, which act at right angles to each other, and are equivalent, respectively, to the normal force and the frictional force of the surface against the foot. R is thus the result of the forces N and F.

The relationship between the frictional force and the normal force can be expressed by the law of friction:

$$F \leqslant f N$$

in which F is the frictional force, f is the coefficient of friction and N is the normal force (the force at right angles to the contact area).

The coefficient of friction is a number between 0 and 1, a smooth surface having a small, and a rough surface a large, coefficient of friction. The equation is a mathematical representation of the statement that frictional force cannot be greater than the product of the normal force and the coefficient of friction.

In sporting activities, different frictional properties of soles and playing surfaces are required in different situations. In the run-up before jumping or heading, for example, high static friction is required between the sole and the surface, but when someone running at high speed stops dead the friction between sole and surface must not be too great or the knee and ankle joints will be subjected to stress as the foot grips the surface.

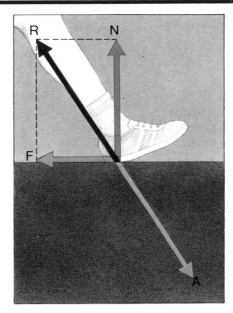

The relationship between the action/reaction force, the normal force and the frictional force.
A = action force
R = reaction force
N = normal force
F = frictional force

When a subject is standing still, all his force is directed vertically through the length of the leg and the foot on the ground. When he is about to run, change direction during running or stop, the leg is held at an angle and consequently the force applied through the foot is directed at an angle to the surface. As has already been mentioned, the force can be divided into two components: N which is equivalent to the normal force and F which is equivalent to the frictional force and is parallel to the surface. When the relation between these forces (F/N) exceeds the coefficient of friction f, the shoe loses its grip and starts sliding. In order to avoid this situation it is best to take short steps on a slippery surface to reduce the angle at which the foot strikes the floor.

Equilibrium

When a body is at rest or moving in a straight line with constant velocity, certain laws of equilibrium apply. One relates to the equilibrium of the centre of gravity and the other to the equilibrium of rotational motion around a point. According to Newton's Second Law a body is in equilibrium if the forces acting on it fulfil the following conditions:

— the sum of all external forces acting on the body is zero (the condition for static equilibrium);

— the sum of all external torques acting on the body is zero (the condition for rotational equilibrium).

Some examples of calculations of equilibrium are given in the following section.

The law of the lever and its importance in the mechanism of injuries

Two girls, Anne and Lisa, are going to play on a seesaw (see diagram on page 77). Anne weighs 30 kg (67 lb) and Lisa 20 kg (44 lb), roughly equivalent to 300 N and 200 N respectively. The seesaw is 6 m (6 yd) long and is balanced on a central support. Lisa is sitting at one end. How great is the force on the support, and where should Anne sit for the seesaw to balance?

The weight of the seesaw itself can be ignored. Let us assume that the force on the support is x newtons and that the distance between the point where Anne is sitting and the central support is y metres.

If the upward force is regarded as positive, it follows from the law of equilibrium that:

$$x - 200 - 300 = 0$$
$$x = 500$$

Therefore, the force on the support is 500 N.

According to the law of movements it follows that:

$$300 \cdot y - 200 \cdot 3 = 0$$
$$y = 2$$

Therefore, Anne should sit 2 m (2 yd) from the fulcrum. The latter equation can also be written $300 \cdot y = 200 \cdot 3$, stating in effect that the moment of rotation, that is, the product of each force and the distance from its line of action (the pivot of the seesaw), is equal. This is called *the law of the lever*.

The law of the lever implies that a small force can have a large moment of rotation if its lever is long. Similarly, the force must be large to achieve the same moment of rotation if the lever is short.

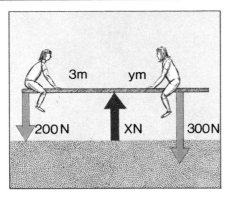

The laws of equilibrium: an example of the law of the lever.
x = the force on the support
y = the distance from the fulcrum

The law of the lever can be used to explain why certain sports injuries such as sprains occur near joints or as a result of tackles. Ligaments and muscle attachments near a joint usually have short levers compared to those of the external force. According to the law of the lever, the force acting on these body structures is greater than the external force. The strength limit can easily be exceeded if the relationship between the levers is unfavourable. In the following section this relationship will be illustrated with some typical examples of injuries caused by sporting activities.

Sprained ankle   A common type of sprain occurs when the foot is 'twisted', stretching the lateral ligaments of the ankle. Suppose that the force at the surface is U with the lever u to the fulcrum V. For the force L in the ligament and its lever l to have an equivalent moment of rotation to U it is necessary that:

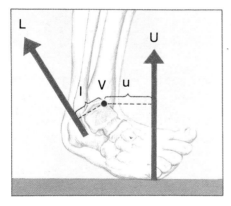

The forces at work when an ankle joint is sprained.
L = the force in the ligament
U = the force from the surface
l = the lever of the force in the ligament
u = the lever of the force from the surface

$$L \cdot l = U \cdot u$$

$$L = \frac{u}{l} \cdot U$$

In unfavourable circumstances the muscles do not have time to protect themselves from sprains. The ankle is twisted so far that u may be up to five times as great as l. Consequently force L can be five times as great as U and in this situation it can easily tear the ligament.

Tackle against knee

The ligament L on the inner (medial) side of the knee joint (see diagram below) is affected in a similar way if a violent tackle with force T is made against the outer (lateral) side of the knee. This is particularly true if the foot adheres to the surface with a force M and if the force from the surface is roughly equivalent to the tackling force T. The fulcrum in this case is K. According to the law of the lever it follows that:

$$L \cdot l = M \cdot m$$

$$L = \frac{m}{l} \cdot M$$

The force M with which the foot adheres to the surface has a lever m which is roughly five times as long as the lever of the ligament l. The ligament can therefore be torn easily unless the force of the tackle against the knee joint is compensated by muscular defence, knee bracing or parrying movements.

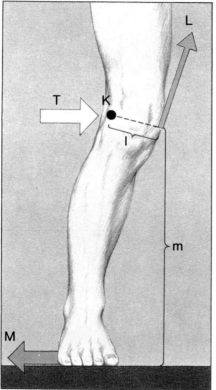

The forces at work when a tackle is made against a knee joint.
T = the tackling force
K = the fulcrum
L = the force in the ligament
M = the force from the surface
l   = the lever of the force in the ligament
m = the lever of the force from the surface

External and internal forces

Part of the load to which the human body is subjected results from external forces such as gravity and reaction forces arising from the environment. Part is the result of internal forces, that is, the effect of the muscles on tendons, muscle attachments, the skeleton and joints. The external and internal forces are partly interdependent and can act together, or oppose each other, with a more or less favourable outcome.

Consider, for example, the combined effects of gravity and muscular force on the knee joint. If the bent leg supports the full body weight, the load on the knee joint will be several times that body weight and only the action of the musculature prevents the knee joint from collapsing. A similar condition applies to other joints in the lower limbs.

This illustration demonstrates the important protective function of the muscles and their role in contributing towards the active stability of joints. If there is good co-ordination between muscles and nerves, the risk of injury is reduced. Experience also shows that the risk of injury increases if muscle defence and function are impaired by fatigue or excess strain.

Some muscle groups act across several joints, with various muscles in the group having similar effects on joint movement. By interaction between different muscles the load can be kept low. This load-reducing function varies with the type of movement performed. People with knee disorders usually find it more painful to descend than to ascend stairs, and this difference can be explained by examining the techniques used. When climbing stairs, the load on the leading knee joint, which is bent at a more acute angle than the other knee, can be reduced by forcefully straightening the ankle of the trailing leg when pushing off. The knee joint of that leg is then almost straight. This technique cannot be used when walking down stairs since braking is applied by bending the knee further, thus subjecting it to a greater force. Also there is a natural tendency to lean backwards when walking downstairs. The thigh muscles are flexed to counteract this tendency and this inflicts further stress on the knees.

MECHANICAL EFFORT — ENERGY

In spite of its stationary existence, an apple hanging from a branch possesses a potential force which manifests itself when it falls to the ground. The height of the apple above the ground is one of the factors which determines the size of the force. It may be considered to be an energy resource for the apple, which is therefore said to possess potential energy. This energy is equal to the mechanical effort required to lift the apple back onto the branch after it has fallen. The effort is equal to the weight of the apple multiplied by the difference between the two distances.

During its fall from the tree, the velocity of the apple increases rapidly, and the potential energy is converted into kinetic energy. The kinetic energy is $\frac{1}{2} mv^2$ where m is the mass of the body and v its velocity. It is the height which determines the velocity of the fall at the moment of impact, but it is not the velocity which determines the force of impact. This force is instead determined by the mass and the deceleration (that is, the rate of change of velocity) on impact, as demonstrated by Newton's Second Law. The deceleration on impact from a pole-vault of, say, 5 m will be considerably reduced by filling the pole-vault pit with foam rubber. Thus, despite the fact that the impact velocity (about 10 m/s) is great enough to cause serious injury if landing takes place directly on the ground, the foam rubber will reduce the risk.

The above example illustrates one of the main principles employed in preventing a certain type of injury due to trauma, namely impact load. By prolonging the braking distance, and thus the time over which the change in velocity occurs, the force, and consequently the risk of injury, can be reduced. A similar principle is that of distributing force over a large area. Modern safety equipment constructed with these two safety principles in mind should be used in all instances whenever there is any risk of bodily injury from blows, collisions and falls.

> By decreasing velocity, prolonging braking distance and distributing force in time and space, the risk of sports injuries can be reduced.

LOADS — STRENGTH

Traction

A wire will break if it is pulled hard enough, and a thicker wire of similar material will withstand greater forces. In the latter case the greater strength of the wire is related to its cross-sectional area. If this area is twice as great, the wire will resist twice as strong a pull. The tension in the wire when it breaks is, however, the same in each case and is equal to the force per unit of cross-sectional area. The tension at the breaking point indicates the limit of so-called 'tensile stress'. Tensile stress occurs in muscles, tendons and ligaments and exceeding this limit will cause tears and sprains (see diagram opposite).

An example of tensile stress in a tendon.

Muscle

Tensile stress

Tendon

Bone

Compression

Thin ice will break under the feet of a person standing on it, while the same ice will support him if he lies down on it with his legs and arms outstretched. The total force acting on the ice is the same in each instance, but in the latter case the force is spread over a larger area, and the compressive stress, that is, the compressive force per unit area, is smaller. Compressive stress acts on the cartilaginous surfaces of joints (see diagram below). If a ligament injury leads to instability of a joint, parts of the articular cartilage can be subjected to more compression than normal, increasing the risk of wear. A similar situation exists when a meniscus is injured or removed at operation.

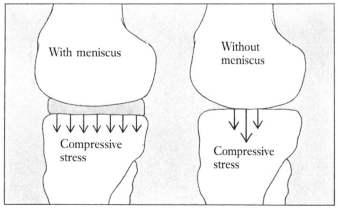

With meniscus

Without meniscus

Compressive stress

Compressive stress

Compressive stress on a joint surface of, for example, the knee joint.

Bending

A branch which is being bent is subjected to a combined load, tensile stress on the outside of the curve and compressive stress on the inside. If the branch is old it can snap transversely, beginning on the convex surface at the point where the tensile stress first exceeds its strength. A young branch does not break in the same way. It is more flexible and may become creased or folded as a result of the compressive stress on the concave surface of the curve. Whatever the age of the branch, however, the load is the same, and it is the properties of the material which will determine the nature of the injury sustained. The older branch has less

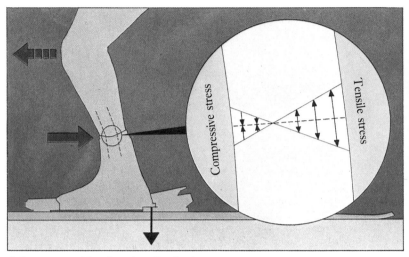

A fracture resulting from bending load.

tensile strength than the younger, but the compressive strength does not differ greatly between the two.

It is the type of mechanism described above which causes the so-called 'ski-boot fracture' of the lower leg. This fracture is caused by failure of the safety binding to release the ski boots during a fall forwards. The bone always breaks on the tensile side because bone is weaker under tension than under compression. Children have more resilient skeletal tissue than adults which is why they may suffer from 'greenstick' fractures (see page 409); these can be compared to fractures of the type that occur in a young branch when it is bent.

Twisting (torsion)

Twisting stress is exerted by a screwdriver used to tighten a screw. If the material of the screwdriver is brittle, a spiral fracture may occur in the shaft. The shape of the surface of the fracture is then determined in part by the direction of the greatest tensile stress. The lower leg of a skier, as shown on page 83, can break in a similar fashion if the foot is twisted violently during a fall without binding release.

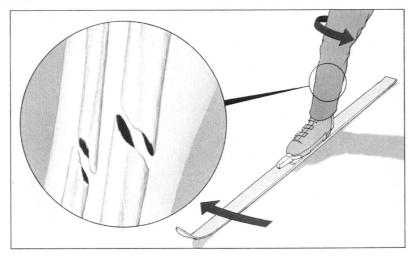

A fracture resulting from twisting load.

Shear stress

The blades of a pair of scissors which are cutting paper subject it to shear stress. The stress acts over the cross-sectional area and is measured in the same way as tensile and compressive stress, that is, in force per unit area. The force that is the result of the shear stress on a cross-sectional surface is reminiscent of frictional force; shear stresses occur in the material underlying the contact area when such a frictional load is applied.

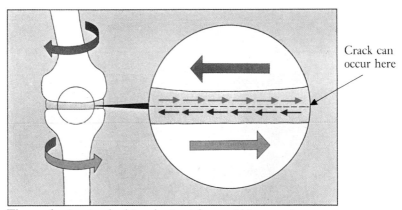

Crack can occur here

The mechanism involved in a horizontal tear within a meniscus.

In the body, major shear stresses occur in joint surfaces and menisci. Such stresses may cause flaking of the tissues in areas where the tissue strength is exceeded, and this is the mechanism of certain types of meniscus injury (see diagram above).

Shear stress also occurs in the lordotic segments of the lumbar spine. Certain athletes, such as gymnasts, have a higher rate of spondylolisthesis as a result.

Repeated load — fatigue

The commonest cause of tearing or breaking of body tissue is the application of a single load which exceeds the tissue's strength limit. Similar injuries can result, however, from repeated smaller loads, the size of which, with respect to the strength limit, will determine the number of load cycles required to cause damage (see diagram below). The smaller the load, the greater the number of load cycles that can be tolerated.

Any part of the body which is subjected to repeated mechanical loads is liable to develop an injury and the likelihood of such injury, caused by wear or fatigue, depends not only on the size but also on the frequency and the duration of the load. Individual factors such as build, age, training level, previous injuries and illness are also relevant.

There is one essential difference between fatigue occurring in biological

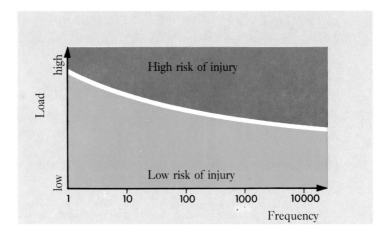

tissue and that occurring in non-biological material. Body tissues have the ability to adapt to the strains to which they are subjected but metal, for example, does not. Adaptation of the body to repeated physiological loading results in improved performance. Its adaptation to repeated over-loading, however, can cause sore muscles, pains in the legs, peritendinitis, and so on as a result of an inflammatory response. Such discomforts are warning signals, and if they are not taken seriously, the body may not have time to repair an incipient injury. If, on the other hand, a suitable training level is chosen, the inflamed tissue can repair itself and gradually adapt to tolerate the higher load.

There are several parts of the body which are at risk from repeated overuse. The skeleton is often affected and the stress fractures which occur in army recruits who are unused to strenuous exercise are examples of the possible results.

A well functioning and strong musculature can reduce the risk of fatigue injuries in the skeleton by preloading it. The tensile stress resulting from the application of a further load will therefore be well below its fatigue limit.

Injuries due to overuse also occur in the soft tissues of the locomotor system; in fact they are probably commoner here than in the skeleton itself. Even minimal tears in tendons and muscle attachments can cause irritating pains which can make sporting activity impossible for months or even years, if they are not given the opportunity to heal. *The healing process may even be prolonged by increased tensile stress placed on the fibres in the immediate neighbourhood of the injury in combination with weakening of the tissue by the normal inflammatory processes.*

Some examples of injuries due to overuse of soft tissues include 'tennis elbow', Achilles tendinitis, 'jumper's knee' and groin strain. Many athletes have been forced to take long breaks from training and competition because, in their enthusiasm to improve their performance, they have come dangerously close to exceeding the strength limit of their body tissues. Children are particularly prone to this type of overuse during certain periods of their growth. The protracted pains in the quadriceps tendon attachment just below the knee joint in individuals who suffer from Osgood-Schlatter's disease can be explained in part by fatigue at the tendon attachment. Inflammatory reactions in other parts of the body where strong muscles are attached, for example heels and groins, can arise from the same cause.

Sports injuries due to fatigue and overloading are very frequent, and may run a chronic course. Many heal with so-called 'active rest' during which the injured area is not loaded beyond physiological limits.

An increased knowledge of the biomechanical background to the origins of sports injuries may lead to a reduced incident of injuries in general.

Preventive Measures

TRAINING AND PREPARATION FOR COMPETITION

Training in general

Only thorough training leads to good results, enabling the athlete to build up his muscles, strengthen his joints and bone structure and improve his co-ordination. Active training will eventually produce enhanced performance, provided it is accompanied by a generally healthy life style and a balanced diet.

It is important that the body parts that are loaded during training should be given the opportunity to rest and recover. The harder the training the longer the break needed for full recovery. Exercising repetitively with a heavy load, for example, would require between 1–3 days' recuperation before the next session. Running and other less strenuous forms of training, on the other hand, can be practised daily. Daily training, however, is of little benefit to those who have either had a long break from training or are physically unfit. Instead they should break themselves in gently with 2 or 3 days' training per week.

Every athlete should analyze the demands of his chosen sport before deciding on a training programme. Apart from the specialized techniques of individual sports, there are other factors which influence performance, and he needs to ask himself the following questions:

1. What factors influence performance in my chosen sport?

2. Which of these factors can I influence and improve by training?

3. How should I train in order to influence each of these factors to best effect?

4. How much time should I devote to training in order to influence each specific factor and when should the training be carried out?

5. Considering all these factors, how should I train in order to reduce the risk of injury to a minimum?

Training intensity and load should then be adapted by the athlete to correspond to the level of physical fitness he or she has achieved.

Basic physical fitness

It goes without saying that good physical fitness is of the utmost importance in avoiding injury. Those whose basic fitness is below normal are more prone to injury both from accidents and from overuse.

After a period of inactivity, the ability of the body tissues to absorb oxygen decreases noticeably. In one experiment, five healthy test subjects stayed in bed for 20 days without any physical activity whatsoever. This relatively short period of inactivity reduced their capacity to absorb oxygen by 20–45 per cent. This and similar experiments demonstrate how quickly the body adapts to the physical demands made on it. When the demands are reduced there is a corresponding decrease in the cardiac output, muscle mass diminishes (atrophy) and blood volume decreases. The body is less efficient in transporting oxygen from the lungs to the tissues and, as a result, the energy supply of the muscles is reduced.

A basic physical fitness can be achieved by exercises and general physical activity carried out throughout the year. All training aimed at achieving good basic physical fitness should be progressed gradually and this applies above all to those who are no longer young. During the period of rehabilitation following illness, injury, or a break in training, it is important that a reasonable level of basic physical fitness is reached before competition is resumed.

The warm-up period

Warm-up exercises are designed to prepare the body for the ensuing sporting activity. They have two functions: to prevent injury and to enhance performance.

In a body at rest the blood flow to the muscles is relatively low, and most of the small blood vessels supplying them are closed. When activity begins, the blood flow to the muscles increases as the vessels open. At rest 15–20 per cent of the blood flow supplies muscles, while the corresponding figure after 10–12 minutes all-round exercise is 70–75 per cent. A muscle can achieve maximum performance only when all its blood vessels are functional.

Physical work increases the energy output and the temperature of the muscles, and this in turn leads to improved co-ordination with less likelihood of injury.

A progressive warm-up leads to a marked decrease in the risk of injury and an enhanced performance, while at the same time providing some psychological preparation for the task to come.

Warm-up exercises should begin with movements of the large muscle groups as these are the main areas to which blood is redistributed. After this general warm-up, more specialized exercises can begin. Runners, for example, should concentrate their warm-up on the muscles and joints of the lower limbs. Stretching of muscles and joints is essential, but heavy loads at the outer limits of joint movement should be avoided. The final stage of warm-up concentrates on technique, perhaps checking a run-up or practising a sport-specific movement. The pace of the exercises can be gradually increased, and the warm-up sessions should last for at least 15–20 minutes, depending on the sport involved.

After a warm-up, a fresh shirt should be put on to prevent the muscles

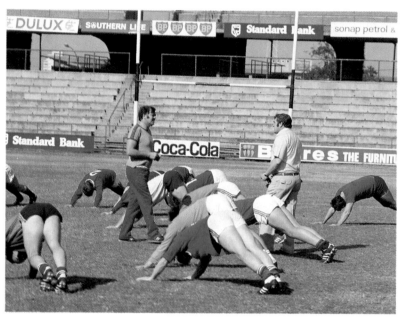

Warming-up exercises are essential before training and competition. *Photo: All-Sport/AdrianMurrell.*

cooling too quickly as sweat evaporates, and a tracksuit is also advisable for warmth. The effect of the warm-up soon starts to wear off and ideally the time delay before competition should be no longer than 10 minutes.

> Warm-up exercises should be completed before both training and competition, and clearly represent a major factor in preventing injury and enhancing performance.

After training or competition, cooling-down exercises, such as gentle jogging, are desirable. Stretching should also be part of the cooling-down process if maximum benefit is to be achieved.

PREVENTIVE AND REHABILITATIVE TRAINING

The effect of training on the musculo-skeletal system

The musculo-skeletal system, upon which locomotion depends, comprises the bones and their associated joints, ligaments, muscles, tendons, nerves and blood vessels. The load placed upon these tissues by exercise and physical work can influence their development, the degree of the influence varying with age.

Skeleton

The skeleton consists of outer, hard bone (compact bone) and inner, soft bone (spongy bone). The compact bone is covered by a membrane (periosteum). Studies of the bone structure of patients who have been bedridden for some time or have been immobilized in plaster show that bone tissue which is not exercised becomes decalcified and weakens with increased risk of fracture.

If the bone structure is exercised regularly by physical training, it adapts to the increased demands and becomes stronger and more robust, though those parts which are subjected to least stress may still undergo some weakening and degeneration. These changes take place relatively slowly, but they must be borne in mind during the rehabilitation period after an injury and, most importantly, during prolonged and unbalanced training of children and young people. They can cause permanent alterations in the skeleton (see page 406).

Cartilage

Articular cartilage covers the ends of the skeletal bones and has a smooth, resilient surface. It is nourished and lubricated by fluid secreted by the synovial membrane which lines the joint and covers those surfaces unprotected by cartilage. Physical activity keeps the articular cartilage strong, whilst inactivity makes it soft, thin, and easily damaged.

The central parts of the joint surfaces are least susceptible to strain, but overloading the joints at their outer limits of movement, should be avoided. For example, any attempt to squat, hop, or do the splits, should be delayed until these extreme positions have been incorporated gradually into the regular training programme. The best way of keeping the articular cartilage in good condition is by means of gentle exercise, as any repetitive, unbalanced, extreme load can damage it.

Connective tissue

Ligaments, joint capsules, muscles, tendons, muscle sheaths and fascia are formed by connective tissue (collagen). The ligaments are strong and rather inelastic. They give the joints stability and govern their movements. The joint capsules consist of a fibrous, outer tissue for stability and a thin, inner synovial membrane which secretes the synovial fluid. The joint capsules are very susceptible to overuse and irritation, and react by secreting more synovial fluid than usual, resulting in an effusion in the joint.

Regular exercise can preserve the strength of the connective tissue and delay degeneration which occurs with age. It also increases the mechanical properties (material composition) and the structural properties (hypertrophy) of the tendons. Inactivity weakens ligaments and joint capsules; ligaments have been known to shrivel and shrink, impairing mobility and putting inappropriate strain on the joints.

Muscles
Each muscle consists of a number of contractile fibres. With exercise, a muscle increases in size (hypertrophy). With ageing, the total mass is maintained but the muscle's strength diminishes as some of the muscle fibre volume is decreased and replaced by fat.

Inactivity affects muscles in various ways. Their stamina and strength declines, and co-ordination and proprioception deteriorates, thus increasing the risk of injury. On the other hand, a healthy and active muscle structure can protect the joints from some injuries by reducing the load imposed by external impact.

Training of the musculo-skeletal system

The training of the musculo-skeletal system includes muscle training, mobility and flexibility training, co-ordination, proprioceptive training and sport–specific training.

Training of the musculo-skeletal system

Exercises are the key to both the prevention of injuries and to a successful rehabilitation programme. An inelastic scar with decreased ability for contraction is often the end product of an injury to muscles or tendons. This will increase the risk of further injury. After an injury, therefore, therapy should aim to limit the amount of scarring and preserve the strength, elasticity and contractibility of tissue components. Repeated exercises will improve the mechanical and structural properties of the tendons.

Muscle contraction is the basis for all movement and exercise. There are three kinds of contraction; *isometric* (or static) work involves contraction without a change in the length of the muscle (for example, holding a weight stationary in an outstretched hand); *concentric* work implies the muscles contract and shorten in length simultaneously so that their attachments are drawn closer together (for example, the contraction of quadriceps muscles when climbing stairs); *eccentric* work implies that the muscles contract and lengthen simultaneously so their attachments are drawn apart (for example, the contraction of the quadriceps muscles when walking downstairs).

During activity that involves change from eccentric to concentric muscular work, or vice versa, there is a risk of tearing a muscle or tendon.

Concentric work mainly accelerates a moving object; eccentric work decelerates it. Injuries often occur during deceleration.

Different types of muscle training

1. Isometric or static muscle work

Isometric or static exercises are those in which the muscles are contracted without moving the body. The leg, for example, can be held at right angles to the body with the knee joint rigid, or a weight can be held in the hand with the arm outstretched.

During isometric training the muscles work constantly in a contracted position. The increase in strength is highest around the angle at which

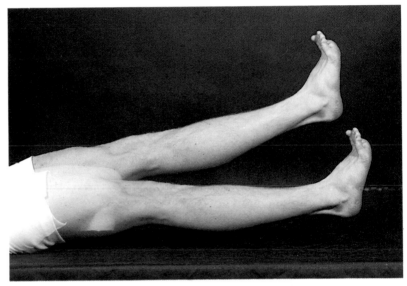

An example of isometric or static muscle training of the extensors of the knee joint.

the training is carried out. Therefore the muscles should be trained at different angles. For maximal effect, maximal contractions are needed. Pressure can build up to such an extent that the blood flow, and thus oxygen supply, to the muscle is restricted. This creates an anaerobic environment and the formation of lactic acid (see page 142). As the amount of lactic acid in the muscle increases, its working capacity is diminished. For this reason isometric exercises are often considered to be strenuous and very tiring, but they are, nevertheless, effective and safe for anyone wishing to build up muscular strength.

Isometrics can increase the circumference and the strength of the muscles in the area which is exercised. The increase in strength, however, is also related to and influenced by the angle of the joint across which the isometric contraction occurs. Long periods of isometric training impair speed, indicating that this training method has its limitations with regard to preventive and sport-specific training. However, it does have an *important role to play in the initial training after an injury.* During training after a knee injury, for example, isometric exercises are very useful as they can be carried out on a knee joint immobilized by a plaster cast or similar support.

2. Dynamic muscle work

Dynamic muscle work means that the distance between the origin and attachment of a muscle varies, either shortening (concentric) or lengthening (eccentric) the muscle.

Dynamic isotonic training

The term, 'isotonic training' implies that the entire movement is performed at a constant level of muscular tension. The speed of a movement can vary according to the load, for example, training using the weight of a leg

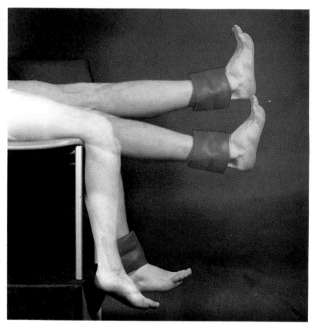

An example of dynamic isotonic muscle training of the flexors and extensors of the knee joint.

alone or placing a weight on the ankle. Typical dynamic exercises include knee bending with or without weights on the shoulders, bending the elbow with or without a weight in the hand (concentric work) or extending the elbow with or without a weight in the hand (eccentric work).

When dynamic isotonic training method is used, the weight remains constant, but the lever arm (the distance from the joint centre of rotation) and torque (the product of the force produced by the muscle and its lever arm) vary during the range of motion resulting in the production of varying strengths. For the same reason the load on the joints will vary. This applies to most athletic events but some situations call for special care and attention (for example, the joint between the patella and the femur during knee bends with weights on the shoulders) if injury is to be prevented.

The most commonly used isotonic training exercises include concentric work. The importance of exercises using eccentric work has been increasingly recognized as eccentric contraction is common to many preloaded situations in sport, for example, kneeling before jumping. Eccentric contraction results in greater increase in strength and is less energy demanding. The athlete should be aware of the increased risk of injury using these types of exercise.

A combination of eccentric and concentric contraction is common in

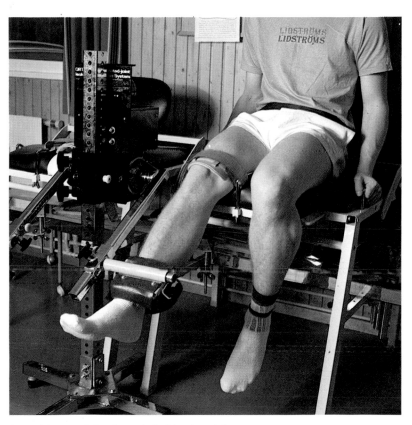

A machine used for dynamic isokinetic training.

sport and can be used in sport-specific training. Such training is called *plyometrics*, and includes jumping, running and throwing.

The aim of plyometrics is to develop power in these movements and to improve the strength of the muscles and tendons, both properties being important in the prevention of injury. Examples of plyometric exercises include hops, bounds, depth jumps and medicine ball exercises.

Dynamic isokinetic training

Dynamic isokinetic training implies that the body acts against an adjustable resistance taking into consideration the changes in the lever arm during the range of motion. The training can be performed at different speeds but the speed of movement chosen remains constant during the range of motion; the higher the speed, the lower the resistance. The training is speed-specific, that is the main effect is achieved at the training speed.

93

This means that, for maximum effect, the training should be carried out at different speeds dependent on the demand of each sport. The resistance can be adjusted by choosing different speeds for training in order to compensate for variations in bone or muscle capacity caused, for example, by pain or weakness.

Isokinetic training is the most effective method of active muscle training. It has numerous advantages and the risk of injury is low since there is little chance of the muscles, joints and connective tissue being overloaded when the appropriate speed is chosen. It is especially useful in rehabilitation, for, if movement over a certain range is painful, the resistance at that point can be reduced while being maintained at a higher level elsewhere. Long training periods at high speed are possible using isokinetics. The combination of maximum speed and maximum resistance is not only conducive to increased strength but also improves the so-called explosive force ('high-speed strength') of the muscle. In other words, isokinetics are extremely effective during all training, including preventive and sport-specific training. Special apparatus is, however, necessary (see photograph on page 93).

Training with a variable resistance

Training with a variable resistance, for example, with a traction rope running over a cam shaped like a nautilus shell, means that resistance is varied to correspond to the difference in strength at various points during the range of motion. This type of training is very useful for building up strength.

Special equipment is again required, and variable resistance training should not be used in the early stages of rehabilitation because the resistance cannot be adjusted to a pain-free range of movement. Its advantages include the ability to isolate particular muscle groups for individual training, and to allow muscles to work eccentrically.

Ranges of application

During dynamic isotonic or isokinetic work the muscles are contracted and relaxed alternately so that blood can pulsate regularly through them. These training methods are therefore considered to be less tiring than isometric (static) training. Dynamic training is included in the sport-specific training for most sports.

Summary

To sum up, isometric (static) training is used particularly in the early stages of rehabilitation of muscle-tendon injuries or when an injured limb is immobilized. Dynamic isotonic training is used in the later stages of rehabilitation but can also be used to increase and maintain a certain level of strength in preventive training of some risk areas. Dynamic isokinetic training is less arduous since, by choosing a higher speed of motion, provision can be made for reducing resistance at any points which are painful in one range. In addition, isokinetics induce a marked increase in strength, whether performed at high speed or at low speed with maximum resistance. Training with a variable but not adjustable resistance allows particular muscle groups to be isolated for individual training and facilitates eccentric muscular work and mobility training.

Mobility and flexibility training

No matter what sport is involved, it is of the utmost importance to maintain and improve speed, strength and technique by means of training. It is equally important to keep the joints sufficiently mobile to cope with the movements and the load to which they are subjected during training and competition.

There are several factors that restrict the mobility of joints (that is, the range of movement they can normally achieve). They include:
— the temperature of the tissues and the efficiency of warm-up;
— the neural receptor system present in all the muscles and around the joints;
— the flexibility of muscles, tendons, ligaments and joint capsules;
— muscular strength and degree of exertion;
— the configuration of the articular surfaces;
— age;
— psychological features.

Joint flexibility is not uniform for all joints but is joint-specific, that is, unique for each joint. It declines after growth has ceased and is generally better in women than in men; it bears no correlation to body type or weight and can develop very variably during different activities. Improved joint flexibility can last for 6–8 weeks after special flexibility training has finished. It is enhanced by good warm-up sessions, and both improves performance and prevents injury. Flexibility exercises should be an integral part of all training and warm-up and cool-down sessions before and after competition.

The flexibility required by a number of sports is a combination of joint mobility, strength, co-ordination and proprioception, and should be adjusted to the activity involved. Flexibility must be maintained at the level demanded by the sport, but training must not be overdone in growing individuals; over-mobility can result, and be a contributory factor in causing overuse injuries (for example, during back extension exercises in gymnastics) and permanent changes in the musculo-skeletal system, for example, tennis elbow.

During periods of intensive training, certain muscle groups may be exercised more consistently than others so that the natural muscular balance of the joints is upset. This is when flexibility training becomes important

Flexibility can be divided into two main types:
— *active (dynamic) joint flexibility* which is the maximum range of motion that can be achieved in a joint by voluntary contraction of muscles;
— *passive (static) joint flexibility* which is the maximum range of motion that can be achieved in a joint, with the aid of apparatus, a colleague or body weight. Passive joint flexibility is limited by the structure of the joint and its surrounding tissue.

The aims of flexibility training are:
— to maintain and/or improve joint mobility;
— to reduce the risk of the joints being subjected to great load at their

outer limits. Good joint flexibility provides a safety margin;
— to prevent injury by co-ordinating the various parts of the musculo-skeletal system;
— to adapt the musculo-skeletal system to the special demands of a particular sport.

The word 'stretching' is often used incorrectly as a synonym for 'mobility' or 'flexibility'. Stretching is, however, one of the methods of flexibility training in current use. Flexibility training is more effective if it is carried out when the muscles are well warmed-up and relaxed. Several methods, including 'stretching', are used:

Dynamic stretching – a ballistic and bouncing movement in which the muscle is extended to its limits and then relaxed; this type of stretching is also called ballistic, spring, bounce or rebound stretching;

Static hold stretching – a full, passive extension is reached and sustained for 10–30 seconds; this type of stretching is also called static, prolonged, plain and hold stretching;

Static contract-relax-hold stretching – the muscle is fully extended by active movement, then further extended passively; this type of stretching is a modification of the PNF technique (proprioceptive neuromuscular facilitation) which is often used by physiotherapists.

Here follows a description of these three different methods of flexibility training.

Dynamic stretching exercises

Using slow relaxed movements, the muscle is gradually extended further and further. Sudden jerks and violent stretching should be avoided. The exercise should be repeated 4–8 times, and for maximum effectiveness the muscle should be held fully extended at its outer range on the final repeat. Dynamic stretching will activate the stretched reflex which, in turn, will counteract the effect of the stretching by initiating a contraction.

This method should suffice to maintain normal mobility. It can be used as a warm-up exercise to activate the tissues around the joints, stimulate the articular cartilages and raise body temperature. However, it should not be used in training after an injury.

Static contract-relax-hold stretching

The muscle in question is first stretched to just below the pain threshold or to the end point at which there is a marked increase in its tension. In this position a maximum isometric contraction is sustained for 4–6 seconds. This contraction is carried out in order to fatigue the stretch reflex so that the effect of the stretching is maximal. The muscle is allowed to relax for about 2 seconds and then extended further and held in the new position for about 6–8 seconds. The whole process is repeated 3–5 times or until the muscle's limit has been reached. The isometric contraction should be as strong as possible in order to benefit the muscle.

This method improves passive as well as active flexibility and is especially useful after an injury. It can be used to increase flexibility to meet the special demands of any sport.

Static hold stretching

This technique is based on maintaining a muscle group in an extended position for 10–30 seconds. Over this period the muscular tension is gradually decreased. After this first 'easy' stretch the muscle group is further extended and the new position is again sustained for $10-30$ seconds. Few published scientific data support the efficacy of this method but practical clinical experience has shown good results.

A technique called the '3S system' (Scientific Stretching for Sport) was first introduced in Canada and claims to improve the following factors: range of motion, retention of flexibility and muscle strength. This method, however, requires the assistance of another person, to hold and stretch the leg, for example.

If a muscle tendon or its attachment has been completely ruptured, it is wise to take care when stretching. If the muscle tendon has been inflamed or otherwise injured in the past month, the stretching exercises should consist of a slow, cautious extension of the muscle to a painless position in its outer range and holding for $8-10$ seconds.

When carrying out stretching exercises, it is easy to check that the correct muscle group is in action and that it really is working in its outer range. Stretching is an excellent method of maintaining and increasing flexibility and should be used both as a method of preventing injury and in rehabilitation.

Co-ordination and proprioceptive training

It takes a long time to learn how to perform movements in an economic and functional way.

Injuries impair co-ordination. Even after the injury itself has healed, it usually takes some time before the interaction between nerves, muscles and joints returns to a satisfactory level. Co-ordination training should start soon after other training has been resumed; there should normally be at least 6 months of special co-ordination training after an injury. Aspecial type of co-ordination training is proprioceptive training. Proprioception is the interaction between the nervous system, muscles, tendons, ligaments and joints.

Sport-specific training

Every sport makes special demands on its participants. Athletes, coaches and trainers should be aware of which muscle groups are most used and thus subjected to the greatest load and risk of injury in their particular sport. These muscle groups should undergo sport-specific training before active sport is resumed after injury. For the principles of weight training, see page 102. Sport-specific conditioning can be achieved by training within the sport itself, for example, soccer players running with the ball instead of running on a track.

Principles of training after injury

Rehabilitation and training after muscle injuries or damage to tendons or joints require special knowledge on the part of both the injured athlete and his trainers and advisers; if the strength of the injured tissue is overestimated, healing may be impaired or the injury may recur.

The objective in training muscles, tendons and joints after injury is to:
— regain good mobility of the joints;
— stretch the connective tissue fibres of the tendons and muscles to an optimal length;
— increase the strength and stamina of the muscles;
— increase the strength of muscle and tendon attachments;
— improve co-ordination and proprioception.

Biomechanical considerations

The range of movement of a joint is normally limited by the articular surfaces, the ligaments and the joint capsule and by the length and flexibility of muscles and tendons. The ligaments and joint capsule are comparatively inelastic and are responsible for maintaining passive stability, while muscles and tendons control active stability.

Muscles, tendons and ligaments all contain collagen fibres. A tendon, for example, consists of 90 per cent collagen fibres and 10 per cent elastic fibres. The collagen fibres run parallel in tendons, in tendon attachments, and in the areas where they merge with muscles. They are under no tension at rest but are loaded and stretched during muscle contraction. Collagen tissue can be elastic (resilient) or plastic (pliable), and has a high viscosity (internal friction). The fact that it is both viscous and elastic means that the speed with which it is loaded is of importance. The faster a tendon is loaded, the stiffer (less elastic) and less pliable it becomes. During slow loading, on the other hand, there is an increase in its elastic and plastic properties.

The collagen in tendons must be subjected to extension for at least 6 seconds for its plastic properties to change. At temperatures of about 39–40°C (100–101°F or just above normal body temperature) there is an increase in the elasticity and plasticity of collagen fibres, so a careful and thorough warm-up should be carried out before any flexibility training begins. Localized warming of tendons followed by slow stretching to the pain threshold results in extension of the collagen fibres of the tendons to their maximum length. The stretching should be carried out within 15–20 minutes of the application of local heat treatment, otherwise the warm-up effect will be lost.

1. Muscle training after injury

Muscle strength is proportional to the cross-sectional area of the muscle (that is, to the diameter and number of muscle fibres). The larger the cross-sectional area, the greater the force that the muscle can generate. The degree of force generated varies inversely to the speed at which the muscle contracts. Maximum force is generated by isometric contractions in which a large number of motor units are used. The faster a muscle contracts, the less force it can generate as fewer motor units are used.

Strength training increases the strength not only of the muscles but also of their attachments. The strength of tendons, ligaments and the skeleton does not increase as quickly as that of the muscles since their metabolism is slower, and this fact should be borne in mind in training growing individuals. During rehabilitation after injury, strength training should be carried out to the pain threshold. In order to shorten recovery time, training of muscles in the injured area can begin along the following lines.

Static (isometric) training

After many joint and muscle injuries, isometric training can start immediately. For best results the muscle contractions should be as strong as the pain allows. A slow isometric contraction increases the load on the injured tissue gradually, so that it is easier to avoid going beyond the pain threshold and the strength limit. The training starts with relatively few muscle contractions per day and increases gradually. *An increase in the number of muscle contractions should precede an increase in the load.* Rest should be taken between successive isometric muscle contractions so that the lactic acid formed in the tissue can be dissipated. If possible, a physiotherapist should check constantly that no further problems develop as a result of the training.

Once isometric training can be carried out without pain, the dynamic training should start.

Training of this type is suitable for the extensors and flexors of the knee joint, for example.

Dynamic training

After bandaging has been removed and medical permission has been given to move the joint, dynamic training can start, at first using only body weight or weight of a limb as the load. Subsequently the load can be increased gradually by the addition of weights. In dynamic training with weights (that is, isotonic training), maximum loading of a joint can only be achieved during part of the range of motion. This leads to the risk of overloading the joint at its weaker points. This risk is reduced in isokinetic training, though this, of course, requires the use of special apparatus (see photograph on page 93). Isokinetic training, as described previously, involves working at constant speed against maximum resistance throughout the range of motion. The risk of further injury is small because the resistance is adjusted at every stage of the movement, according to the strength of the injured tissues.

Dynamic training should start with a low load, and in the early stages the training programme should be expanded by increasing the frequency of the exercise rather than the load. This enables the stamina and the blood flow of the muscle to improve before it is stressed further. When load *is* increased, it is important to remember that the force to which a joint is subjected can be great. Placing a weight over the ankle joint during training of the knee, for example, increases the load on the knee joint by ten times.

Dynamic training has a limited effect on the isometric strength of a muscle, except when it is carried out at low speed, in which case it resembles static training. Similarly, static training has only a limited effect on the dynamic strength of a muscle. In other words, all training should be relevant and designed specifically to work on those elements used in the sport in question.

In summary, *an exercise programme after injury* should begin carefully with a gradual increase of load to the pain threshold. Careful isometric exercises are recommended initially, to be performed without load. It is often sufficient to use the athlete's leg alone, as load. Gradually increased strength training with loads can then be applied.

As soon as healing permits, the athlete can start dynamic exercises, including both eccentric and concentric contractions. Eccentric contractions will maximize time delays and energy expenditure. These exercises should not exceed the pain threshold as pain signifies overuse of the tendon or muscles.

After an initial period of rehabilitation the pain limit can be exceeded during the final few contractions in the exercise programme in order to increase the pain threshold.

It is important to consider the following points before commencing strength training after an injury:

— All strength training should begin with warm-up exercises.
— All training should begin without load and should not exceed the pain threshold.
— There should be a gradual increase in load but it is better to increase the number of repetitions with one load before proceeding to greater loads.
— Asymmetrical exercises should be avoided.
— Rest and recovery are important in all types of strength training.
— Strength training should be combined with flexibility training.

2. Mobility training after an injury

One factor which determines the overall length of a muscle is the stretchability of its connective tissue component. If this is to be increased, the tissue must be subjected to stretching for at least 6 – 10 seconds while the muscle tension is low. The tension developed within a muscle determines the degree to which it can increase in length and is dependent on the activity in the nerve fibres which supply it. Pain increases this activity and results in shortening of the muscle.

Flexibility training can be active as well as passive and an appropriate programme could consist of some of the different types of stretching exercises previously described (see page 96). Dynamic (ballistic and bouncing) stretching is a swinging movement in which the muscle is extended to its outer range and then immediately returned to normal. This type of exercise should be carried out slowly and in a relaxed fashion as too great a pace causes the muscle to contract due to reflex action and it becomes impossible to stretch. This method should *not* be used in training after an injury.

During each stretch the range of motion should be increased, if possible, without the muscle springing back to its rest position.

Static stretching involves passive stretching of a muscle already in a stretched position. The origin and insertion are situated at a maximum distance from each other. This type of training influences the tissues around the joints and should be repeated until flexibility increases. The technique is described on page 96.

Extension training (static stretching) should be an integral part of the rehabilitation programme following an injury. In most cases, it can begin relatively soon after the injury occurs, though in cases of muscle or tendon rupture, it should be postponed until a doctor gives approval. As a rule, static stretching can start when there is no local tenderness in the injured area and when static muscle contractions can be performed without pain. However, static stretching can be used to evaluate the healing progress in an injured muscle or tendon by using the level of pain as a measure of the state of the healing process.

3. Co-ordination training after an injury

Any injury impairs co-ordination, which must be regained before resuming competition. A soccer player with a knee injury, for example, should not take part in further football matches without first having trained with the ball and regained his co-ordination (or 'timing').

Co-ordination training leads to an improvement in proprioception, which is the interaction between the central nervous system and muscles, tendons, joints and ligaments. As co-ordination improves, movements can be made with more confidence and less energy expenditure. Imperfect co-ordination, on the other hand, can result in faulty execution of movements during training or competition which can often lead to overuse injuries.

Good co-ordination training enables steady and controlled movements to be made without their being hampered by activity in those muscles which exert an opposite effect. It should be adapted to suit the techniques of the individual sport, and should be carried out at the beginning of the training period without going beyond the threshold of fatigue. It should be pointed out that it often takes a long time, sometimes 6 months or more, to achieve good muscle co-ordination and proprioception.

In all rehabilitation, thorough training of large muscle groups is essential. As muscular strength, endurance, joint flexibility, co-ordination and proprioception return, sport-specific training can be resumed.

4. Sport-specific muscle training

Athletes, coaches and trainers should be well aware of those muscle groups which are used in their own sport and of the maximum loads and possible injuries to which they may be subjected. These muscle groups should undergo specialized training before sporting activities are resumed after an injury.

In any rehabilitation programme, the injured and healthy sides of the body should be trained in parallel. This means, for example, that it is also necessary to train the non-racket (idle) arm in racket sports. The results are best evaluated by comparing one with the other.

Training should be regular and adapted to suit the individual. It should adhere to the following guidelines:
— All training after an injury should first be carried out without a load. Subsequently the frequency of the training movements is increased before any load is added.
— Asymmetrical training should be avoided.
— Strength training should be combined with co-ordination and static stretching exercises.
— Any muscle groups of particular importance in the sport in question should be specially trained.

Conditioning after injury

Running should not be resumed after injury until static and dynamic training, both with and without a load, can be accomplished without problems. As a rule, physical fitness training should begin again with non-vigorous cycling, swimming or similar, less strenuous exercises. A doctor or physiotherapist should be consulted before running is resumed. In addition, the following points should be noted:

— Running puts great strain on the musculo-skeletal system.
— Conditioning after an injury should recommence with slow running on an even and soft surface, for example grass.
— Running should initially be over short distances, and interspersed with periods of jogging or walking over short distances.
— Clothing (especially footwear) must be appropriate.
— Track training should be combined with all-round muscle training.

Weight training

Regardless of the sport involved, most athletes need general muscle training to reduce the risk of injury to the muscle-tendon unit itself and to the joints protected by muscle activity.

The aim of such training, besides prevention of injury, is to improve the strength and performance of the muscles. As 'muscular strength' is not a standard concept, 'weight training' is only a collective name given to the various types of training aimed at increasing in some way the strength and functional capacity of muscles.

The strength requirements of a particular sport should form the starting point for weight training. Each sport requires a special programme aimed at precisely those muscle fibres which are used most intensively in competition. However, it is not sufficient for a thrower, for example, to train only the strength of his arm. If his body is to develop comprehensively he should also devote time to general weight training.

The following factors should be considered when a programme of weight training is planned:

— type of strength required (dynamic, see page 92 or static, see page 91);
— potential use of strength (occasional maximum effort or repetitive sub-maximal effort);
— pace of movements (explosive, rapid or slow).

General advice *All weight training should begin with warm-up and flexibility exercises* which should be continued for at least 15 minutes.

If weight training is to be effective it must be carried out *regularly and methodically*. It results in a fairly rapid increase in muscular strength, but a slower increase in the strength of the skeleton, ligaments and tendons, and caution is recommended, particularly in young people and beginners. *It is important that intensity and load are increased slowly* so that muscular strength does not exceed the strength of tendons and ligaments and their attachments.

During weight training, all movements should be performed in a similar

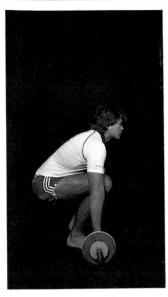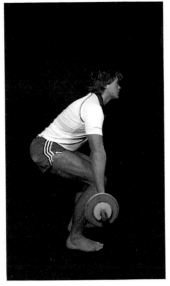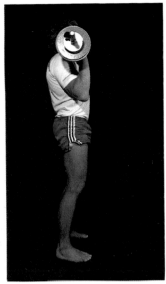

The correct technique for weight training with a barbell.

way on each occasion. In order that this should be achieved, the correct movements are practised, at a slow pace and using light loads, during a preparatory learning period. Then, the variety and period of training are gradually increased. Too rapid an increase can lead to injuries and impaired results. In the case of weight-lifting for example, training should start with a low load and then the *number of lifts should be increased gradually* before increasing the load. During the training periods the particular movements that are relevant to competition should be practised during training periods.

Rest and recovery are important elements in weight training. Recovery time varies both from individual to individual and according to the intensity of training. At the end of the session there should be a cool-down phase, which should also include some flexibility exercises.

Lifting technique

The correct lifting technique must be used if athletes are to train with heavy loads without being injured. The correct way to lift a barbell from the floor must be learned carefully and practised regularly as the wrong technique can cause back injury, including disc damage. The best advice is to begin using the bar only as a load and to lift 'with the legs', keeping the back straight and placing the load as near to the centre of the body as possible.

When leg-strengthening exercises involve knee-bends with a barbell on the shoulders, the knees should not be bent to more than a right-angle as persistent, exaggerated knee-bends greatly increase the risk of meniscal or other knee injury.

Weight training programmes should be drawn up individually and with regard to the subject's age, sex, build, physical fitness and sport. Great caution is advisable in the preparation of strength training programmes for growing youngsters.

Technique and co-ordination

It takes a long time to achieve good interaction between the muscles and the nervous system, that is, good muscular co-ordination, lack of which can result in faulty execution of movements during training and competition with resultant injury and poor results. Injuries due to wear (such as cartilage damage) are also sometimes caused by repeated incorrect muscle loading, that is, by faulty technique.

Co-ordination is believed to be at its peak between the ages of eight and fourteen years, and it can be improved by technique training which athletes should start while still young. The training brings about a rapid

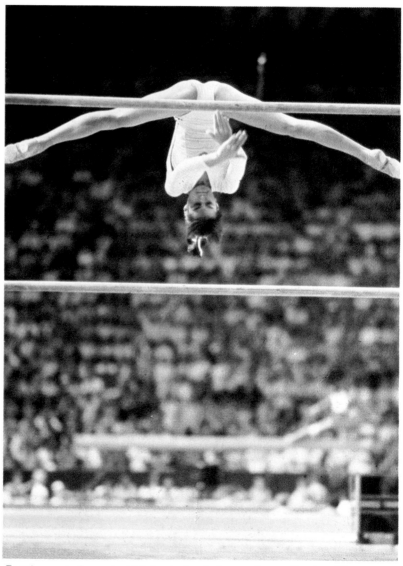

Certain sports demand a high level of technique and co-ordination. *Photo: Pressens bild.*

initial improvement followed by a plateau, which may last for some time and during which performance remains unchanged. However, if training continues, further improvement will be achieved by similar stages.

Movements in technique training must be performed correctly right from the start as it can be difficult to correct a faulty pattern later. When a runner suffers injuries resulting from wear and tear, for example, his running technique should be analyzed. Is the strike made with the whole sole or too far in front of the body and too hard? If he uses the correct technique, striking close to the body on the outer edge of the sole first in order to load the whole foot thereafter, his running is more effective and economical and the risk of injury is reduced.

Achieving optimal co-ordination requires constant repetition of the various elements of the movements. Technique training should be assigned to the beginning of the training session when it is easier to concentrate and the body is well-rested, and it should alternate with other types of training so that sessions are not monotonous.

All athletes should have learnt the correct technique before taking part in competition.

PSYCHOLOGICAL PREPARATION

Good psychological balance and harmonious team-work are often the basis for achievement. With this in mind, various methods of psychological training have been developed in recent years.

The relationship between athlete and coach

Group unity

In all team-work, the team as a whole is influenced by the mood of its individual members, each of whom has his or her own personality. Team players prefer to pass the ball to team-mates they like rather than dislike.

Certain personality traits may be overrepresented amongst participants in particular sports and at particular levels. In many studies athletes have been characterized as successful if, as a group, they have scored higher marks than average in personality tests identifying traits such as aggression, dominance, psychological rigidity, courage, rapport and self-confidence.

In order to assimilate a variety of personalities it is important that the team as a whole should have a feeling of affinity and that each of its members should be accepted by the rest of the group. This enhances team loyalty which is a characteristic that should be allowed to develop over a long period and which can be intensified before important contests.

When members of a group have clearly defined roles and common aims, a sense of unity develops, and with it improved efficiency. Active

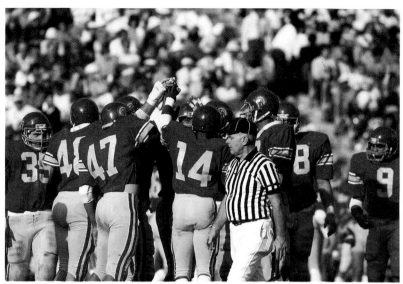

A strong feeling of team spirit. *Photo: All-Sport/Tony Duffy.*

athletes who are given the opportunity to define their own roles and aims, and to discuss questions relating to training and competition, will achieve much more than others in this respect.

Older players can be valuable links in the team, but in spite of their experience, if they have lost the incentive to win, they can have a negative influence on the team in a purely psychological sense.

Coach and team captain A good relationship between the coach and players is essential for success in sport. The coach should have the confidence and respect of his players, something that often rests on his expert knowledge and teaching skill. He should also be able to provide a sense of security during a match and, when necessary, have a calming effect on the players. A good coach should be aware both of the psychological and emotional mood of the group as a whole and of the interactions between individual players.

The importance of the coach increases during visits abroad and on long tours when many athletes can suffer from 'hotel boredom' during periods of inactivity. It is then up to him to try to keep the players occupied both physically and mentally.

The team captain's function is also very important, as he is the man who has to encourage and stimulate the team to perform well. For this reason, he is often chosen more for his psychological qualities than for his athletic ability, and he has usually proved his qualities as a leader before being elected captain.

Coach, team captain and team members should be made aware of the fact that players who do not perform as well as expected need encouragement. If the world around him reacts negatively to inadequate performances, the player under scrutiny may respond with hesitancy or uncertainty, which, in turn, may cause his performance to deteriorate further. An atmosphere of positive and constructive criticism, and spontaneous and positive encouragement, is the best basis for success.

Mental tension

Heightened mental tension leads to faster heart and respiratory rates, increased blood pressure, expansion of the blood vessels in muscles and increased release of sugar from the liver, amongst other effects. As a result the body acquires a higher state of readiness for activity and at the same time increases energy consumption.

The requirement for some degree of mental tension varies from sport to sport. Sports which are technically simple and require strength and speed, demand a high degree of mental tension for the athlete to reach maximum performance. Typical examples of such sports are cycling, long-distance running and cross-country skiing. In sports such as gymnastics, diving, table tennis, badminton, soccer and American football, which are technically more difficult and demand finer co-ordination and greater concentration, too high a degree of mental tension is counter-productive. Orienteering is an example of a sport with mixed demands, as the running component demands a high level of mental tension, while the orientation itself demands a lower level.

Raised mental tension can cause reactions such as lack of appetite, headaches and, occasionally, defective co-ordination which can lead to an increased risk of injury. If an athlete performs less well in competition

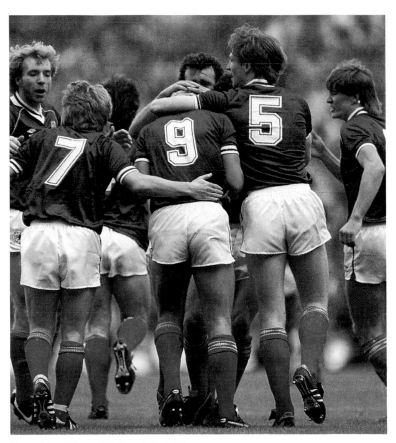

Shared joy. *Photo: All-Sport/David Cannon.*

than in training, his degree of mental tension is probably too high, and his training should be adapted to the situation, perhaps by including competitive elements in the training itself or by more frequent competition.

Preparation before a contest   In general, physical activity has something of a dampening effect on mental tension, and warm–up exercises can therefore be of benefit. A long warm-up period may be advantageous to an athlete who wants to lower his level of mental tension, but only if he does not watch his fellow competitors during that time. Heat in the form of a hot shower before competition can also have a relaxing effect, as can massage.

With regard to team sports, the coach can try to divide the warm–up session into three sections: a warm–up period common to the whole team, a longer period during which everyone chooses his own activity and a concluding warm–up period for the whole group again. One should not forget that the members of a team are also individuals all of whom have their own particular desires and needs. Athletes should not be forced to change established habits as this increases mental tension.

Should an athlete, either consciously or unconsciously, feel too self-confident, he may fail to develop the mental tension required to produce a good performance. It is, for example, easy to underestimate an opposing team which is playing in a division far below one's own. When this is a possibility, the trainer may try to encourage a certain degree of tension by changing the usual routine, for example by making surprise positional changes in the team.

To sum up, those athletes who wish to reduce too high a level of mental tension should try to raise their expectations in training and lower them in competition. Most athletes suffer from nervousness to a greater or lesser extent before a match. In such a situation it is probably best for them to discuss their feelings with others and to know that they are accepted by their coach and trainer.

Concentration

Training the ability to concentrate   It is important for athletes to have good concentration, especially in sports demanding advanced techniques. Mental tension adversely affects concentration, and anxiety is probably the reason for those inhibitions that sometimes affect athletes during technique training.

Training can improve the ability to concentrate, particularly over protracted periods. Intense and prolonged concentration demands energy and depletes the athlete's mental resources. Concentration training should therefore be rationed and begun only at the appropriate time.

During the day before an important competition the manager should assist in diverting the concentration of the players *away* from the competition.

Biofeedback   Biofeedback can achieve improved mental and muscular relaxation and enhanced concentration. It is based on the recording of a physical measurement, such as pulse rate, which the subject can monitor himself and modify by his own efforts. The technique is based on the following assumptions:

1. Mental processes have some effect on the physiological functions of the body. Changes in these functions can therefore be achieved by intense concentration.
2. A relaxed state achieved in one part of the body tends to spread to other parts of the body and become generalized.

In practical terms, biofeedback aims to teach the athlete to relax and to experience a state of rest and warmth with the aid of mental concentration. Each session follows a specified pattern and can be time-consuming. (For additional information please refer to specialist literature, see page 463.) It can, however, be used whenever and wherever required. In sports where reaction speed is decisive and strength and stamina are not limiting factors, it can be effective when used, for example, immediately before and during breaks in competition.

As this technique may have certain negative effects on those who are too tense, experts in the field should be consulted before it is used.

Meditation

Meditation implies passive, effortless concentration. The thoughts that emerge are neither controlled nor checked, but simply registered. It has been discovered that practising this technique can lower the rate of metabolism, reduce the level of lactic acid in the muscles as they relax and slow down the heart rate. The resting pulse rate, which does not fall during ordinary relaxation, is lower during meditation.

The supporters of meditation maintain that it produces superior physical relaxation and thus reduced cardiovascular load, even during activity. It is claimed that those who meditate experience a certain tranquillity and acquire the ability to relax, while athletes who have tried the method say that it improves their concentration.

Meditation is practised for two 20-minute periods per day. The person meditating concentrates on a special word ('mantra').

The method is controversial and can, in rare cases, cause psychiatric problems, but the positive results which it seems to achieve cannot be completely disregarded.

'Pep' talks

'Pep' talks aim to inspire athletes before competition with the additional help of slogans, shouting, stamping on the floor, and similar behaviour. The phenomenon should be seen as part of the overall process of psychological preparation. Sessions such as these may have stimulatory effects, and athletes who suffer high mental tension should not indulge in them.

With regard to team sports, 'pep' talks should be used with some discretion as the reactions of individuals may differ according to their mental state and ability to channel their feelings.

> Physical and psychological preparation are both important before training sessions and competition, and each has a major contribution to make towards reducing sports injuries.

KIT (EQUIPMENT)

Footwear

Normal daily activities make considerable demands upon the feet, which are required constantly to support the entire body weight. These demands are far greater during sporting activities. Running is an obvious part of training in most forms of sport. During running, when the foot makes contact with the ground, a load equivalent to 3–4 times the body weight must be distributed through the limb, shoe and running surface, so the relationship between them is of major relevance with regard to possible injury. In most sports, shoes are by far the most important item of clothing (equipment).

When choosing shoes, several factors must be taken into consideration, including the sport involved and the surface used. Today's market offers shoes specially designed for most sports. It is always wise to choose the best fitting and most suitable shoe, even if it is more expensive than other models.

General points on sports shoes

A sports shoe must be designed around the resilient arches of the foot. The twenty-six bones of the foot are connected by joints and ligaments and form a longitudinal and a transverse arch. When load is applied to the foot these arches adopt a comparatively flat configuration and resume their original positions as soon as the load is removed.

Use the correct shoe for the right purpose. A number of factors have to be considered when choosing sports shoes, including the proposed training programme, the surface to be used, the anatomy of the foot, previous injuries and the requirements of the particular sport concerned. A football player who is improving his fitness by training on asphalt, for example, should not wear studded boots or shoes.

Shoes should be designed orthopaedically if they are to protect the various tissues of the feet from damage, and, in some cases, arch supports may be required. These can be ordered from an orthopaedic workshop after consultation with an orthopaedic surgeon.

Sole

The sole of the shoe determines the amount of shock absorption that the shoe provides, and thus a sports shoe should be constructed of layers with different properties.

The *outer sole* should insulate from cold and be water-repellent and hardwearing as it is this surface which determines the durability of the shoe. Worn soles affect the application of the load and reduce the amount of friction against the playing surface. Anyone who runs on soft surfaces or on open ground should buy shoes with grooved or studded soles. The studs should not be too deep and should extend across the entire width of the sole so that the load on the shoes and feet is even.

The outer sole should be constructed of different shock-absorbent materials — leather, rubber or synthetic materials — on the multi-layer principle. When choosing the appropriate thickness of the sole, body weight should be taken into consideration. The heavier the athlete, the

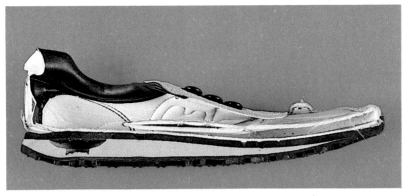

Cross-section of a shoe showing how the sole is constructed for optimum shock absorption.

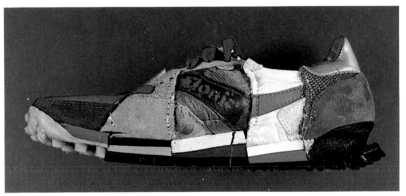

The 'ideal' shoe.

more shock-absorbent the sole should be.

At the initiation of a running movement, that is, at the moment of take-off, the toes are bent. It is essential that the sole should allow for this movement, and the front of a running shoe should be so flexible that it allows bending to an angle of at least 45° with no great effort on the part of the runner. A runner who has to make a great effort to bend his shoe could easily find himself suffering from overuse injuries.

Tennis players often turn when there is a load on the ball of the foot. The soles of tennis shoes must therefore be provided with a strong pad at this point.

Beneath the hard outer sole of a sports shoe lies the *mid-sole*, a layer of soft material which should also be shock-absorbent. Manufacturers have tried to improve the shock-absorbent qualities of the soles of their shoes in several ways, including incorporating air cushions into wedge-shaped heels. These innovations have not as yet been evaluated scientifically.

The *inner sole* of a sports shoe should be constructed of a firm material as it supports the longitudinal and anterior transverse arches. Anyone who needs arch supports should have them fitted expertly, as the soft insertions in most of today's sport shoes are of little value.

The inner sole should be covered with a soft, elastic and absorbent material which prevents the formation of calluses and blisters.

Raised heels	Athletes training for long distance races who have problems with Achilles tendinitis should wear shoes with heels ½–¾ in (10–15 mm) higher than the rest of the sole. A wedge heel relieves the tension on the tendons and can be used for the same purpose by anyone who is recovering from an Achilles tendon rupture. Unless tendon problems exist, shoes with raised heels are unnecessary, and they can sometimes cause problems arising from the toes and anterior arches.
Heel counter	The heel counter of a sports shoe should be made of a firm material, cover the whole of the heel area and fit well around the heel. A well-fitting heel counter should give improved lateral stability, with restriction of the movements of the joints below the ankle. The inside of the counter should be smooth and soft and covered in leather to prevent blisters and pressure on the foot.
Uppers	The uppers should be flexibile but firm. A soft, flimsy upper can give the foot too much lateral mobility and increase the risk of sprain. In some sports it is an advantage for the uppers to extend over the ankles. The tongue and the border of the upper should be padded. The shoe should lace over the top of the foot without affecting the movements of the ankle and toe joints. The shoe should fit firmly without pressure on the foot, perhaps by means of lacing in two sections in order to achieve the desired effect.
Vamp	Most shoes provide little room for the toes, though ideally they should be wide at the front so that the toes can move freely and so that there is room for movement of the foot during take-off. The toes should be protected from bumps and similar hazards, possibly by replacing the sole at the front of the shoe with a fitted toe cap with padding on the inside.
Weight	In long-distance running the weight of the shoes can be of importance. They should not, however, be so light that their stability is impaired.
Shoe care	A man's foot normally produces about 1·5 fl oz (40 ml) of perspiration a day while a woman's produces just over 1 fl oz (20 ml). Socks and shoes should therefore be changed frequently. Shoes keep their shape better if they are stored using shoe trees. Their useful life is also prolonged if they are occasionally rested and are kept clean and polished. Do not let the shoes dry near a radiator or other source of heat, as this will stiffen the leather. Shoes should be bought at the end of the day when the feet are a bit larger.

> Shoes are the most important items of clothing in most sports, and the right shoes are a good investment.

Clothing

Appropriate clothing keeps the body at a comfortable temperature and protects it from wet and wind.

Humans function best at a body temperature of about 99°F/38°C, and, in order to maintain this temperature, we can lose heat by conduction, radiation, convection and sweating. Overheating as a result of strenuous physical exertion can be avoided by wearing loosely fitting clothes with good ventilation.

Heat loss by evaporation takes place mainly through the clothes, but is insufficient to allow sweat to evaporate completely. This is important, as clothes which have become moist with sweat can lose up to 99 per cent of their heat-insulating properties.

The 'cold spots' of the body, that is, those through which most heat is lost, generally coincide with openings in clothing and, by adjusting these, body heat can be regulated.

During prolonged physical exertion, especially in winter, athletes should dress according to the *multi-layer principle*. Several layers of thin clothing retain body heat better than fewer layers of thick clothing.

The innermost layer

The innermost layer of clothes may consist of a vest which allows sweat to evaporate easily, and prevents contact between damp material and the skin. A suitable garment is the so-called 'thermal' vest which is made of cotton woven into vertical channels which absorb drops of sweat and disperse them quickly. Between the channels are thin terylene threads which further distribute the sweat and enhance its evaporation by the circulation of air.

In winter the vest should have long sleeves, reaching well below the waist, be roomy and have no tight seams. The accompanying long underpants should have angle-cut legs with no tight seams in the crotch where the skin is sensitive, and should be made of cotton which is soft and absorbent.

One of the latest items on the market is so-called 'super' underwear which is made of a water-permeable but non-absorbent material. Body heat forces sweat out through the underwear so that the body is kept warm and dry. The 'super' underwear is an important step forward and is of particular use, for example, during events such as long cross-country skiing races.

The intermediate layer

The intermediate layer of the clothing should contribute to heat insulation and may consist of a shirt or jersey of wool or cotton. In winter it is advantageous to wear wool since it has a good insulating capacity and moisture permeability. A shirt is best worn one or two sizes too big, so that it is long and wide enough, and the collar should be soft.

When the weather is cold many athletes wear V-neck or polo-neck sweaters while warming-up. If the cold is severe the sweaters should be long-sleeved and reach down to thigh level.

The outer layer

The outermost layer of clothing may consist of a long, windproof coat, preferably waterproof and double-breasted so that ventilation can be regu-

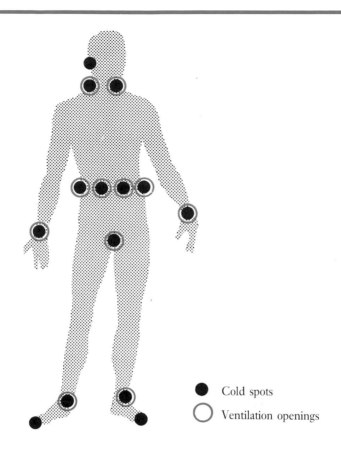

● Cold spots

○ Ventilation openings

lated. The coat should allow moisture to evaporate and should fit loosely around the waist. In rain or strong wind a nylon jacket can be used.

Track suits   Track suits (or 'warm-up' suits) vary from sport to sport, depending, among other things, on heat insulation requirements.

Socks   Socks should be of cotton, terry towelling or wool, all of which absorb moisture better than synthetic materials. They should be free of holes and should fit sufficiently closely not to crease. By preference, choose socks that reach up to or above the knee. Socks should be changed and washed frequently for comfort and hygiene.

Headgear   An ordinary, double-knit hat is suitable headgear. Sometimes, a peaked cap with protectors for ears, forehead and neck can be of value.

It should be noted that the head is the part of the body that suffers the greatest heat loss, so headgear should not be neglected, especially in cold weather.

Gloves and mittens   The hands can be protected by gloves or mittens with loose cuffs.

Other remarks   The market now offers clothes tailored to the requirements of particular sports — quilted jackets and trousers and windproof garments for downhill skiing, wet suits for wind-surfing, and so on.

> Clothing should be adapted to the requirements of the individual sport. It should be comfortable and appropriate.

The requirements of protective clothing (equipment)

Any protective device should prevent, or at least reduce, both long– and short–term injuries to the part of the body for which it is designed. This it achieves by relieving the relevant part of the body of the full force of the impact and redistributing it over as large an area as possible.

Protective clothing should not hamper the athlete's activity or technique, but man's ability to adapt is quite considerable. There may be certain restrictions in movement when, for example, a guard is first being used, but the athlete's adaptability will soon overcome any problems.

In many fields of sport there is no standard design or specification for protective clothing, so it is left to the individual athlete to evaluate its effectiveness. Poorly designed guards give a false sense of security which may have disastrous consequences.

Athletes and spectators alike often have preconceived ideas of what athletes should wear. If this attitude can be changed by enlightened and objective information, the use and range of protective clothing could be increased with a corresponding reduction in the number of injuries suffered.

Protective helmets
(For head injuries see page 376)

Safety helmets are used by, among others, boxers, American football, lacrosse and ice hockey players, cyclists, riders, Alpine skiers and racing drivers. Different sports have specific safety and design requirements relating to helmets, but the principles are generally similar for those used in ice hockey, cycling, riding and American football. Considerably higher safety standards have to be met by the helmets used in Alpine skiing and motor racing because of the potentially much greater speeds of impact in these sports.

The head must be protected from contact with other players, the ground and surrounding objects and from blows from sticks, pucks and balls. Safety helmets are usually made of a hard outer shell that is separated from the skull by a softer lining, for example American football helmets. When the helmet is subjected to a violent impact the energy is transferred to the softer lining. In those helmets in which the outer shell is softer, for example ice hockey helmets, it can be partially deformed without coming into direct contact with the skull. The force of the impact is moderated by the change of shape and the remaining energy is both distributed over a larger area because of the soft lining of the helmet and further moderated when the lining is compressed.

For a protective helmet to fulfil its task properly, it must be fastened securely so that it does not fall off or fall down in front to block the player's vision.

115

Important

In the sports in which the wearing of safety helmets is compulsory, serious head injuries have become rare. The injuries that have occurred in spite of the helmets have been less severe.

Face guards
(For facial injuries see page 380)

Face guards are used, for example, by players of American football and youth hockey, by goalkeepers in ice hockey and by fencers, cricketers and Alpine skiers. Facial injuries can occur as a result of a blow from a stick, puck or ball, or through a collision with surrounding objects or with other players. It is essential that face guards are designed with due regard for

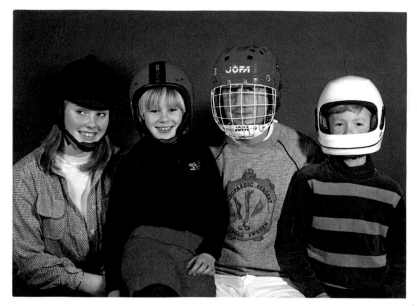

Safety helmets should be used for certain types of games and sports, such as riding, downhill skiing and ice hockey and American football.

the shape and size of the equipment used in the sport concerned. Standards have been laid down for the design of face guards for ice hockey and American football players.

A *visor*, made of plexiglass (perspex), covers the upper half of the face and serves mainly to protect against injuries to eyes, nose and temple bones. A *mask* is made of steel wire, covers the whole or part of the face and protects against eye injuries, fractures of facial bones, cuts and gashes to the face and dental damage. Protective eye frames or glasses are essential for squash and other racket sports. Ski goggles are valuable protectors against snow, sun and wind.

Important

Face guards, above all, prevent eye injuries which may cause permanent disability, cuts, gashes, bone and dental injuries. Their success is borne out by the fact that virtually no injuries have occurred in athletes who wear those which completely cover the face. There is a strong case for their compulsory use in sports such as ice hockey.

Gum shields
(For dental
injuries see page
384)

Dental injuries are serious and expensive and can present a great problem, particularly in contact sports such as rugby, boxing, ice hockey, and American football. As the loss of a tooth can influence the development of the jawbone and maxillary bone, a dental injury must be considered more serious in a young, growing athlete than in an adult. In boxing it is compulsory to use gum shields, which may be designed in one of two ways. An *intraoral* gum shield is made from a cast of the upper teeth and is worn inside the mouth, while an *extraoral* shield is worn in front of the mouth. The surest protection against dental injuries is probably using both types of protection in combination.

Standards for extraoral gum shields have been established.

**Shoulder
padding**
(For shoulder
injuries see page
174)

At present shoulder padding is used by ice hockey, American football and lacrosse players and in motor racing. Similar padding could probably also be used in other sports such as riding, cycling, Alpine skiing and ski jumping in which injuries to the shoulder area often occur.

Above all, shoulder padding protects the front and outside aspect of the shoulder from impact. The padding should cushion the ball-and-socket joint and distribute the energy of the impact over the more robust surrounding tissues. The commonest causes of shoulder injuries are falls on to the outside of the shoulder, shoulder-to-shoulder tackles or collision with the board in ice hockey. Such injuries can be prevented by shoulder padding. In American football, the tackle often hits the shoulders from above. These areas are especially protected with shoulder pads.

Important
Shoulder padding designed according to the principles mentioned above can prevent many common injuries to the shoulder area. These are often difficult to treat and take a long time to heal.

Elbow guards
(For elbow
injuries see page
207)

Elbow guards are used in sports such as basketball, team handball, volleyball, ice hockey, American football and lacrosse. The commonest cause of elbow injuries is falling and landing on the tip of the elbow. The guard should completely cushion this area and prevent it from hitting the surface.

Important
In the short-term, elbow guards prevent injuries to the bursa and the tip of the elbow, and in the long-term, cartilage injuries in the elbow joints.

**Genital
protectors**
(For injuries to
the lower
abdomen see
page 387)

Boxes (cups) are used by ice hockey and soccer players, cricketers, boxers, and sometimes by American footballers, team handball players and others. A box should enclose the penis as well as testicles and protect them against direct impact.

Important
In the short term, a box protects against the acute pain caused by a direct blow to the genitals. As these organs are invested with a good blood supply, they are very susceptible to bleeding after a blow to this area. The bleeding can be difficult to treat and may cause recurrent problems.

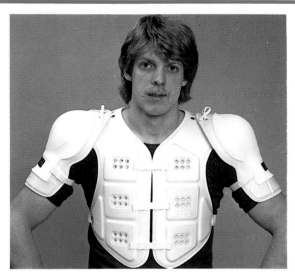

Shoulder padding.

Hip or thigh guards
(For hip injuries see pages 259 and 281)

At present, hip or thigh guards are used by cricketers, ice hockey and American football players and by goalkeepers in team handball and field hockey but they should be used more extensively. Currently, there are only a few hip guards on the market and they are generally badly designed. A hip or thigh guard should cushion the upper end of the femur and thus unload the hip joint itself.

Important
In the short-term, hip or thigh guards prevent the pain and bleeding that may occur after falls and during tackles by an opponent. In the long term, the guards prevent cartilage injuries in the hip joint by diverting direct impact.

Knee pads
(For knee injuries see page 283)

The knee pads in use today protect the knee joints only during falls, and not when they are subjected to blows from the side or to twisting, which may cause meniscus or ligament injuries. Combined knee and shin pads are used by ice and field hockey players, while separate knee pads are used by basket-ball, team handball and volleyball players and by American footballers, cricketers and soccer goalkeepers.

The pads should cushion the force of the impact from falls as well as from blows to the knees and shins. The patella is especially sensitive and should be completely cushioned from impact, so that a blow to the knee is redistributed over the surrounding tissues.

Important
It is important that the knee joint is cushioned to avoid cartilage injuries to joint surfaces, especially in the patello-femoral joint.

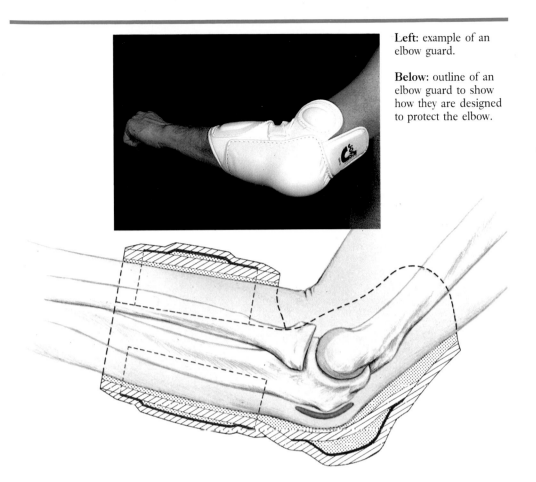

Left: example of an elbow guard.

Below: outline of an elbow guard to show how they are designed to protect the elbow.

Shin pads
(For leg injuries see page 317)

Shin pads are used to protect the shin from kicks and painful contact with the surroundings. Further development and research is needed to improve the shock absorption required of shin pads and ultimately to reduce the risk of injury to bone and soft tissue.

Important
Shin pads should be capable of preventing the occurrence of bone and soft tissue injuries, or at least of reducing their severity, by distributing the force of the impact on the shin over a larger area.

Ankle and foot protection
(For ankle injuries see page 340)

For many athletes, shoes or boots are of prime importance since they protect against overuse injuries and sprains. The development of the protective properties of shoes, however, has been neglected, and we have, for example, only a limited knowledge of the relationship between the playing surface, the shoe and the foot and of the importance of the design of the sole with regard to studs, profile, resilience, and so on.

The skating boot offers ice hockey players a built-in protection against injuries to the ankle and foot; Alpine skiers have a similar protection in the ski boot. Skating and ski boots protect the ligaments and bones in the foot and ankle.

119

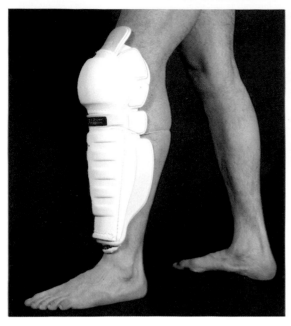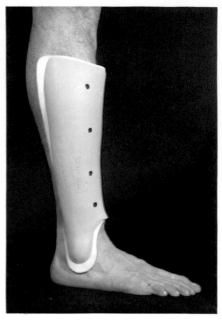

Left: example of a combined knee and shin pad used, for example, in ice hockey. The kneecap and the shin are cushioned against impact. **Right:** example of a shin pad designed to give good protection to sensitive areas. Such pads are used in soccer and American football, for example.

Ski-binding

A further safeguard which is of importance in preventing injuries to foot, ankle, knee and leg in Alpine skiing is the safety-release binding of the ski, providing that it has been correctly designed and set. Some injuries occur because the release bindings are poorly designed and adjusted. The release can be in a one-way direction, for example rotation, in a two-way direction, for example rotation and forward release, and multimode, for example rotation, forward and backward release. Multimode release ski bindings are recommended.

Important
Well-designed equipment prevents injuries to ligaments and bones and injuries due to overuse caused by sports activities on different surfaces.

Gloves
(For wrist and hand injuries see pages 223 and 230)

Gloves protect against fractures of the bones of the hand and painful bruising. They are used mainly by ice hockey and American football players, cricketers and boxers.

Important
Gloves protect against fractures of the bones of the hand and painful bruising. Injuries to the ligaments of the thumb and wrist may also be prevented.

General advice
It should be in the interests of every athlete to protect himself in the best possible way in order to prevent injury. Each should form his own opinion

about the risks of injury in his particular sport and should then test the protective clothing available. If this advice were followed more widely it would be possible to reduce the injury rate in many sports, especially in sports like rugby in which traditionally little or no protection is employed.

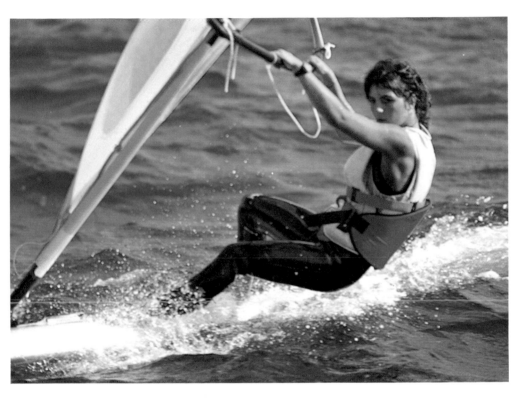

A life jacket used in watersports provides protection and buoyancy. A protective and insulating wet suit can allow the athlete to train even in cold weather. *Photo: Dan Ljungsvik.*

Braces

Braces are increasingly used in sport. They can be divided into three types: prophylactic, rehabilitative and functional. Knee braces are the commonest form of brace, designed to help reduce the high incidence of serious knee injuries in many sports. Braces are, however, also available for other joints, notably the elbow and the ankle. (The principles behind knee braces will be discussed in accordance with the American Academy of Orthopaedic Surgeons' Sports Medicine Committee.)

Braces are available in two basic designs:
1. Hinges, posts and straps
2. Hinges, posts and shells

The hinges may be monocentric, bicentric and polycentric.

Prophylactic knee braces

There are two types of design:
1. Lateral bar with all three types of hinge
2. Medial and lateral bars with polycentric hinges and plastic cuffs that encircle the thigh and calf.

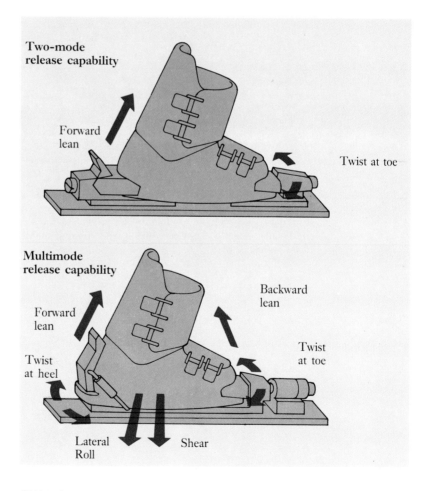

Ski bindings with different release modes (Johnson and Pope, 1982)

Few clinical studies have been made on the effectiveness of these braces but some short term studies indicate a trend in the reduction of serious medial collateral ligament injuries, while others have been shown no reduction.

This type of knee brace has no effect on anterior cruciate ligament injury. They are designed to protect against contact loading and valgus stress. Limited research indicates increased stiffness to valgus loads by the brace, with highest efficiency at lower flexion angles (around 20°). These braces can, however, cause 'preloading' of ligaments, resulting in increased susceptibility to injury.

Rehabilitative knee braces

This type of knee brace consists of four components: leg supports of plastic shells or velofoam, side arms, monocentric, bicentric and polycentric hinges, and foot plates to control tibial rotation and brace migration.

Rehabilitative braces have been shown to be as effective as a plaster cast in treatment of total medial collateral ligament injuries. They are also valuable during the first weeks of conservative treatment of knee ligament injuries and as an alternative/complementary treatment to plaster casts after knee ligament surgery.

Functional knee braces

These braces are valuable in supporting the functional stability of the knee. In this dynamic condition, the knee joint can function without 'giving way'. The brace operates by interacting with ligament, meniscus and muscle function. Functional knee braces support the following:

— *varus/valgus instability* with medial and lateral side posts.
— *Anterior tibial translation* by preventing hyperextension with moulded tibial piece, post strap, hinges loaded in flexion, and condylar pads.
— *Rotational control* with straps, tibial piece and condylar pads. This is, however, extremely difficult to achieve and at present no brace can really control rotation.
— *Suspension* with thigh and calf straps, condylar pads, moulded shells, neoprene sleeves, and Velcro straps.

Biomechanically, these functional knee braces provide some degree of control of anterior/posterior laxity at low forces. But, in general, it is impossible to make any valid clinical conclusions on their effectiveness in providing functional knee joint stability because no control studies have been carried out. However, even if the brace cannot guarantee the protection of knee ligaments, it may have some psychological effect on the athlete.

In summary, there are many braces used in sport today but, at present, we only have a limited knowledge of how they function and how they should be designed and constructed.

EQUIPMENT AND RULES

Rapid technical developments during the last few years in the field of sports equipment have had both advantages and disadvantages for athletes. Performance is improving at the expense of an increase in the risk of injury. Modern Alpine skis and boots, for example, have contributed both to improved results and to a changed pattern of injuries. The design of the ski boot is such that injuries now occur not in the area immediately above the ankle but mainly at mid-shin level and especially the knee joint level. The injuries have therefore become potentially more serious than before. To counteract this development, the safety-release bindings are gradually being improved but more research is still needed. Technical developments have also contributed to better results in athletics, as, for instance, in pole vaulting where a change in design and material has resulted in a change in the technique of vaulting and the achievement of greater heights.

When new equipment is being designed, it is of great importance that medical opinion concerning its requirements should be sought at an early stage. This would enable the designer to avoid errors which could lead to an unforeseen increase in the number of injuries. At the time of writing, a survey of the sports equipment currently available and of its design and use is urgently needed so that attempts can be made to improve it. If there are obvious elements of risk, then safeguards should be incorporated into the equipment from the outset. A change in one type of equipment can affect the functioning of another and this should be borne in mind when designing equipment; for example, the shape of a ski boot sole markedly affects the functioning of the ski binding. Or the openings in the faceguard used by both goalkeepers and players in ice hockey, for example, should be adjusted with the design of ice hockey sticks in mind.

— Equipment often causes serious injuries, especially if the rules governing its use are not followed. It is the duty of every athlete and coach to adhere to the rules of the game.
— If the rules of the game are thought to contribute to increased risks of injury, they should be changed.
— When new rules are being considered, due attention should be given, before they are finally approved, to the fact that they could lead to further risk of injury.

HYGIENE AND PERSONAL CARE

Parallel with the rise in our standard of living, personal hygiene has also improved considerably. Hygiene should be an essential part both of keeping fit and of day-to-day life. A great deal of what is said on the following pages will seem obvious to most people, but there can be no harm in stressing its importance.

General hygiene The skin secretes sweat and grease in which dust and dirt become trapped. If the dirt is allowed to accumulate it becomes a breeding ground for bacteria which break down the dirt, and produce unpleasant odours. Rashes, irritation and pimples can occur as a result. Soap dissolves grease and thereby removes bacteria.

Most athletes have access to showers, and *it should be a matter of course to have a shower and wash with soap after every training period or competition*. Regular use of soap and water may cause dehydration of the skin in some people, in which case, the body should be rubbed down with unperfumed skin cream or something similar after the shower.

Cycling is often an excellent form of exercise, and cycling to work daily, for example, improves fitness. After such exertion, however, there is a natural tendency to perspire and it would be a great advantage if all working premises were to provide shower facilities and locker rooms.

Most people make an effort not to smell unpleasant, as the extensive use of deodorants and anti-perspirants testifies, but these expensive preparations are no substitute for the frequent use of good, honest soap and water.

Foot hygiene Inadequate foot care can allow dirt to collect between the toes and under the cuticles and become a breeding ground for bacteria and fungi. Preventive measures, such as daily washing with soap and water and subsequent careful drying, are very important. Anyone using public swimming pools should be extra careful with foot care. If fungal infection occurs, visits to swimming pools and similar places should be avoided as infections are easily transmissible to others.

For ingrowing toenails, athlete's foot, calluses, etc., see page 374.

Groin hygiene One area of the body that perspires easily is the groin which should be washed daily with soap and water. Underwear should also be changed often, preferably every day.

Pants that are too tight or made of unsuitable material may, along with poor hygiene, result in the skin of the groin becoming irritated. Loose-fitting underwear in natural fibres is best. Skin irritations that persist in spite of careful hygiene and frequent changes of underwear call for a visit to the doctor.

Hand hygiene It is a matter of course to wash one's hands with soap and water after visiting the lavatory and before every meal. Nails should be cleaned frequently and cut every week.

Oral hygiene Good oral hygiene prevents dental decay and bad breath. Teeth should be brushed with toothpaste for at least 3 minutes morning and night, and toothpicks or dental floss should be used in addition.

Hair care Hair should be washed with a shampoo and the scalp massaged when showering. High standards of cleanliness should be maintained, particularly by those with long hair.

Good physical hygiene increases well-being and prevents illness.

Care of clothing and equipment In daily life it is automatic to wash clothes that have been worn and are sweaty and dirty. Some athletes prefer to use the same trousers, shirt or vest during every training period and competition as they think this gives them psychological support. However, this can lead to the clothes not being properly cared for, and everyone should have more than one set of sports clothes so that they can be washed often.

Good shoe care prevents foot complaints. Shoe trees prevent creases and keep the heel counters straight, thus preventing blisters. Clean shoes 'breathe' better than dirty ones. Leather shoes should be regularly rubbed with grease in order to keep them soft and water-repellent.

Socks should be stretchable and of the right size. Bad darning and creases may cause irritation. Socks should be changed frequently. If they are sweaty they lose heat insulation and this may be a contributory factor in fungal infections and verrucas.

Hygiene in training and competition abroad

In order to reap the anticipated benefits of training and competition abroad, certain aspects of foreign travel should be considered before departure.

When a journey abroad is planned, information should be obtained on the prevailing local weather and humidity at the time in question. Details about the height above sea level, time differences and so on should also be ascertained. On the basis of this information the time of departure can be arranged so that the need to acclimatize oneself on arrival can be accommodated. Other important factors to be aware of before arrival are the standard of living and sanitation of the areas to be visitied, the diseases prevalent and the medical care available.

Changes in the daily rhythm Considerable time differences between home and destination can disrupt the daily rhythm of the body, affecting sleep, body temperature, cardiovascular functions, mental performance, appetite, bowel activity and certain hormone levels.

Sleep disturbances result in lack of initiative and lethargy. If the flight goes westwards, for example, from Europe to the United States, the time changes by 5–8 hours, and it will be 2–4 days before sleep patterns return to normal. The time needed for adjustment is shorter in younger people.

Changes in body temperature influence metabolism and may possibly affect performance.

The *ability to concentrate* is impaired and can sometimes be reduced for 4–6 days.

A *change in eating habits and reduced appetite* can also affect bowel activity, with resultant diarrhoea or constipation.

Hormone balance takes 4–10 days to be restored to normal during which time performance is probably impaired. In women there can be changes in the menstrual cycle and menstruation may either fail to occur or do so earlier or later than expected.

In general terms, 1 day's physical disturbance occurs for every hour's time change.

The complaints that result from disruption of the daily rhythm can be prevented by adjusting the rhythm by 2 hours per 24 hours during the week preceding departure. Alternatively, if adjustment is to start at the destination, departure should be timed so that arrival is well before the competition (at least 6–10 days before if the Atlantic is crossed).

Disease prophylaxis

Before travelling abroad it is essential to find out in good time which inoculations are compulsory for the countries in question and which are recommended. Inoculations against certain diseases, such as typhoid fever and cholera, must be given well before departure so that the body will have time to build up the necessary resistance. As far as malaria is concerned, it is necessary to take precautions, in the form of tablets, against the disease before, during and after visits to an area where there is a risk of infection. A gammaglobulin injection given a few days before departure provides protection against epidemic jaundice for 4–6 weeks and is particularly desirable for travel to underdeveloped areas.

Travellers abroad come in contact with a different bacterial and viral environment from that at home, and may therefore be more susceptible to infections, including stomach, bowel complaints and colds. Meticulous personal hygiene is therefore essential. In many countries ordinary tap water is unsuitable for drinking and bottled mineral water should be used instead. If there are doubts about the standard of hygiene, hot, cooked or fried dishes should be ordered, and cold dishes, salads, pastries and desserts — in some places even ice cream — should be avoided. All fruit should be peeled before being eaten. If this is not possible the fruit should be rinsed in mineral water. Drinks accompanying meals should be mineral water, bottled soft drinks, pasteurized milk or boiled beverages such as coffee and tea.

It is important to find out whether the local water supply is clean enough for bathing, and in hotels of doubtful standards it is preferable to shower rather than to bath. If a team member falls ill while abroad, he should be isolated and a doctor consulted.

GENERAL RISK FACTORS

Heart and lung function

The human body is built for physical activity, not for rest. Throughout the ages man has had to work hard using his muscles in the fight for survival and working hours, as well as leisure time, demanded physical effort. Today much of our life is sedentary. A human heart at rest pumps out 7–9 pt (4–5 l) per min of blood; during physical effort the volume might increase to between 18–70 pt (10–40 l) per min. When breathing normally at rest 6 l per min of air is exchanged, but the volume can increase to over 100 l per min if necessary, and a well-trained athlete can exchange up to 200 l per min.

There is very little risk of sporting activity leading to serious medical complications. The likelihood varies, however, with the age and physical constitution of the athlete and with training methods. Factors which increase the risk of suffering a heart attack (myocardial infarction) are above all thought to be smoking and high blood pressure. Anyone who is fifty years old, has high blood pressure and is a heavy smoker (more than 25 cigarettes a day) runs a 100 per cent greater risk of suffering a heart attack than a non-smoker of the same age with normal blood pressure.

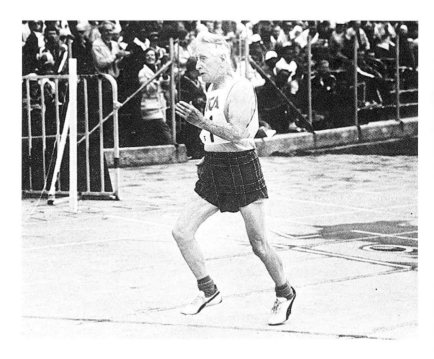

Regular physical activity can be carried out by all ages, even at the ripe old age of 92.

It is impossible to say with certainty whether any of the many positive effects of a physically active life (for example, improved cardiovascular performance and metabolism) provide protection against cardiovascular and other diseases. There are several studies, however, which show that the incidence of heart disease and subsequent death is lower among the physically active than among the inactive. Exactly how great an effect physical activity has cannot be evaluated, but, along with other aspects of the individual's lifestyle, it is probably significant. Frequency of exercise is important, and it has been shown that regular physical training reduces the amount by which blood pressure rises for a specified expenditure of effort. The percentage of some blood fats (which may influence the development of heart attacks) can also be reduced by training twice to three times a week.

> Available evidence indicates that even very moderate physical activity, provided it is regular, is valuable in preventing cardiovascular disease.

Sudden death Cases of sudden death during sports competitions are reported occasionally.

A number of factors are probably relevant. Several studies have shown, for example, that the number of sudden deaths increases in cold weather. A cold shower or a cold bath may cause a severe rise of blood pressure which can have disastrous effects on untrained people. Hard physical work in hot weather can result in large losses of body fluid and thereby increase the risk that the circulation and sweating system will not be able to cope with the stress placed upon them.

Medical factors that should be considered in this connection are chest pains (regardless of type), a previous heart attack, irregular heart rate, disorder of the heart valves, inflammation of cardiac muscle and high blood pressure. All may constitute risk factors as do smoking and consumption of alcohol. A number of cases of sudden death have also been described in connection with doping.

> Pains in the chest and abnormal fatigue during sporting activity are serious warning signals. If they appear, the sporting activity should be stopped immediately.
>
> Sports competitions should never be run in very hot or very cold conditions. Competitors should always be given the chance to warm-up properly in cold weather. Sport should be carried out regularly, the extent and intensity of training being increased gradually.

High blood pressure Anyone suffering from high blood pressure (hypertension) should only take part in sport after consultation with a medical doctor. In general, however, some forms of high blood pressure benefit from physical activity.

Other medical risk factors as far as sporting activities are concerned, for example diabetes, asthma and epilepsy, are dealt with on page 402.

Physical checkup If sporting activity is taken up after the age of forty or if physical activity produces symptoms such as abnormal fatigue, obvious breathlessness or irregular heart rate, a doctor should be consulted. Even if irregularities are present, they do not necessarily preclude sensible sporting activities. It is worth pointing out that even after the most careful physical examination, a doctor cannot always predict a potential cardiovascular disorder of sudden onset.

Studies have shown that people who do not smoke, drink little alcohol, take food and exercise regularly and are of normal weight, live longer on average than people with less healthy habits. *Everyday habits are more important than medical measures when it comes to preventing illness and death.*

Infections

The word 'cold' is used in everyday terms to cover a variety of respiratory infections. These are, as a rule, transmitted by direct contact or via the air, as, for example, when an infected person sneezes.

The warning signs of an impending upper respiratory tract infection include feeling feverish, tired and generally unwell. There may be aches and pains in the muscles, similar to the stiffness felt after training; headache, runny nose, sore throat, coughs and sneezes are often present. When these symptoms last for 3–4 days and are accompanied by a temperature of 100.5–102°F (38–39° C), the cause is likely to be a virus. Resting quietly at home for the duration of the illness is recommended. Fever can be controlled with the help of a proprietary aspirin or paracetamol preparation and plenty of fluids. Sporting activities should not be resumed until the temperature has been back to normal for a week.

A doctor should be consulted if:
— symptoms and fever persist for more than about 4 days;
— the temperature rises again after it had settled;
— the patient has chest pain or difficulty in breathing;
— a productive cough develops;
— pain is felt in the sinuses, ears, etc.
Any of these symptoms suggest that a bacterial infection may have occurred and that antibiotics may be necessary.

A doctor's advice and antibiotic prescription may similarly be needed if tonsillitis occurs. This is likely to be indicated by red, swollen, tonsils (sometimes covered or spotted with a white exudate) and tender enlarged glands in the neck.

Some upper respiratory infections are so mild that they pass almost unnoticed and neither athlete nor coach feels the need to discontinue training. It should never be forgotten, however, that any feverish illness can be complicated by the development of myocarditis (*inflammation of cardiac muscle*) which might lead to serious consequences, including sudden death. It may pass with very insignificant symptoms which are the same as those of a general infection – fatigue, a feeling of discomfort, and so on. Chest pains and palpitations may also occur.

Urinary tract infections include infections of the urethra, bladder, ureter, renal pelvis and kidneys. The symptoms include pain on urination, frequent urgent urination and sometimes fever. (The latter occurs particularly when the renal pelvis is inflamed, in which case it is also likely to be accompanied by pain in the lower back). Anyone who suspects that he has a urinary tract infection should consult a doctor as soon as possible for diagnosis and treatment.

In men, the prostate gland may become inflamed, causing vague discomfort over the bladder, an urge to pass water frequently, pain on urination and sometimes a fever. Again a doctor should be consulted for diagnosis and treatment.

The same rules apply to urinary tract infections as to other feverish illnesses.

> No sporting activity should be resumed until all symptoms have resolved and the temperature has been normal for at least a week. There is no place, in this respect, for acts of heroism.

Anaemia and iron deficiency

The capacity of the body to transport oxygen is one of the factors which limits physical performance. Oxygen is transported in the blood by the pigment of the red blood cells (haemoglobin). If the concentration of haemoglobin is reduced, the oxygen-transporting capacity of the body is correspondingly diminished, the maximum ability to absorb oxygen is impaired, and therefore the capacity to exercise falls.

Anaemia is said to occur when the concentration of haemoglobin falls below that specified as normal for the individual's age and sex. Athletes who subject themselves to prolonged, strenuous exertion (for example, by long–distance running every day) may develop some degree of anaemia. The reasons for this have been discussed at length and a number of possibilities have emerged. One is that the red blood cells may break down more rapidly than usual as a result of the mechanical effect of repeated contact of the runner's feet with a hard surface during training. Such effects are known to vary with the type of footwear used. Another possibility is a dilutional effect. Blood is composed of blood cells and fluid (plasma), and it is known that during training the volume of the plasma increases comparatively more than that of the red cells.

Iron deficiency can also be a factor in causing anaemia. Iron occurs in small quantities in the body, totalling about $1\frac{1}{2}$–$1\frac{3}{4}$ oz (4–5 g) in the adult. It is required not only for the manufacture of haemoglobin, but also for that of the related compound, myoglobin, found in muscle tissue. Both these substances bind oxygen and play an important part in its transport.

When an untrained individual begins hard training he produces both an increased number of red blood cells and a greater muscle bulk, and this extra demand for iron may result in a slight deficiency.

In many areas of the world, insufficient food is the commonest cause of anaemia. This is hardly the case in the Western world, but single young athletes in particular sometimes do not bother to eat a well-balanced diet and may then find themselves short of important nutrients.

During prolonged running on a hard surface, and above all in marathon races, small amounts of iron may be lost from the body in the urine as a result of cellular damage. Under normal circumstances, the body should be able to compensate for these losses by an increased absorption of iron from food, provided the diet is adequate.

During strenuous physical exertion, sweat production is considerable, but most recent studies indicate that the amount of iron lost by this route is insufficient to cause iron deficiency.

Approximately one-fifth of women of childbearing age in developed countries have some degree of iron deficiency because of blood loss during menstruation. Obviously the risk is greater when menstrual flow is heavy — 3 fl oz (more than 80 ml) per period — and this is particularly significant in those who have had contraceptive coils (loops) fitted which may increase loss by over 50 per cent. It may, therefore, be advisable for sportswomen in the relevant age groups, and particularly those with coils (loops), to have their haemoglobin count checked regularly.

Young people usually have only a small amount of stored iron in their bodies, and the requirements imposed by active growth combined with sporting activities mean that they should be considered a high risk group for anaemia.

Diagnosis

Anaemia can be confirmed by measuring the haemoglobin content of the body. An iron deficiency can be identified by blood cell analysis and by determining the serum ferritin level and, if necessary, the amount of haemosiderin in the bone marrow. Young people store only small quantities of iron, and low serum ferritin levels are therefore normal in individuals under about twenty years of age. The examining doctor needs expert knowledge in order to be able to decide whether or not an apparent iron deficiency is really significant. Generally speaking, it is not very common for well-nourished adult athletes to suffer from iron deficiency.

Views on treatment

The daily requirement of dietary iron is about 15–20 mg for women and 10–15 mg for men. Usually only 5–20 per cent of the iron ingested in food is absorbed by the body.

The best way to avoid iron deficiency is to follow a well-balanced diet, with meat and bread included in suitable proportions. Certain foods, notably meat products, enhance the ability of the body to utilize iron, while tea and eggs, for example, reduce this ability.

Top-level athletes with low serum ferritin levels may in some cases be prescribed treatment 'just to be on the safe side'. The upper limit for iron supplementation can be quite high for these athletes, and the daily dosage might be 100–200 mg of iron in tablet form for up to 2 months. At the end of the period of treatment the haemoglobin concentration should be checked again. An obvious rise indicates that there was a significant iron deficiency before treatment began. Iron supplements, prescribed as outlined here, not only normalize the haemoglobin level but also enable a store of iron to be built up. After a course is completed, the serum ferritin level should be checked again within one year.

Iron-containing preparations *can* be bought over the counter, but should only be used when they have been prescribed by a doctor. They may produce side-effects such as nausea, diarrhoea or constipation and an overdose of such preparations can be extremely dangerous.

To sum up, it can be said that athletes in general, and casual enthusiasts in particular, do not run any risk of developing an iron deficiency. For this group, the great majority, there is no reason to take iron supplements. Women with heavy menstrual losses and younger athletes should, however, have their blood counts checked regularly. As long as the counts are normal there is no need for iron supplements.

Menstruation

First menstruation (menarche) usually occurs between the ages of twelve and fifteen years, but some girls have their first period as early as the age of ten or as late as sixteen years. About two years before menarche, growth of the breasts and pubic hair begins and continues for about four years. Menstruation ceases (and the menopause occurs) anywhere between the ages of forty and fifty-five years. The average menstrual cycle is 27–30 days long but variation from one woman to another can be considerable, although in an individual woman the length of the cycle does not generally vary by more than 2–3 days.

Each period normally continues for 3–5 days, though in young girls they may last a little longer and are often irregular.

The effect of menstruation on the body

The effects of menstruation vary tremendously from one woman to another and physiological as well as psychological effects may influence sporting performance.

Various symptoms, including tension, headache, general malaise, nausea, abdominal pain and fluid retention may occur shortly before the onset of menstruation, during its first days and sometimes also at the time of ovulation (mid-cycle). They tend to be commoner in those women whose menstrual cycles are irregular.

The amount of blood lost during a period can be very variable, and when it is large, iron deficiency and anaemia may result (see page 131).

From the psychological point of view, there is evidence that stress can influence the length of the menstrual cycle and menstruation itself, and that in some women emotional and behavioural disturbances occur at certain points in the cycle. Physical activity seems to enhance the ability to cope with menstrual symptoms and so can have a positively beneficial effect.

Amenorrhoea (the absence of menstrual periods) occurs in women who indulge in strenuous and prolonged long-distance training or jogging and also in dancers. When training is reduced, menstruation returns spontaneously.

Travel abroad may either delay or advance menstruation, but the normal cycle is restored on return home.

Treatment

The *sportswoman* should:
— get to know her own menstrual cycle. Not everyone is affected by menstrual symptoms to the same degree;
— keep a careful record, noting variations in performance and relating them to the different phases of the menstrual cycle. (Some women actually maintain that they achieve their peak performances during the menstruation itself.)

The *doctor* may:

— relieve disturbing menstrual symptoms by prescribing medication;

— in exceptional cases (for example, for an important competition) change the time of the menstrual period with hormone treatment but this type of treatment should be avoided, if possible. The optimum time for peak performance is highly individual, but often falls immediately before or immediately after ovulation. If the menstrual period is to be brought forward or delayed because of a particular competition this should be done as early as possible.

Pregnancy

Physical activity has no adverse effect on a normal pregnancy, but it should be adjusted, of course, as the pregnancy develops. Physical fitness can make both pregnancy and delivery easier. Most active sportswomen stop competing in the fourth or fifth month of pregnancy and are content with only a limited training programme. Caution, however, is advisable, particularly in contact sports and in those sports where a large increase in core body temperature may occur.

After delivery, sporting activity should not be resumed for 6–8 weeks, when any discharge has ceased and the uterus has returned to its normal size. During the 8 weeks after delivery pelvic muscle exercises will help to prevent possible future problems such as uterine prolapse. Other training and competitive sporting activities can then be resumed gradually.

Many women breast-feed their babies, and milk production is adversely affected by heavy physical training. During the breast-feeding period the breasts are also relatively enlarged and thus more easily damaged by physical activity.

Doping

The word 'doping' implies attempting to improve sporting performances in an artificial way with the help of drugs. The number of cases of doping has increased greatly in recent years, and a number of deaths has occurred, as a result of which controls have been tightened.

Drugs prohibited by doping regulations

Hormones

Anabolic steroids (substances closely related to male sex hormones) are abused by some international top-level athletes, mainly those involved in strength-orientated sports.

Most scientific documentation indicates that anabolic steroids have no effect on muscular strength, but recently some publications have produced results to the contrary.

During short-term treatment (4–6 weeks) with anabolic steroids, side-effects such as headaches, dizziness, nausea and reduced sexual potency may occur in men and increased sexual potency in women. In addition, women may suffer masculinization with excess facial hair, increase in muscle size and deepening of the voice. The risk of injury, to the musculature for example, increases. Long-term treatment with anabolic steroids involves a risk of serious damage to internal organs, such as the adrenal glands and liver, and serious side-effects may occur. In men, sperm production is nearly always reduced, and in either sex growth may be affected; in children, in particular, growth may cease prematurely, resulting in permanent short stature. Overall, the side-effects are potentially so serious that the use of anabolic steroids cannot be defended on any other than well-documented medical grounds.

> Anabolic steroids should definitely not be used to improve performance in sport.

Decongestants and bronchodilating drugs

One of the drugs which causes shrinking of mucous membranes and widening of the bronchial passages is ephedrine. Ephedrine is present in ordinary cough mixtures and hay fever preparations which can be bought over the counter. Competitors should be cautious in their use.

Drugs that stimulate the central nervous system

Certain drugs of this group can increase the working capacity of the heart by dilating the blood vessels which supply it. Some of the important mechanisms that regulate body temperature and blood pressure are affected by these drugs to the extent that they fail to respond to the demands of hard physical exertion.

Amphetamines

Amphetamines are the drugs most often used for doping in top-level sport. Amphetamines alleviate fatigue in the short-term, but judgement is impaired and there is a marked increase in the risk of injury. By elimination of the body's usual defence mechanisms, amphetamines have, on a few occasions, been the cause of death in sport.

Narcotics   Morphine and closely related substances such as codeine are constituents of cough mixtures and analgesics (pain-killers). Codeine as such is not regarded as a narcotic drug, but since 10 per cent of codeine ingested is broken down into morphine in the body, the two cannot be distinguished in doping tests. Cocaine is used as a doping drug in many sports. It decreases the experience of pain and gives a feeling of well-being (euphoria). Side effects inlude physical destruction and mental deterioration with hallucinations. The addiction is strong. The use of marijuana and hashish must also be avoided, as sooner or later it will lead to addiction to stronger drugs.

Blood retransfusion (auto transfusion or 'blood doping')

The physical capacity of the human body depends on how well it is able to transport oxygen. This depends, in turn, upon the haemoglobin content of the blood, which raises the question of whether increasing the haemoglobin concentration could increase oxygen absorption and thus physical performance.

During research at the College of Physical Education in Stockholm, subjects were transfused with their own blood which had been stored in a blood bank for 4 weeks, and it has been demonstrated that this has enabled them to attain a 9 per cent increase in their previous maximum ability to absorb oxygen. Some effects of blood retransfusion can persist for up to a week, and are thought to result not only from the increase in haemoglobin content, but also from the increase in blood volume.

Blood retransfusion is doping, and is covered by a 'general clause' in the doping regulations which states that 'anyone having taken a substance in abnormal quantities and/or in an unnatural way with intent to increase performance is doped'.

There are as yet no practical means of ascertaining whether blood doping has taken place, but, theoretically, it is possible and viable methods will undoubtedly be evolved.

All types of doping must be avoided, not least out of respect for the individual's health, and should be opposed by means of more widespread information and research. Doping is cheating.

Alcohol

Alcohol in moderation is socially acceptable and can be a pleasurable experience, but prolonged alcohol abuse can cause damage to the liver, nervous system and heart.

Effects on the central nervous system

Even very low alcohol concentrations in the blood impair the co-ordination of muscular movements and delay reactions, and these effects are seen even in subjects who do not otherwise appear to be under the influence of alcohol. When the blood alcohol concentration reaches 0.3 g/l, its effect is seen in impaired memory, difficulties with co-ordination and changes of mood. At a concentration of 0.6 g/l, reactions are further delayed, and there is difficulty in controlling emotions and movements.

In small amounts, alcohol has a stimulating effect on the central nervous system but larger amounts are inhibiting. In each case, these effects are probably due to the fact that nerve pathways are blocked. Alcohol, initially, causes relaxation, and a desire to experience this sensation may tempt a person to start drinking alcohol more and more regularly. After a time, increasing quantities are needed to achieve the intended effect, leading to a degree of habituation. At this stage the use of alcohol seems to the drinker to be a pleasant habit, but psychological dependence may be developing, and, if consumption continues, physical dependence can follow. The pattern is an easy one to fall into and coaches have an important task to fulfil in counteracting the tendency. It is unnecessary to celebrate a sporting victory by drinking to excess.

Other effects

Alcohol consumption causes blood vessels to expand, resulting in a sensation of skin warmth. The loss of body heat is increased and the temperature reduced. This means that, contrary to popular belief, drinking alcohol in cold weather is not conducive to keeping warm. Alcohol also increases excretion of urine, mainly because of high fluid intake, and reduces blood sugar levels, causing an increased desire for food and drink.

Alcohol is eliminated from the body by metabolism and excretion. The former is by far the most important, more than 95 per cent of alcohol being handled in this way. Excretion in the breath and urine is much less significant. It is not possible to accelerate the elimination of alcohol from the body by perspiring profusely (another common myth), and physical exercise and sauna baths consequently have no effect.

Alcohol is metabolized mainly in the liver. Breakdown occurs at a constant rate of 0.1 ml of alcohol/kg body weight per hour. So, in a person weighing 154 lb (70 kg), the liver can metabolize 7 ml of alcohol in an hour. An alcohol intake equivalent to only two single measures of spirits impairs liver function for up to 2 days, and physical performance, especially during prolonged exertion, is impaired for a similar period after alcohol consumption.

> Consumption of alcohol impairs performance and causes a marked increase in the risk of injury. The breakdown of alcohol in the body occurs at a constant speed and is not influenced by such measures as physical exercise or sauna baths. Sport and alcohol do not mix.

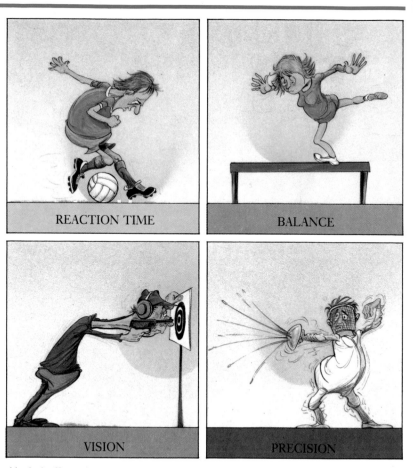

REACTION TIME	BALANCE
VISION	PRECISION

Alcohol affects the vital functions.

Tobacco

**Tobacco
smoking**

A World Health Organization report in 1970 stated that 'diseases associated with tobacco smoking have such a grave importance as the cause of disease and premature death in the industrial countries that a reduction in cigarette smoking would mean more for improving health and prolonging life in these countries than any other single activity within the field of preventive public health care service'.

As a group, cigarette smokers have a 30–80 per cent higher mortality rate than non-smokers. The rate rises along with cigarette consumption, and is higher for those who start smoking early in life.

Tobacco smoking damages the mucous membranes as well as the cilia (mobile, hair-like structures) which remove particles of dust and other foreign material from the upper respiratory tract. At the same time it causes an increase in mucus secretion, and this combination of factors causes irritation in the air passages and 'smoker's cough'; resistance to infection may also be lowered. Cigarette smokers often suffer from breathing difficulties and fits of coughing during exertion.

One of the most important and potentially harmful ingredients of tobacco smoke is *carbon monoxide*, the amount of which varies between 4–22 mg per cigarette depending on the brand. If smoke is inhaled, a larger amount of carbon monoxide is retained. Although most of the gas is eliminated in the exhaled air, it is potentially very harmful. The ability of carbon monoxide to combine with haemoglobin is 300 times greater than that of oxygen, and consequently carbon monoxide displaces oxygen from the blood. Studies have shown that, in people who smoke 15–25 cigarettes a day, 6–7 per cent of their available haemoglobin is combined with carbon monoxide, and therefore not available to transport oxygen. Since a person's physical performance is dependent, as we have already explained, on his body's capacity to transport oxygen, this significantly reduces the smoker's capacity for exercise. The 'blocking' of haemoglobin as a transporter of oxygen does not cause any problems as long as the smoker is at rest, but during physical exertion the effects are noticeable. Regular cigarette smoking can reduce maximum absorption of oxygen by 9–10 per cent.

The smoke of a cigarette also contains 0.5–2.4 mg of *nicotine* which is absorbed into the body through the oral cavity, the alimentary canal, the respiratory passages and the skin. In smokers who inhale, 90 per cent of the nicotine is absorbed by the body, in other smokers about 20 per cent. About 80–90 per cent of nicotine absorbed is metabolized, mainly in the liver but also in the kidneys and the lungs. Together with its breakdown products, the nicotine is then quickly and completely eliminated, mainly in the urine.

Nicotine causes the amounts of circulating stress hormones (adrenaline and noradrenaline) to increase, which in turn results in a rise in oxygen consumption. Adrenaline constricts the blood vessels supplying the skin which therefore becomes pale and cold. By its effects on hormone production, the nicotine causes a rise in the pulse rate of 10–30 beats per min as well as a rise in blood pressure. The effects of nicotine continue for several hours after smoking has ceased and can influence physical performance. Moreover, nicotine is addictive.

In summary, cigarette smoking impairs physical condition because carbon monoxide reduces the capacity of the blood to transport oxygen and nicotine affects hormone production and thus increases the pulse rate. *Since the effects of nicotine last for several hours, and it may take more than 24 hours to purge carbon monoxide from the body, there should be no smoking during the 24 hours before a training session or competition.*

Cigarette smoke also contains *tar* of which the smoker absorbs (6–33 mg) per cigarette depending on the brand. Tar has a strong irritant effect on respiratory passages and mucous membranes and is also highly carcinogenic. Cancer, not only of the lung but also of other organs such as the urinary tract and throat, is commoner in smokers than non-smokers.

Passive smoking (that is, the inhalation of another person's cigarette smoke by a non-smoker) is now known to pose health hazards as well and can affect performance. For this reason, smoking in the locker rooms should be strongly discouraged, and team managers, coaches and others should refrain from the habit during sporting activities.

Athletes should avoid smoking, mainly because the benefits of training are partly negated by the effects of tobacco. Furthermore, it impairs appetite, the senses of taste and smell, and sleep, all of which are important to athletes.

How to give up smoking

It is generally more successful to give up smoking by stopping completely than by trying to cut down gradually. Those who cannot manage to stop smoking on their own should consult their doctor who will either help and advise them himself or may refer them to an anti-smoking clinic. Giving up is not always easy and some people complain, especially in the early stages, of symptoms such as irritability, poor concentration and insomnia. Weight gain, too can be a problem. Despite this, it is well worthwhile persevering.

Results of giving up smoking

The immediate positive results of giving up smoking are obvious even after a week. They include:
— a better sense of taste and smell and sweeter breath;
— improved physical fitness;
— diminished cough.

The long-term benefits are:
— a reduced risk of cardiovascular disorders;
— a reduced risk of various forms of cancer;
— a reduced risk of chronic bronchial disease.

Common decency demands that smokers consider those around them who are non-smokers, especially now that the dangers of passive smoking are understood. There is now a general move towards the prohibition of

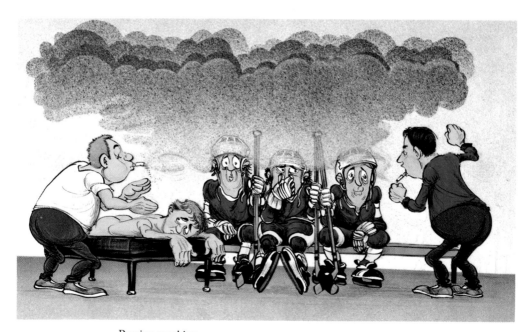

Passive smoking.

smoking in public places including restaurants, theatres and various forms of transport. A similar ban could be applied with benefit to sports arenas and conference rooms.

Goethe voiced the opinion of many when he said:

'There is a coarse impoliteness in smoking, an affront to the company present. Smokers pollute the air and choke every individual who cannot bring himself to smoke in self-defence.'

Chewing tobacco

Unlike the situation in many countries, the habit of chewing tobacco is unusual in Britain, although there has been a recent advertising campaign presumably in response to the falling rate of cigarette consumption.

Unlike the smoker, the tobacco-chewer does not ingest tar and carbon monoxide. On the other hand, he ingests a larger amount of nicotine, since it is absorbed into the blood through the mucous membranes of the mouth. Nicotine constricts the blood vessels, which impede the circulation and hence the blood supply to the musculature. The heart rate is increased and the nervous system is affected. The sum of these effects is a reduction in the tobacco-chewer's physical performance.

Chewing tobacco affects the mucous membrane lining of the mouth, and may cause small blisters to appear. The membrane in the area in which the tobacco is first placed becomes wrinkled and then hardens and turns whitish in colour. A sensitive mucous membrane is susceptible to the development of cracks and ulcers and, rarely, malignant changes.

After a long period of chewing tobacco the gums may deteriorate. Tobacco-chewers should be particularly careful about cleaning their teeth as poor oral hygiene increases the risk of tooth decay and loss. Even when oral hygiene is good, the tobacco-chewer suffers from bad breath.

Chewing tobacco is as addictive as cigarettes and other tobacco products but the so-called psychological need, is perhaps not so strong in the tobacco-chewer. Widespread tobacco-chewing especially in North America among adult athletes is probably one of the causes of increased tobacco chewing among young people.

Tobacco-chewing is becoming more and more of a hygiene problem. Chewed 'quids' are thrown or smeared onto walls and ceilings in toilets, locker rooms, shower rooms, and so on. Apart from the unpleasantness of having 'quids' scattered about everywhere, they give off an unpleasant smell.

Overweight and obesity

The overweight are usually less physically active than their lighter fellows and hence tend to have a less robust musculo-skeletal system. This, combined with the greater load they have to support, increases the risk of injury and can accelerate joint degeneration.

Obesity is a significant, though probably comparatively minor, risk factor for the development of cardiovascular disease. Its main cause is a surplus of unused calories; an underlying physical disorder is the exception rather than the rule. The calorie surplus, whether supplied by dietary fat, carbohydrates or protein, is ultimately converted into fatty tissue.

A person who has a sedentary job and does no physical exercise in his spare time requires 2,000–2,500 kcal (8,000–10,000 kJ) every 24 hours. Most people's diets, however, are not ideal, so that in order to ensure a sufficient intake of important nutrients, they have to consume the equivalent of 2,500–3,000 kcal (10,000–12,000 kJ) daily, which for many people is far more than they need. The problem can be solved by:
— eating smaller quantities of food, but making sure that the diet is well-balanced;
— eating at the right time of day. There is more chance of calories being used up when meals are taken in the early or middle part of the day when people are at work and active, than when large meals are eaten immediately before going to bed.
— increasing the rate of metabolism by exercise or other physical activity.

A combination of these three methods is more likely to be successful than one used in isolation.

A sensible diet comprises mainly lean meat, fish, potatoes and other root-crops, bread, vegetables and fruit, with only limited amounts of fat and sugar. Saturated fats are as fattening as polyunsaturated fats, because they contain the same amount of kJ/g but the latter are preferable in terms of their effects on blood fat content and therefore on cardiovascular disease.

A brief example will demonstrate the importance of physical activity in preventing accumulation of fatty tissue: 2.2 lb (1 kg) of fatty tissue corresponds to about 6,000 kcal (25,000 kJ). An excess intake of 50 kcal (210 kJ) a day amounts to 18,000 kcals (75,000 kJ) a year, which is equivalent to 6.6 lb (3 kg) of fatty tissue. The daily excess 50 kcal (210 kJ) may be the result of eating only four sugar lumps or one chocolate, but it would need a 2 mile (3 km) walk or jog to dissipate it. So, in a nutshell, this means that anyone who wishes to control his weight has to choose one of two alternatives: he can lead a sedentary life and feel hungry or lead a physically active life and eat more freely.

The table below shows how many minutes' exercise is necessary in order to use up 100 kcal (400 kJ), which is the energy derived from about 25 g of carbohydrate. The figures apply to a person of average exercise capacity, able to absorb about 3 l/min of oxygen.

1.	Running	8–10 min
2.	Skiing at a fast pace	8 min
3.	Cycling	11 min
4.	Swimming, skating	12 min
5.	Badminton, squash	12–15 min
6.	Gymnastics	15 min
7.	Football, ice hockey	15 min
8.	Tennis, fast walking	15–18 min
9.	Gardening	20–25 min
10.	Slow walking	25–30 min

OTHER POINTS

Sweating and fluid supply

During physical exertion the body's core temperature increases. The cooling effects of wind and heat loss by radiation are insufficient to prevent it rising dangerously; they are supplemented by the production and evaporation of sweat. Sweating begins after 1½–3 minutes of work and increases steadily before levelling out after 10–15 minutes, or longer in a humid environment.

70 per cent of the human body is composed of water, most of which is contained inside the cells. When sweating, fluid is drawn mainly from this intracellular supply with a resulting adverse effect on cell metabolism. Fluid loss therefore results quickly in impaired performance, which usually becomes apparent when 1–2 per cent of the body weight has been lost as sweat. When the fluid loss amounts to 4–5 per cent of the body weight the capacity for hard physical work is reduced by nearly 50 per cent. Further fluid losses are likely to lead to collapse and this does occasionally

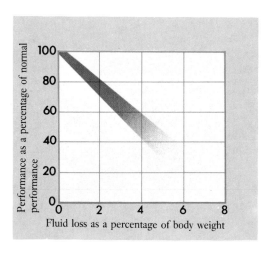

This diagram shows the relationship between fluid loss and impaired performance.

happen during sporting competitions, especially long events conducted in warm weather.

Fluid supply

In order to maintain physical performance, especially during prolonged training sessions, an adequate fluid supply is essential. When a match or competition continues over a long period and the resulting fluid losses are considerable, it is almost impossible to replace all the lost fluid during the session itself. It is important, therefore, to ensure copious fluid intake during the days before the competition and during the preliminary warm-up so that hydration is adequate from the outset. If the period of competition lasts for less than 30 minutes it is generally unnecessary to stop for fluid intake during that time.

The sensation of thirst is not an accurate guide when it comes to replacing fluid lost by sweat. Slaking one's thirst generally provides only about half the amount of fluid required, and anyone who indulges in strenuous physical activity would be well advised to drink considerably more than he thinks he needs.

The fluid used for replacement should be of an appropriate composition to replace those substances lost by the body during strenuous physical exercise. Water is the most important component, but sugar too is needed. Sugar is absorbed from the intestinal tract into the bloodstream and transported to the muscles, brain and nervous system. If the blood sugar level sinks too low, performance is reduced. Sensations of faintness, dizziness and hunger are likely to occur and collapse can ensue. Judgement and reaction time may be affected so that the risk of injury is increased.

Although some sugar is necessary in the replacement fluid, too much should be avoided as, in high concentration, it is retained in the stomach (sometimes causing discomfort) and is absorbed only slowly into the bloodstream.

Except at very intense levels of exercise, the absorption of fluid into the body is independent of intensity of activity, so that it is immaterial in this context whether the body is at rest or hard at work. The rate at which the stomach empties is, however, a limiting factor on absorption and is reduced by strenuous physical activity. Thus, if fluid high in sugar content is drunk during this type of activity, emptying of the stomach virtually stops, and the fluid is no longer transferred into the intestinal tract from which it would normally be absorbed. All this points to the fact that athletes should take their fluid replacement during the less strenuous parts of competitions or drink plain water without sugar.

The replacement fluid chosen should be palatable (flavoured with lemon, for example) and at a temperature of 77–80°F (25–30°C). As it is difficult to drink more than 4–8 fl oz (100–200 ml) of liquid in one go, this amount should be supplied at frequent intervals (for example, 15–25 minutes) and, consistently, every 3–4 miles (5–6.5 km) in, for example, orienteering, cross-country running and skiing. The hotter the weather, the more fluid is required, even during training sessions. This is partly to establish the habit of taking frequent fluid before the competition itself and partly to keep up a good pace which is at least as important. In all training lasting more than 20–40 minutes, sugar solution should be drunk frequently.

A suitable solution can be made by dissolving ¾–2½ oz (25–75 g) of granulated sugar or glucose in 1.76 pt (1 l) of water. This constitutes a sugar content of 2.5–7.5 per cent which is as high as that of most of the sports drinks at present on the market.

Advice

— *During warm-up periods*, ½–1 pt (200–500 ml) of fluid should be drunk.

— *During sporting activities* sugar solution should be drunk regularly and often. In winter its sugar content should be 5–15 per cent, and in summer 2.5–5 per cent.

— *After sporting activities* large quantities of fluid should be consumed, including 1–1.76 pt (0.5–1 l) before retiring to bed. The precise nature of the drink is unimportant.

— Weight can be checked every morning as changes are most often due to alterations in fluid level.

Nutrition

Diet — fuel

Muscles need energy in order to work. At rest, energy supplied by the metabolism of substances within the body is used primarily to maintain a temperature of 98.6°F (37°C) and to fuel the vital functions of the internal organs. During effort, energy production in the musculature is 50–100 times greater than during rest.

Fatty tissue, of which an average man has 22–33 lb (8–10 kg) distributed in various parts of the body, is the largest of our fuel stores and provides 8–9 kcal/g (35–40 kJ/g) of energy.

The carbohydrates that we eat (for example, bread, rice and potatoes) are stored as glycogen in the muscles and liver. Normally muscle contains ¼–½ oz/lb (10–15 g/kg) of glycogen, and combined muscle and liver glycogen totals 14–17 oz (400–500 g). Glycogen provides 4.1 kcal/g (17 kJ/g) of energy, or 1,500–2,000 kcal (6,600–8,300 kJ) in total. This is approximately the amount of energy used by a top-level skier or cyclist during one hour's hard competition, so it follows that glycogen is a limited energy reserve.

Choice of fuel

When pure carbohydrate is metabolized, 5.1 kcal (21 kJ) of energy are released for each litre of oxygen consumed, and the corresponding figure for fat is 4.7 kcal (20 kJ). In competitions in which the pace is so fast that the athlete's oxygen absorption is maximum or nearly maximum, carbohydrate is the fuel consumed first. Fatty acids, however, provide an equally good fuel source, and the more highly trained the muscles, the more fat is metabolized. Fats are broken down more slowly than, for example, glucose and the presence of oxygen is required for this process. Reduced to everyday terms, the energy conversion of carbohydrates is more efficient than that of fats.

At rest and during moderate muscular work with minimal load on oxygen-transporting mechanisms, the body chooses fat as its principal fuel. When the pace of muscular work increases to more than 75 per cent of the maximum, carbohydrates become the predominant energy source.

Carbohydrate (glycogen) is the most important fuel for athletes during competition, whether of long or short duration. As the glycogen is depleted, the body gradually begins to burn fat and as it does so the pace is reduced. The results of a competition may be directly influenced by a lack of glycogen.

Under normal circumstances, the body's glycogen stores are sufficient to supply energy for competitions lasting up to one hour. Before more prolonged efforts, some dietary loading of carbohydrate is recommended.

Short competitive period	Before competitions which last for up to 1 hour, no particular dietary adjustment is necessary, as the body's normal glycogen stores are sufficient. An unnecessarily high carbohydrate intake results in a weight increase as considerable quantities of fluid are bound in muscles and liver during glycogen storage (1 g of sugar binds 3 ml of water).

At least 3–4 hours before every competition a light meal should be eaten. There is no time for this to be stored as glycogen and its main purpose is to stave off hunger pangs during the run-up to the competition. |
| **Long competitive period** | Before competitions of 1–3 hours duration, some consideration should be given to dietary preparations. Sports such as walking, running, orienteering, cycling, skiing and canoeing, which depend upon physical fitness, are liable to use up the available glycogen during the course of the competition. Therefore in the days leading up to it, meals should include food rich in carbohydrates. As it takes about 48 hours for glycogen stores to be built up, no prolonged or hard training which would deplete the stores should take place in the 48 hours prior to the competition. |
| **Prolonged competitive periods** | In competitions which last for more than 3 hours, for example, marathon races, the final result is to some extent dependent on the glycogen content of the body at the outset.

Seven days before the competition, a 2-hour intensive training session should take place, after which the glycogen stores will be almost exhausted. During the next 2 or 3 days fairly long training sessions continue, even though the athlete may feel that he is physically and mentally unfit to cope with them. During this time the diet should be mixed, but should not be excessively rich in carbohydrates.

Three days before the competition, the loading starts. At this time the diet should consist mainly of carbohydrates, and extra fluid should also be taken. By this method, the glycogen stores will be doubled or trebled in comparison with normal levels (see diagram on page 148). The glycogen lasts for longer than usual, and a good pace can be maintained throughout most of the competition. The increase in weight due to fluid retention may upset some athletes and a modified form of carbohydrate loading may be of benefit.

Optimum glycogen stores are achieved if the 3 days immediately prior to the competition are spent resting. If any training does take place it should be short and gentle. |

> Depleted glycogen stores and low blood sugar levels impair physical as well as mental performance and increase the risk of injury.

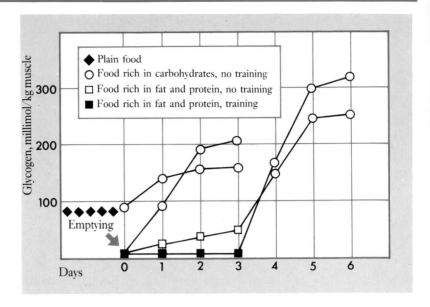

The concentration of glycogen in the muscles of athletes on different diets. The highest level of glycogen was achieved on a fat and protein diet lasting for three days with daily training, followed by a carbohydrate diet for three days without training. This extreme and specialized diet should only be used occasionally each season when extra high levels of glycogen stores are desirable.

Salt

The function of cells during muscular work may be dependent on the body containing sufficient salt. Very large salt losses may result in impaired performance. The salt concentration of sweat is considerably lower than that of blood (0.2 per cent compared with 0.9 per cent), so the salt concentration in the body is actually increased by sweating, though it can be reduced by an ample fluid intake. Though the normal diet usually contains more than enough salt, to be on the safe side, extra salt may be added to the food during the days before a long race and after long periods of training and competition.

Top-level athletes involved in prolonged races do not usually need salt supplements, but less experienced athletes who drink considerably more liquid may need some extra salt in the fluid towards the end of a long race. No one should ever eat salt tablets.

Vitamins

A certain amount of each vitamin is necessary if the body is to function normally, but an excess serves no useful purpose. A normal Western diet should, as a rule, provide all the necessary vitamins, and special vitamin preparations are therefore superfluous.

Proteins

It has already been emphasized (see page 86) that rest is an important part of training. During breaks from activity some cells will be broken down and replaced by new ones, and in order for this to take place the body must be supplied with protein. In adults the requirement is about 1 g/kg body weight per day (about 40–80 g): in children it is somewhat higher. It is higher, too, for an athlete engaged in hard training, but the belief that 'if I eat twice as much protein I will be twice as strong' is not true. When protein intake is increased, the body has to adapt to a new rate of turn-over and it can only utilize a daily protein intake of 150–200 g at most. The surplus is stored as fat or is eliminated in the urine as nitrogen. Knowing this, it is a complete waste of money to buy food supplements in the form of expensive protein preparations, as many athletes do, particularly as the protein in such preparations is usually not superior to that in cheese, eggs, milk, fish and meat.

5 Methods of Treatment

If injuries are to heal satisfactorily they must be treated in the right way at the right time. The treatment must be based on accurate diagnosis, for which the main responsibility lies with the doctor, but close co-operation between patient, trainer, doctor and physiotherapist is of crucial importance, as each complements the others with his own expertise. As a rule, good team work leads to the best results.

Sports injuries are often acute and caused by violent impact on the sports ground. When this is the case, urgent action is needed in order to limit bleeding and swelling. The more promptly treatment is begun, the swifter the healing process. Guidelines are given on page 64.

Other sports injuries are caused by overuse, and their treatment must follow certain patterns if it is to be successful. Various alternatives for the treatment of sports injuries are given in this chapter.

Rest and relaxation

After any injury it is usually necessary to rest the affected part, and sometimes confinement to bed is justified. In cases of overuse injuries and in certain ligament injuries accompanied by swelling, adhesive strapping or tape may be useful to give the injured athlete relief. Rest is also recommended after an operation. It is usually continued until pain and swelling are negligible on loading the injured part.

Rest in an elevated position, that is, with the injured part positioned higher than the rest of the body, is often necessary in the acute phase. This reduces blood flow and improves drainage, so that swelling is minimized, as well as relieving load on the damaged part.

Rest without load but with active muscle contraction (*active rest*) is permissible in certain cases, such as ligament injuries or muscle haematoma, either immediately after the injury has occurred or after an interval of 1 or 2 days.

In knee injuries, for example, the athlete should try to flex the hamstring muscles as soon as possible after medical treatment and continue in order to minimize any weakening. Quadriceps muscle exercises should also be started early depending on the injury. These muscles have an antagonistic effect on the anterior cruciate ligament and should therefore be exercised only after consultation with the doctor.

Resisted exercises often follow on automatically from rest and free exercise as a part of the rehabilitation process. They may entail gradually increasing the load on an injured leg, for example, or, in cases of shoulder injury, training the mobility as well as the strength of the joint.

150

Active rest

Complete rest after an injury is, as a rule, unnecessary. The injured part should be rested and unloaded while other parts of the body are trained by active muscle exercises and conditioning.

Advice to an injured athlete in plaster

Even when an injury necessitates a plaster cast, other parts of the body can still be trained and muscle exercises and conditioning carried out. A lower leg in plaster does not prevent physical fitness being maintained by activities such as cycling. The part in plaster should be held in an elevated position and exercised by repeated static contraction.

If the immobilized limb feels painful, numb or cold, medical advice

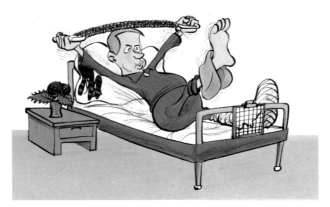

Active rest.

should be sought in case the cast needs adjusting or replacing. When the plaster has to be worn for a long time, a water-resistant preparation can be used so that showering is still possible.

Cooling (cryotherapy)

Cooling is a common and important method of treating acute soft tissue injuries. Its aim is to minimize the bleeding and swelling which are an inevitable accompaniment of such injuries and which interfere to a variable degree, depending upon their extent, with the healing process. Cooling is also used in the treatment of pain, and in overuse injuries.

If it is to have any effect, the cold must penetrate well into the injured tissue. In general terms, the larger the injured muscle or joint, the longer the treatment should continue, and it is an advantage to use special ice packs with a long-lasting effect. There is a risk of local cold injury (frostbite) being inflicted during this treatment, so the skin over the injured area should be protected. This protection may take the form of a single thickness of elastic bandage placed between the ice-pack and the skin.

The principal effect of cooling is that of reducing blood flow by constricting blood vessels, but it also acts as a local analgesic. The pain-relief, however, must definitely not encourage an immediate return to the sports field, for the true extent of the injury may have been masked. A premature return to sporting activity will aggravate the injury and prolong the healing process.

> After cooling the injured part, the athlete must not return immediately to his or her sporting activity as the severity and extent of the injury may have been masked by the analgesic effect.

Cooling is beneficial in sports injuries because:
— the patient quickly feels an improvement in his symptoms;
— the treatment is easy to carry out and is well-tolerated;
— there are few contraindications;
— it is inexpensive.

Cooling brings about the following effects:
— relief of pain and attendant muscle spasm, ensuring that blood flow in adjacent, undamaged tissue is unimpaired;
— constriction of blood vessels with a consequent reduction of blood flow and thus less bleeding. Minimal bleeding in the injured area shortens the healing process;
— reduced capillary (small vessel) blood flow and therefore less swelling;
— reduced metabolism in the tissues and so less risk of extending tissue damage because of local lack of oxygen.

Ice massage

This is a form of treatment which encourages local constriction of blood vessels followed by a reflex dilation (widening) with increased blood flow. It is used in the treatment of injuries and in rehabilitation, and its effect can be enhanced by alternating it with heat treatment.

> Cooling, used with discretion, is of great value in the treatment and rehabilitation of sports injuries.

Heat treatment (thermotherapy)

Heat has been used for thousands of years in the treatment of different types of pain. Experience shows that it has a beneficial effect on pain arising from inflammation which is the body's defence mechanism in cases of injury due either to accident or to overuse (see page 18). Injuries caused by trauma or overuse, such as ligament injuries and muscle ruptures, are often treated during the acute stage by cooling and bandaging so that the bleeding in the injured area is limited. After the initial 48 hours, heat treatment can be introduced to help the healing process, which, once the risk of haemorrhage is over, is aided by increased blood flow.

Perhaps the most important effect of heat treatment is its influence on collagen (connective tissue) fibres. A tendon is composed of 90 per cent collagen fibres and 10 per cent elastic fibres. Collagen has viscous and elastic properties, which means that the more rapidly a tendon is loaded, the stiffer (less elastic) and less extensible it becomes. Heat increases elasticity and plasticity, so after its application the collagen fibres become more extensible and more capable of rehabilitation exercises. Heat also decreases joint stiffness and relieves muscle spasm. This reduces the risk of injury.

Heat can be used in both the prevention and rehabilitation of overuse injuries and to combat the after-effects of torn muscles and tendons. It can be valuable during warm-up before training sessions and competitions and in cold weather, increasing, as it does, the mobility of joints.

> Heat treatment provides pain relief, makes collagen fibres more extensible and is of great importance as a means of both preventing and rehabilitating injuries.

Heat lamp, sauna

Heat lamps, heating pads, hot baths and sauna baths increase blood flow and may have a beneficial effect on stiffness after training amongst other things.

Short wave

Short wave treatment involves a high frequency alternating current passing through the body and generating heat in the deeper tissues. It is used to treat pains in joints, muscles and tendons, but its benefit is doubtful.

Ultrasound

Ultrasonic waves with a frequency of more than 20,000 cycles/sec generate heat by means of vibration. The effect penetrates into the treated area. The method is also believed to provide pain relief, especially for the treatment of pain in tendon attachments and for tendinitis.

There is a possibility that the injudicious use of ultrasound can damage nervous tissue. Interferential treatment consists of a varying medium frequency current which penetrates into the tissues.

Heating pad (heating pack)   Heating pads contain a gel which has the capacity to store both cold and heat. They are immersed in hot water before being applied to the area to be treated.

Heat retainer   A heat retainer is a support made of synthetic material which generates and retains heat in the parts of the body which it encloses. Those available can be used effectively at rest as well as in training and competition.

Heat retainers are made of a fine porous material with low fluid absorption and good heat retention. Retainers have an elasticity which keeps them in place without hampering movement in the bandaged part of the body. In addition, they give some support and exert counterpressure which may be of value when there is swelling. They are available in versions suitable for most joints and most types of injuries.

Heat retainers have been tested clinically to assess their effect on prevention as well as treatment of sports injuries – results have been good. By relieving pain, improving tissue elasticity and maintaining and extending

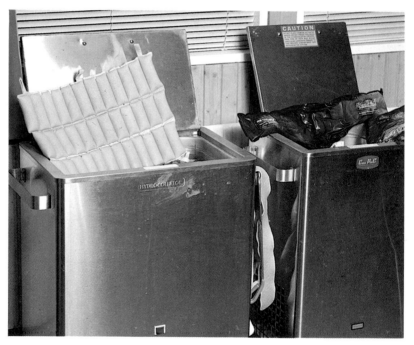

A heating pad which is warmed in hot water. The pad is put into a terry towelling cover before use.

the range of mobility, they assist not only the rehabilitation of ligament injuries in the knees and ankles but also the treatment of pain arising from muscle injuries and osteoarthritis, amongst other things.

Heat retainers can be used as a simple form of heat treatment and are a valuable addition to the other means of treatment available. They can be useful at rest as well as in training, prevention and treatment of injuries due to overuse and trauma, both in sporting and other activities.

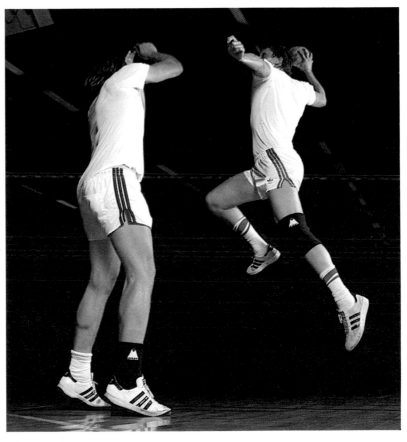

A heat retainer.

Bandages

Support bandages

Different types of support bandage are used depending on the degree of stability required.

Elastic bandage

An elastic bandage comprises cotton woven together with strands of rubber. It can be used for securing dressings or ice packs over injured areas and also provides compression in acute injuries, such as ankle sprains.

The elastic bandage is flexible and stretches after use, which makes it unsuitable for long-term support. It has the advantage of being washable and can be re-used.

Adhesive elastic bandage (Elastoplast)

This type of bandage is firm and flexible and its adhesive properties provide a strong hold. It is particularly useful for injuries of the knee, ankle and wrist. Adhesive elastic bandages can also be used for taping as a preventive measure.

A disadvantage of this type of bandage is that it is bulky and cannot be re-used.

Tape

See page 158.

Self-adhesive elastic bandage

Self-adhesive elastic bandage consists of closely-packed unwoven polyester fibres. It adheres to itself but not to the skin. It does not interfere with the normal functions of the skin and is non-allergenic. It remains in place during bathing and dries quickly after getting wet.

Self-adhesive elastic bandaging can be used as a preventive measure as well as during rehabilitation after an injury. It provides a stable but flexible dressing which is not bulky and even fits inside a shoe when applied to the foot. If the correct technique is used when applying the dressing and its elasticity is overstretched, self-adhesive elastic bandage can be used as a permanent support in ligament and other soft tissue injuries.

Plaster cast

When there is a need for rigid support (for example, in fractures and ligament injuries) or complete immobility (for example, in tendinitis), a plaster cast is by far the best solution. Depending on the nature of the injury, some activity, such as isometric exercises, can be allowed on the muscles encased in the cast. In principle, a plaster cast should include the injured area and the joints above and below it.

Waterproof cast

Casts can be made of many synthetic materials; some are composed of fibre-glass fabric impregnated with a plastic compound which hardens in cold water. The plastic cast becomes pliable 5–7 minutes after it has been dipped into cold water and can then be wrapped around the injured part of the body or applied as a splint. After 30 minutes it can withstand a certain amount of load. These casts are suitable as a temporary or permanent support for various parts of the body without the need for any restrictions on bathing, showering or swimming.

During the last few years there has been a rapid development in the field of bandages made of plastic. Various types of plastic bandages with different properties are available.

One type of plastic cast is available in the form of discs which soften and become malleable when heated (by immersion in hot water) and subsequently stiffen at room temperature. This is a good means of temporary support for an injury during its acute stage and can be used to provide temporary protection during healing and rehabilitation.

Dressings for wounds and cuts   See page 56.

Taping

Taping is a very common method of treatment in the sports world. The method was initiated by coaches and trainers about 40 years ago, and is now also used by sports doctors.

Athletes often suffer muscle, tendon and ligament injuries which can take a long time to heal. During the healing process sporting activity must be foregone and training should not be resumed until healing is complete.

After an initial period of rest, gradual rehabilitation begins and continues for a variable length of time depending upon the type and extent of the injury. As a rule, it takes a long time for a ligament or muscle to regain its full strength and mobility.

A recently healed injury is vulnerable and injury can easily recur if training is overenthusiastic or premature. The risk of this happening can be reduced by the correct application of some form of support, such as taping.

The basic idea behind taping is that the tape should *support a weakened part of the body, without limiting its function, by preventing movements which stress the weakened area.* However, this ideal goal is difficult to achieve even when taping is correctly applied.

Ranges of application

1. Acute injury

It can be risky to use tape on acute injuries, and over-tight taping of an area in which swelling and bleeding are occurring may cause serious impairment of circulation. *If an acute injury is to be taped this should only be done by a doctor experienced in the field,* and elastic tape should be used. Before taping an acute injury a detailed medical examination should be carried out, including a careful stability test. If there are any indications of a total rupture, taping should not be used. The taping of an acute injury may unfortunately lull the athlete into a false sense of security, encouraging him to resume his sporting activity and making the injury considerably worse.

2. Preventive taping

There has been some suggestion that taping healthy ankles as a preventive measure could, by changing mechanical conditions, increase the occurrence of knee injuries. Research, however, has shown that this is not the case and has confirmed that preventive taping can decrease the number of ligament injuries to the ankle. It is of particular value in sports in which the ankles are vulnerable to violent impact, for example, soccer, team handball and volleyball.

Ligaments, such as those around the ankle joint, can be subjected to repeated impact and injuries with a result that they become weak and stretched. *In such cases taping plays an important part in contributing to the stability of the joint.* If, despite precautions, progressive instability of the joint is seen, surgery should be considered.

3. Taping during rehabilitation

Taping is most useful in rehabilitation after an injury has been treated surgically or has healed spontaneously. It is becoming quite common for athletes to use taping when they resume their sporting activity after an injury, though the value of the practice has not been proved. Studies have shown that taping the knee joint does not provide stability to any significant degree. In cases of lateral instability of the knee, taping gives virtually no support after 5 minutes' hard physical activity.

> Used correctly, taping can be of value after an injury but it should not be considered to be a miracle cure for all cases.

Different types of tape

The tape in general use is rather inelastic and is available in widths of for example, $1\frac{1}{2}$ and 2 in (38 and 50 mm). It is perforated so that strips can be torn off easily. By stretching the tape before application it is possible to achieve a firm restriction early in the range of movement.

General risks with taping

— In certain situations, for example in acute injuries, taping may restrict circulation.
— Some doctors believe that tape bandages retain their full effect for up to a week, but the long-term effect of taping is in fact probably limited. It can never provide a permanent solution, and there are few justifications for using it continuously for as long as a week.
— Skin irritations may occur if tape is in contact with the skin for a long period. This problem is unlikely to occur in less than a week, but as a rule tape should not be used directly on the skin for more than a few hours at a time. If it is necessary to exceed this limit, a protective material should be worn under the tape.

Tape may cause irritation by mechanical or chemical means or because of allergy, and the effects may be exaggerated by sweating, itching and bacterial infection. In order to reduce the risk of skin irritation some tapes are backed with zinc oxide.

Practical advice

Knowledge of taping is gained first by instruction and thereafter by experience. It is only possible to learn how to tape quickly and safely by constant practice.

— Any bodyhair in the area to be taped must be shaved. If the skin is damaged or infected it is advisable to wait until it has healed before tape is applied.
— The skin in the area to be taped must be cleaned, as grease or sweat will stop the tape adhering. An adhesive spray may also be used.
— Various types of tape underlay in the form of thin plastic foam, adhesive cream or plastic dressing can be applied to the skin. One of these underlays should be used if the tape is to be worn for a long time or if skin allergy occurs.
— A tape bandage must never be applied round a swollen joint as it may impede circulation.
— In principle, application of a tape bandage should begin above the injured part, be built up over the injury and be fastened below it.
— Tape adheres better to itself than to skin, so an 'anchor' of tape should be applied on each side of the injured joint. The injured ligament which is to be supported should be held in a shortened position during taping. If, for example, the ligament on the lateral (outer) aspect of the

ankle is injured, the lateral (outer) edge of the foot should be directed upwards and the tape stretched over the outer side of the joint.

— Folds and creases in the dressing should be smoothed out as they may cause blisters and skin irritation. The effect of the bandage is also reduced if the tape is 'concertina-ed'.

— The tape should be removed with care. It is better to try to 'push' the skin away from the tape rather than to tear or pull the tape away from the skin. The edges of a wound are often difficult to free but it can sometimes be effective to hold the skin tight and pull it from the tape. Alternatively, tape bandages can be removed with the help of tape cutters or tape scissors; solvents are also available.

— The athlete should always be listened to, and if the tape is causing any discomfort, it should be adjusted.

Location

Between the skin and the underlying structures is a variable amount of fat and connective tissue, allowing the skin a considerable amount of mobility which varies from site to site. As the tape is applied directly to the skin, this mobility can make the value of the tape doubtful in certain situations. The value of taping an injured thigh muscle, for example, is debatable.

Taping should be used primarily over joints where the sliding of the skin can be limited to one direction, for example, the ankles, wrists and knuckles. Taping in these areas can provide good support for ligament function. Guidelines for taping these joints are given on page 162. For further information on taping see the bibliography on page 463.

Compression taping using elastic adhesive bandage is useful as a first aid measure to prevent further bleeding. Taping to prevent muscles tearing is of doubtful value.

How to tape an injury to a medial collateral ligament in the knee joint

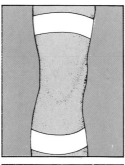

Starting point: Place a 1–1½ in (3–4 cm) wedge under the heel. Attach open anchors of tape 4–6 in (10–15 cm) above and below the knee joint.

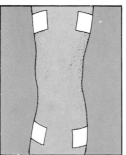

The tape anchors should be open at the back so that circulation is unaffected.

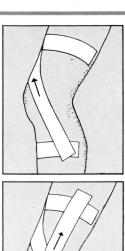

Begin on the inner side of the leg at the bottom anchor and pull the tape diagonally forwards over the top of knee joint – but not across the kneecap – and attach to the outer side of the top anchor.

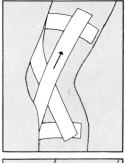

Then start on the outer side of the leg at the bottom anchor, pull the tape just below the kneecap, cross the previous band of tape on a level with the synovial cavity, and secure the tape on to the inner side of the top anchor.

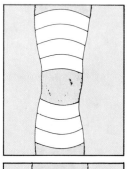

Apply another two or three crossing bands of tape. Make sure that the tape does not touch the hollow of the knee, as it may cause blisters.

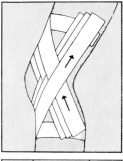

Apply anchors starting below and going up to, but not on to the kneecap. Further anchors are applied above the kneecap.

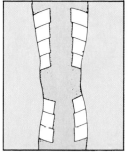

Leave the anchors open and keep the hollow of the knee free from tape.

How to tape an injury to the lateral ligaments of the ankle joint

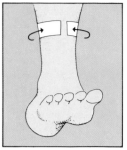

Hold the ankle joint at an angle of 90°. Apply an anchor below the calf muscle.

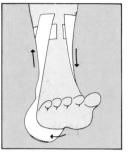

Beginning on the inner side of the lower leg above the anchor, attach a stirrup of tape down across the medial malleolus, under the heel, up across the lateral malleolus and the outer side of the lower leg to above the anchor.
For external lateral ligament injuries, stretch the tape in the direction of the arrows. For internal ligament injuries, attach and stretch the tape in the opposite direction. Apply two to three bands of tape with a displacement of about ½ in (1 cm) forwards and backwards. Secure these with another anchor.

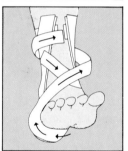

Apply the tape in a figure-of-eight, that is, pull the tape from the outer side of the lower leg diagonally down across the back of the foot and down under the instep. Then stretch the tape up across the lateral malleolus and diagonally up across the back of the foot and finish by stretching the tape round the lower leg.

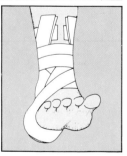

Apply one or two additional figures-of-eight starting below the first. The number of bands and figures-of-eight can be increased if a strong support is needed.

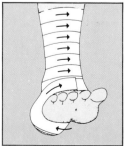

Finally, apply separate anchors from top to bottom, one anchor at a time.

How to tape the hand and wrist

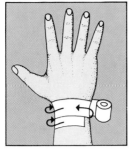

Starting point: bend the hand slightly at the wrist and spread out the fingers. Start taping on the upper side of the wrist and pull the tape twice round the wrist (towards the thumb).

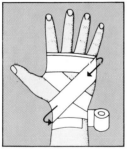

Continue the same band of tape diagonally across the back of the hand between thumb and index-finger and then out across the palm of the hand.

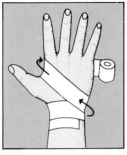

Apply a further one or two bands of tape round the hand with slight displacement between the layers. Then pull the tape diagonally across the back of the hand up to the wrist.

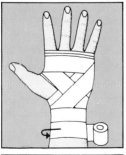

Where necessary, extra layers of tape can be applied around the wrist.

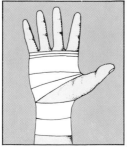

The palm of the hand after taping.

How to tape an injury to the ulnar collateral ligament of the base joint of the thumb

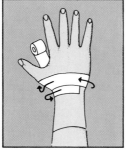

Start taping on the back of the hand on the side of the little finger. Apply one layer of tape round the metacarpus and then pull the tape up between thumb and index finger.

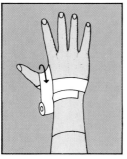

Continue round the base of the thumb and the wrist. Increase the number of layers if greater stability is needed.

Massage

Massage has been used in the world of sport from time immemorial. It was once thought that it increased the blood flow in muscles and thus relieved pain, stiffness and tenderness. Subsequent studies, however, have not been able to prove that blood flow is increased, although massage does bring about symptomatic improvement.

No-one who is untrained should attempt to give massage. Massage should not be too vigorous and should work inwards from the extremities towards the heart.

Carried out by a trained and capable masseur, massage can produce a feeling of general well-being and relaxation.

Water massage Water massage is usually carried out in hot water. The injured part is immersed for about 20 minutes during which time air is injected under high pressure into the water providing an effect very similar to that of manual massage.

Whirl-pool Use of a whirl-pool (jacuzzi) enables the whole body or individual parts to be immersed alternately in hot and cold water which is supposed to stimulate circulation and facilitate healing and rehabilitation.

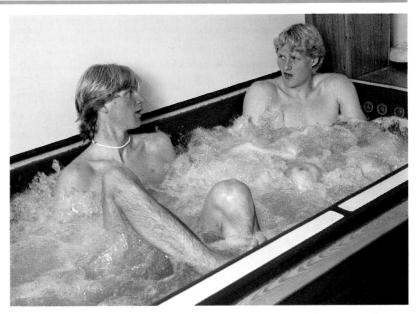

Underwater massage. Air is injected under high pressure into the water and around the body. *From the sports out-patient clinic, Skatås, Gothenburg.*

Movement therapy and physiotherapy

General exercises are part of the athlete's warm-up before training sessions and competition and have an essential function in preventing injuries.

The physiotherapist's role in sports medicine is one of participation in both prevention and treatment. As far as prevention is concerned each sport has its own pattern of movements which subjects various muscle groups to differing types of load. A knowledge of these patterns is vital to the physiotherapist whose task is to emphasize the importance of warm-up, make appropriate suggestions for strength and flexibility training with regard to the requirements of the sport in question and encourage individual training.

When an injury has healed, the aim is to restore original function to the affected part. The physiotherapist's instructions are of the utmost importance in ensuring that the correct muscle groups are trained with the appropriate movements and with a well-balanced load.

If surgery is contemplated, physiotherapy can be valuable both before and afterwards. Prior to a meniscus operation, for example, it is essential for the patient to exercise his thigh muscles as they are responsible for stabilizing the knee, and if they are well-trained before operation, subsequent rehabilitation is facilitated.

Assessing an individual's functional state is part of the physiotherapist's work. By analysing the causes and consequences of a functional impairment, he can draw up a programme for the treatment of muscles, joints and ligaments. The treatment methods used are flexibility, strength and co-ordination training in prescribed proportions, together with encouragement, rest and pain-relief.

The treatment of functional disorders, for example stiff joints caused by muscle damage, is based on neuromuscular stimulation, that is, an improvement in the interaction between nerves and muscles. This interaction is disordered when joints are immobilized, and there is increased tone in the muscles surrounding the joint. Treatment aims to relax the muscles so that an improved range of movement can be achieved (the methods of stretching are described on page 96). The stretching should be carried out slowly and smoothly in order to prevent a rapid reflex muscle contraction.

In all strength training it is essential that the load used is correct. After an injury, training should be appropriate for the type and extent of the damage and to the stage of the healing process reached. No strength training should exceed the pain threshold. The first stage is usually isometric training without load, after which the training frequency and subsequently the load can be increased gradually. When isometric training can be carried out without pain, dynamic training can be started. Muscle training may be supported with electrical muscle stimulation.

Exclusive training of an injured area should be avoided, and a comprehensive training programme should be drawn up to include all the training elements relevant to the particular sporting activity concerned.

It is important to monitor the healing process so that the injured area is not overused and healing delayed. Athletes might not always have the patience to wait for an injury to heal, and it is quite common for intensive training to be started too early. This emphasizes the important role of the physiotherapist who should oversee the training programme during rehabilitation to ensure that it is appropriate in both type and intensity.

Physiotherapists should be involved in the treatment of sports injuries to a far greater extent than is the case at present.

Medicines

Athletes are making increasing use of various medicines and ointments, particularly pain-relieving and anti-inflammatory drugs. The potential advantages of these preparations should always be weighed against their possible side-effects.

The drugs that are generally used for soft tissue injuries can be classified as follows:
— oral analgesics (pain-relieving drugs) and anti-inflammatory drugs;
— muscle relaxants;
— steroids and analgesics for injection;
— ointments and liniments;
— anticoagulants (blood-thinning drugs).

Analgesics and anti-inflammatory medicines

A. *Acetylsalicylic acid (aspirin)* is contained in many proprietary preparations and has been used to help bring down raised temperatures for nearly 100 years. It is effective on mild and moderate pain, particularly that caused by headaches and muscle and joint problems; but is inadequate in controlling severe pain such as that caused by a fracture. It can have side-effects, such as irritation of the stomach lining and allergic reactions. In addition, blood clotting is impaired and the risk of haemorrhage increased. Prolonged use of aspirin may cause permanent kidney damage.

Paracetamol is also a constituent of many proprietary preparations and is as effective as acetylsalicylic acid against some forms of pain, although its anti-inflammatory activity is not great. It is the best drug available for reducing raised temperature. Paracetamol does not damage the lining of the stomach nor does it affect the clotting property of blood; it may, however, in overdose, cause liver damage particularly in women after the menopoause.

B. *Indomethacin* was one of the earliest nonsteroidal anti-inflammatory agents to be introduced. Its pain-relieving effect is, if anything, rather less than that of acetylsalicylic acid. Side-effects are fairly common, but as a rule not dangerous, and include gastrointestinal problems (sometimes with bleeding) and headache. Blood disorders and liver damage are very rare.

C. *Phenylbutazone* and its related compounds are good anti-inflammatory agents but are less effective as painkillers. Their use has decreased because of the possibility of serious side-effects. The incidence of nausea and digestive disorders is high; but, more importantly, serious blood disorders may occur, particularly in women after the menopause, as may liver damage. These medicines should therefore be used in moderation and with caution.

D. Many new preparations with pain-relieving and anti-inflammatory properties have come on to the market during the last few years. Some of them are mentioned below. *Diflunisal* is a preparation closely related to the acetylsalicyclic acid group and has a similar effect. It may have a rather less irritating effect on the stomach lining.

Fenbufen is an effective and well tolerated nonsteroidal anti-inflammatory drug with few side-effects. It can therefore be used in the long-term treatment of, for example, osteoarthritic problems of the knee and hip joints.

Ibuprofen is marketed mainly as an anti-inflammatory medicine. Its effect is of short duration.

Naproxen is the most widely used medicine in this group. It has a relatively good pain-relieving and anti-inflammatory effect which lasts for a comparatively long time; a twice-daily dosage (morning and night) is sufficient. It is often effective in menstrual as well as musculo-skeletal pain. Its irritant effects on the lining of the stomach are similar to those of other preparations in this group. *Piroxicam* provides pain-relief and has a long-lasting effect; one dose a day is sufficient.

Diclofenac sodium is effective against inflammation but has a somewhat weaker analgesic effect than acetylsalicyclic acid. Its effect is relatively long-lasting, and twice daily (morning and night) dosage is sufficient. The tablets do not dissolve until they reach the intestine, so that side-effects such as gastric irritation are if anything rather less frequent than with other preparations in the group.

E. *Combination of peripheral and central analgesics.* Combined preparations usually include one of those medicines mentioned above, together with codeine or the closely related substance, dextropropoxyphene. One example combines dextropropoxyphene with paracetamol, but there are many others.

It should be noted that codeine is included on the doping list, and even the small amount of codeine in some combined preparations may be produce a positive result in a doping test. Moreover, there is little evidence to suggest that these combined preparations are better than aspirin as analgesics and anti-inflammatories.

Peripheral muscle relaxants

Peripheral muscle relaxants sometimes are included with analgesics in combined preparations. They are used primarily for muscle pain, for instance, lumbago. However, it has not been proved that the amount of muscle relaxant included in the recommended dose of these combined preparations has any effect on muscle cramp in man.

Cortisone preparations (corticosteroids) for local injection

Local injections of cortisone preparations *should not be given for acute injuries*. These preparations should be used with caution and only by a doctor.

They can be of great value in overuse injuries such as tendinitis but such injections *should not be given directly into muscles or tendons or into joints* as they may cause weakening and subsequent rupture. They should be given only when specifically indicated and then around a muscle or tendon attachment or into the surrounding sheath. Refraining from exercise with load is recommended for 2 weeks after injection in order to avoid problems.

Ointments and liniments

Several ointments and liniments are used in sports, especially for muscle pain, stiffness and periostitis. Some of the ointments increase the skin circulation and produce a sensation of local heat without affecting muscular blood flow. The psychological effect on athletes of the act of rubbing in ointments and liniments cannot be denied. Applications which contain heparin or an anti-inflammatory substance can have some effect on certain superficial inflammatory conditions, but generally such medications have no effect on any tissue below the skin, including muscle.

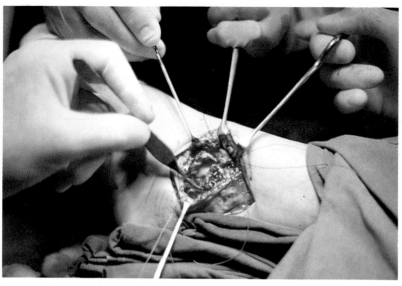
An operation to the external ligament of the ankle joint.

Surgery

The satisfactory functioning of the musculo-skeletal system is essential for an athlete to achieve peak performance. Injuries resulting in tissue damage lead to a disturbance of the function of muscles, tendons and ligaments and the aim of surgery is restoration of the original anatomical relationships.

Emergency operations are often performed in cases of total rupture of tendons and ligaments and muscle rupture with extensive bleeding. Surgery is carried out at a later stage when a torn ligament or injured joint fails to heal completely, or when complications develop. In order to restore function completely, it is sometimes necessary to reconstruct tissue in the damaged area, that is, to perform plastic surgery.

The phrase 'plastic surgery' or 'reconstructive surgery' is sometimes misunderstood and it does *not* imply, for example, that a surgeon who performs a plastic operation on the cruciate ligaments of the knee joints replaces the ligaments with a plastic material.

Some risk of infection is involved in all surgical procedures and risk is greater in an emergency than in a planned operation. Infection in the bone or joints after surgery may need prolonged treatment but is fortunately a rare occurrence.

Acupuncture

Acupuncture is used widely in China where the method was developed and is now being used increasingly all over the world. Traditional acupuncture is based on the assumption that each half of the body has twelve meridians, representing certain organ systems. Along these meridians are a number of points which are connected with particular organs, and these points can be stimulated by needles of varying shape and length, effecting changes in the organs concerned. The connection between the meridians and anatomical nervous pathways has not yet been explained. The effect of the acupuncture needles is intensified by rotating them or connecting them to a low voltage power source (electro-acupuncture).

Scientific evaluation of acupuncture is as yet incomplete and inconclusive, but on an anecdotal basis it does seem to benefit a significant number of people.

Transcutaneous nerve stimulation (TNS)

TNS enhances the body's ability to control pain. A weak electric current is applied to the skin in the painful area by means of superficial electrodes. The response to treatment with TNS varies and some, but not all, patients find it very effective in relieving pain. It probably exerts its effect by activating a 'gate' mechanism in the spinal cord which prevents painful sensations from reaching the brain.

The medical bag

During training sessions and competition a sports club should always have available a bag containing basic medical equipment. The contents of the bag can, of course, be varied according to the needs of the sport concerned.

Similar equipment should be available in larger sports centres and schools, and team doctors should have a reasonable amount of additional equipment available so that they can attend to minor injuries on the spot.

1. The medical bag for sports clubs and sports fields

The following items should be included in the equipment available at a sports club:

A. **Ice packs** with long-term effect. Disposable as well as reusable ice packs are now on the market.

B. **First-aid supplies and wound dressings**:
— gauze bandages;
— elastic bandages
— elastoplast dressings;
— tape;
— cotton wool;
— sterile dressings;
— plaster and surgical tape;

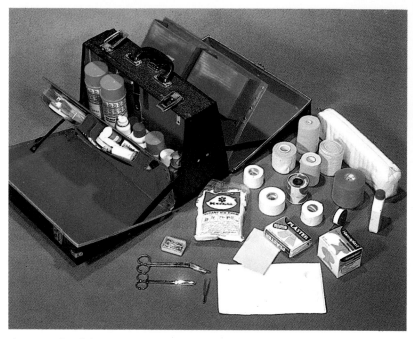

An example of the contents of a sports medical bag.

— solution for washing wounds, for example, saline solution;
— self-adhesive foam rubber and felt.

C. Instruments:
— nail-clippers;
— tweezers;
— scissors;
— safety pins;
— torch;
— disposable plastic gloves;
— thermometer.

D. Medicaments:
— analgesics (pain-relieving tablets);
— soap;
— liniment;
— glucose;
— ointments.

Other drugs available on prescription after consultation with the doctor responsible.

2. The team doctor's medical bag

A. **First-aid supplies and wound dressings**: apart from the items mentioned above the team doctor should have access to suture materials and disposable suture sets.

B. **Instruments**:
— stethoscope;
— sphygmomanometer;
— sterile gloves.

C. **Drugs**:
— analgesics;
— anti-inflammatory drugs;
— antibiotics;
— anti-diarrhoeals;
— cough medicines;
— anti-emetics (travel sickness and vomiting);
— antihistamines;
— topical applications, for example, antiseptic ointments;
— sedatives;
— hypnotics (sleeping pills);
— local anaesthetics with and without adrenaline;
— eye preparations;
— diuretics.
— adrenaline, glycogen;

In special cases, for example during competitions over long distances in extreme heat, intravenous units should be available as should equipment for resuscitation and respiratory support. Adequate rehydration equipment should always be available during events in warm weather.

3. Medical equipment in large sports centres and schools

Apart from the equipment recommended above for sports clubs, schools and large sports centres should have access to:
— stretcher;
— blankets;
— sand bags;
— a pair of adjustable crutches;
— splints.

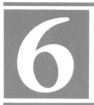

6 Sports Injuries by Specific Area

INJURIES IN THE SHOULDER REGION

The shoulder region includes the following joints.

1. The *shoulder joint* comprises the 'ball' of the humerus and the 'socket' (glenoid) of the scapula. The surrounding capsule is loosely applied and allows a wide range of movement. The articular surface of the socket is enhanced by a fibrocartilage 'collar' – the so-called glenoid labrum which increases the stability of the joint (see diagram below). Four short muscles and their tendons surround the joint and contribute towards its stability. They merge with the capsule and form

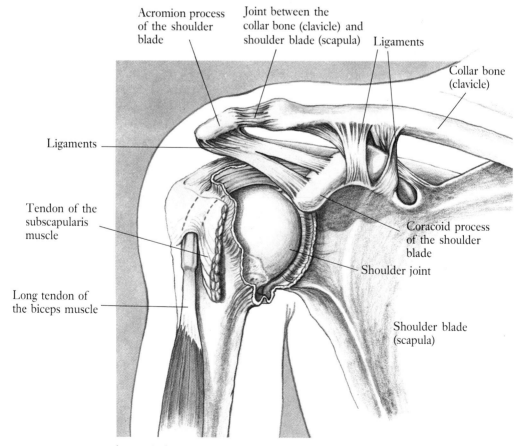

Acromion process of the shoulder blade

Joint between the collar bone (clavicle) and shoulder blade (scapula)

Ligaments

Collar bone (clavicle)

Ligaments

Tendon of the subscapularis muscle

Long tendon of the biceps muscle

Coracoid process of the shoulder blade

Shoulder joint

Shoulder blade (scapula)

Anatomical representation of the shoulder region.

a 'rotator cuff' which encloses the upper part of the humerus on three sides: behind, above and in front. Between the cuff and the deltoid muscle, which partly overlies it, is a bursa.

2. The *joint between the clavicle and the scapula*. The clavicle is a rather flattened and elongated S-shape and is connected by strong ligaments to the scapula.

3. *The joint between the clavicle and the sternum* is surrounded by a joint capsule and strong ligaments.

The total range of movement of the shoulder is very extensive because the shoulder joint itself has a shallow socket and a loose capsule, and it is mainly the muscles and tendons of the rotator cuff (see page 186) which are responsible for stability. Movement at the shoulder joint involves the other two joints mentioned. In some movements, the sheath around the long head of the biceps will be involved, in others the bursa between the muscle on the upper part of the the joint and the bones and ligament above the joint (coraco-acromial ligament); also between the scapula and the chest wall. Twenty different muscles are involved in performing these movements making it difficult to reach a correct anatomical diagnosis in the shoulder region, where combination injuries are, in any case, common.

Injuries which affect the shoulder region include fractures, dislocations, ligament injuries, muscle ruptures and inflammatory disorders.

Fractures of the clavicle

Fractures of the clavicle occur as a result of falling on to the shoulder or the outstretched hand during contact sports and also, for example, during skiing, cycling and riding. The fracture is often located in the middle third or towards the outer third of the bone.

Symptoms
The area over the fracture is extremely tender and swollen and a crackling sensation (crepitus) can be felt between the bone ends when movement is attempted.

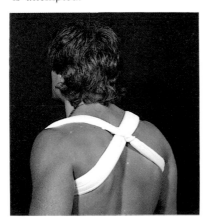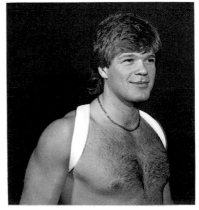

A figure-of-eight bandage seen from the back and the front.

Treatment

A fracture of the clavicle should be treated by a doctor who will use a figure-of-eight bandage to immobilize both shoulders. With the bandage in place, the arms can still be moved freely below the horizontal plane.

This treatment is usually sufficient but surgery may be necessary in certain cases, if, for example, the fracture is situated at the outer (lateral) end of the bone. Here the action of the ligaments may be such that, in circumstances in which a joint dislocation would normally take place, the joint is held together and an oblique fracture through the clavicle occurs instead.

Healing

Fractures of the clavicle generally heal well. Conditioning exercises, such as running, should not be resumed until the fracture has healed (about 4–8 weeks after the injury), but cycling, for example, can be carried out during the recovery period.

Fractures of the scapula

These fractures are not common but may occur in American football, rugby, ice hockey and riding. They can be located at the neck of the scapula and may sometimes extend through the joint surface. Other locations include the coracoid process and the acromion. The main symptom is pain on motion; treatment is usually symptomatic.

Fractures of the upper part of the humerus

Fractures of the upper part of the humerus occur most frequently as a result of falling on to an outstretched arm but may also follow a direct fall on to the shoulder during contact sports, such as rugby and American football, Alpine skiing and riding. Fracture of the upper part of the humerus occurs most frequently through the neck of the humerus. Sometimes they are avulsion fractures of the greater tubercle (supraspinatus tendon insertion) and of the lesser tubercle (subscapularis tendon insertion).

Symptoms

Tenderness and swelling occur over the area of the injury and pain on attempted movement.

Treatment

— The injured person should be taken to a doctor or a hospital for examination and possibly an X-ray.
— A support bandage is applied and kept in position for 10 days, after which mobility training is begun, first with pendular movements and subsequently with the exercises described on page 419.
— Physiotherapy aids the process of rehabilitation. If the displacement of the avulsed tubercle is large, surgery should be considered.

Healing

As a rule, fractures of the upper part of the humerus heal well, and conditioning can be resumed after 4–8 weeks.

Dislocation of the shoulder joint

A dislocation of the shoulder joint is a relatively common injury in sports such as ice hockey, team handball, American football, rugby, riding, Alpine skiing, skating and wrestling.

Causes — When an athlete falls, he instinctively lifts his arm and turns it outwards to protect his body. Dislocation can occur when the arm, held in this position, receives the impact of the fall.

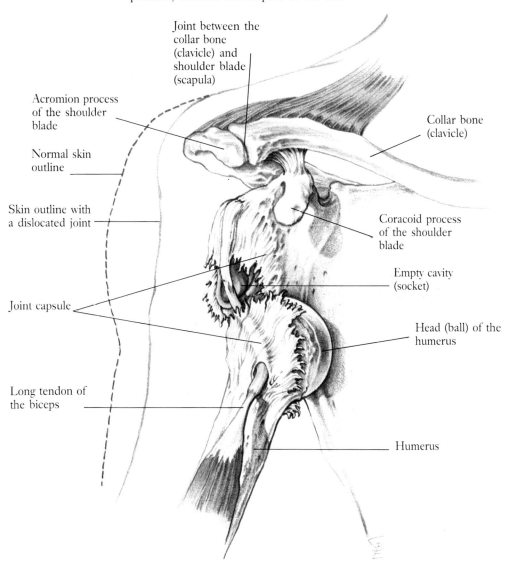

Joint between the collar bone (clavicle) and shoulder blade (scapula)

Acromion process of the shoulder blade

Normal skin outline

Skin outline with a dislocated joint

Joint capsule

Long tendon of the biceps

Collar bone (clavicle)

Coracoid process of the shoulder blade

Empty cavity (socket)

Head (ball) of the humerus

Humerus

Anterior dislocation of the shoulder joint, caused by extensive injuries to the soft tissues surrounding the shoulder joint. Compare this torn joint capsule with the joint capsule on page 180.

— The joint can be dislocated by falling directly on to the outer (lateral) aspect of the shoulder or by violent impact with another player.

— The arm can be caught by another player and pulled vigorously outwards and backwards with a resulting dislocation of the shoulder joint.

Types of dislocation

— *Anterior dislocation (forward and downward)* is commonest and has a tendency to recur.

— *Posterior dislocation (backward)* is unusual and can be difficult to spot and sometimes to treat.

Symptoms and diagnosis

— Pain.

— Lack of mobility. The arm hangs loosely beside the body.

— The upper part of the humerus can be felt as a lump in the armpit, and, where it is normally located, an empty joint socket can be felt.

— The outline of the injured shoulder looks uneven in comparison with the rounded outline of the undamaged shoulder (see diagram on page 177).

— The diagnosis can be verified with X-ray. A posterior dislocation often requires an X-ray examination using special angles.

Treatment

The injured athlete should be taken to a *doctor* for treatment immediately. As a rule, the earlier the joint is realigned, the fewer the complications and the shorter the healing period. It is more considerate to manipulate the joint back into position under anaesthetic. After that, X-ray should be carried out to check alignment and to exclude a concurrent fracture.

After manipulation, the arm is immobilized against the body in order to reduce pain and allow the joint capsule and ligaments time to heal. Should this not occur there is a risk of ligament stretching and joint instability. Three weeks' immobilization is usually sufficient for the older athlete, but this period should be extended for the young in whom the danger of re-dislocation is high, especially if this is the first time dislocation has occurred. In recurrent dislocations, an early, thorough muscle-strength training programme can be initiated.

After the bandage has been removed the injured athlete should train with pendular movements for 1–2 weeks. After that the arm can be lifted above the horizontal plane and cautious outward rotational movements can be made. For a suitable training programme see page 419.

Healing and complications

— If there are no complications a dislocated shoulder heals well. Light conditioning or similar exercise can be resumed after 2–4 weeks.

— Return to sporting activity should not take place until full mobility and strength are regained, usually 2–3 months after the injury occurred.

— Sometimes a dislocation of the shoulder joint is complicated by a fracture of the upper part of the humerus or the scapula.

— In rare cases, nerve and blood vessel injuries and muscle ruptures may occur.

— After a forward and downward dislocation, the shoulder joint is vulnerable to further similar injuries as the joint capsule remains unstable anteriorly and below. Ultimately dislocation may occur during a normal movement, such as raising the arm behind the head. Once dislocation of the shoulder has occurred 3–4 times, surgery to stabilize the joint should be considered.

Separation (dislocation) of the joint between clavicle and acromion process of the scapula

Separation of the acromio-clavicular joint is a relatively common injury in contact sports, riding, cycling, skiing and wrestling. The joint is surrounded by ligaments, one running between the clavicle and the acromion process of the scapula (the acromio-clavicular ligament) and others between the clavicle and the coracoid process of the scapula (the coraco-clavicular ligaments). The joint sometimes contains a cartilaginous meniscus or disc.

Causes

The acromio-clavicular joint can be injured by falling on to the shoulder, elbow or outstretched arm, forcing the joint inwards and upwards. The ligaments and the joint capsule may tear as a result and a partial separation or dislocation (subluxation) occurs. If the strong ligaments joining the clavicle and the coracoid process also tear, separation is total, and the meniscus may also be damaged.

Symptoms and diagnosis

— Depending on the degree of separation, the lateral end of the clavicle is displaced upwards (see diagram on page 180). A partial separation (grade I and II) involves tearing of the acromio-clavicular capsule and ligaments; a total separation (grade III) also affects the coraco-clavicular ligaments.
— There is pain and tenderness over the outer end of the clavicle and pain on moving the shoulder joint.
— The diagnosis is confirmed by X-ray, which is more likely to reveal the abnormality if carried out with the joint loaded. In grade III separation, there is no contact between the articular surfaces.

Treatment

The *doctor* may:
— prescribe early mobility exercises when the dislocation is partial and sometimes, in elderly athletes, when it is total;
— manipulate a totally separated clavicle back into its correct position by pressure. This position is maintained by applying a bandage over the outer end of the clavicle and down round the elbow joint which should be bent at an angle of 90°. The bandage is worn for 2–3 weeks;
— resort to surgery in total separation, especially in young and active athletes, if it is difficult to keep the clavicle in position.

Healing and complications

— Once the supportive bandage has been removed, conditioning exercises, such as cycling or running, can be resumed.
— Strength training can be carried out to increase mobility.

— If a separation of this joint is neglected, it will remain displaced. This will cause wear and tear which, after a few years, can result in permanent discomfort, pain and weakness and impaired flexibility in the joint. When there are persistent symptoms, surgery can be performed at a later stage.

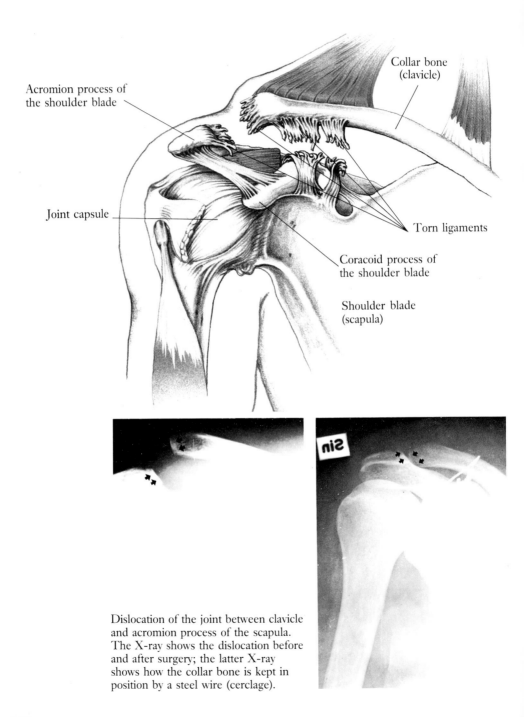

Dislocation of the joint between clavicle and acromion process of the scapula. The X-ray shows the dislocation before and after surgery; the latter X-ray shows how the collar bone is kept in position by a steel wire (cerclage).

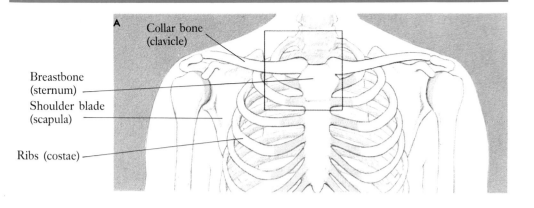

Collar bone
(clavicle)

Breastbone
(sternum)

Shoulder blade
(scapula)

Ribs (costae)

A. Diagram of the shoulder region. The inset picture shows a normal joint
between collar bone (clavicle) and breastbone (sternum).
B. A normal joint between collar bone and breastbone. Note the position of the
large blood vessels that go up to the head and down the arm.
C. Partial dislocation (subluxation) of the joint between collar bone and
breastbone. The ligaments and the capsule around the joint are torn.
D. Total posterior dislocation (backwards) of the joint between collar bone and
breastbone. The ligament between the collar bone and first rib is also torn. In
some cases, the end of the collar bone may pierce blood vessels.

Ligament and
capsule over the
joint between
breastbone and
collar bone

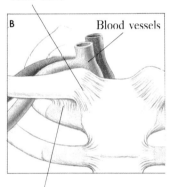

Blood vessels

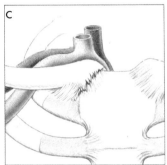

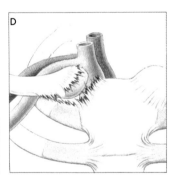

Ligament between
the collar bone and
the first rib

Separation (dislocation) of the joint between clavicle and sternum

The sterno-clavicular joint is seldom separated but it is an important
injury to recognize. The inner (medial) end of the clavicle, and hence the

shoulder, is anchored to the sternum by the sterno-clavicular ligaments and to the first rib by the costo-clavicular ligaments. The joint cavity lies obliquely and contains a meniscus or disc. If the shoulder is subjected to a violent impact, the sterno-clavicular joint can slip and the ligaments tear, causing the inner (medial) end of the clavicle to move either forwards (making it stand out) or backwards.

Symptoms and diagnosis
— Pain may be located towards the shoulder region rather than in the sterno-clavicular joint itself.
— Tenderness occurs when pressure is applied to the joint.
— The injury should be X-rayed by a doctor. The clavicle is usually only partially separated, but its inner (medial) end can be completely detached from the sternum.
— If the end of the clavicle is displaced backwards towards major blood vessels, serious damage can occur.

Treatment
The *doctor* may:
— suggest that the injured person should rest without further treatment if separation is partial;
— operate to realign the joint. This is necessary if the medial end of the clavicle is detached from the sternum and difficult to keep in position;
— treat the injury in hospital in cases of backward separation.

Healing
In cases of partial separation of the sterno-clavicular joint, the injured athlete can generally resume sporting activity relatively early, even if pain and other symptoms remain for several months.

Unstable shoulder joint (subluxation)

Problems can be caused if an unstable shoulder joint slips backwards and/or forwards in the joint although dislocation is not total. The injury is not unusual among pole-vaulters who get too close to the pole-vault pit, ice hockey players, team handball, volleyball, basketball and American football players, and in throwing and racket sports. The slippage in the joint may cause pain during and after sporting activity. The injured athlete often feels as if 'the shoulder has almost slipped out of joint'.

Symptoms and diagnosis
— Pain in the shoulder joint during and after exertion.
— A feeling of dislocation when the arm is lifted above the horizontal plane.
— The diagnosis can be made with the aid of the 'apprehension test'. In cases of anterior instability of the joint the athlete lies on his back, and his arm is moved outwards (abducted) at the same time as it is vigorously turned (rotated) outwards. In this way, the humeral head is lifted forwards in its socket, and the injured athlete feels discomfort and sometimes pain. In cases of posterior instability in the joint the patient's arm is instead rotated inwards [sic].

— An X-ray examination can confirm the diagnosis by showing skeletal changes along the anterior edge of the joint socket. A contrast X-ray can give further support for the diagnosis.
— Arthroscopy of the joint can be of value.

Treatment

The *athlete* should:
— improve the functioning of the joint with active strength exercises.

The *doctor* may:
— operate in cases of prolonged problems.

Glenoid labrum tear

The glenoid labrum is a fibrocartilage rim surrounding the articular surface of glenoid cavity and can be the location of injuries. A glenoid labrum tear is commonly associated with anterior dislocation and subluxation of the shoulder or with a degenerative lesion. An isolated glenoid labrum tear, without instability, can occur in younger throwing athletes, in wrestlers and boxers and in racket players.

Symptoms and diagnosis

— Pain in the shoulder during activity, especially in overhead movements. The pain is often deep and located anteriorly.
— Popping or locking sensation on motion.
— Sometimes there can be a feeling of instability and a slight limitation of motion.
— During examination the doctor can feel a click or locking. This can be felt during overhead abduction and rotation.
— Tenderness to palpation over the joint line.
— The diagnosis is confirmed by shoulder arthroscopy.

Treatment

The *athlete* should:
— rest;
— carry out strength training.

The *doctor* may:
— perform arthroscopic surgery;
— perform open surgery in cases with instability.

Rehabilitation

An early range of motion and strength training, especially overhead rotation exercises, should be carried out. Sport-specific training can start after 2–6 weeks, and the athlete may return to competition after 6–12 weeks.

Throwing injuries

Throwing injuries are of increasing importance in both professional and amateur sport, and affect adults and children alike. Sports prone to throwing injuries include baseball, American football, soccer, tennis and other racket sports, javelin-throwing, team handball, and sports with other overhead motions such as swimming and volleyball.

The throwing mechanism can be divided into three stages: the windup or cocking stage, the acceleration stage, and the follow-through stage. Throwing injuries most frequently affect the shoulder and the elbow.

Windup or cocking stage

During windup, the shoulder is hyperextended, externally rotated and abducted, and the elbow is flexed to an angle of about 45°. At this stage, the anterior structures of the shoulder are under tension and are therefore stressed. Lesions may then occur, most frequently in the anterior capsular structures and the long tendon of the biceps. The flexor and extensor muscles around the elbow are contracted and are prone to overuse injuries.

Acceleration or forward motion stage

This second stage extends from the end of windup to ball release and consists of two distinct phases:

In the first phase, the shoulder and elbow are brought forward, leaving the forearm and hand behind. This creates valgus stress upon the elbow causing distraction of the medial aspect of the elbow and compression of the lateral aspect. Lesions may result.

In the second phase, the shoulder is rapidly rotated inwards with a whip-like action as the forearm and hand are snapped forward. In adults this movement may cause injury to the internal rotators of the shoulder (latissimus dorsi and pectoralis major). Rotational injuries, represented by spontaneous, usually spiral, fractures of the shaft of the humerus, may occur.

In children and adolescents, the second phase may cause injury to the proximal humeral epiphysis. In the shoulder, widening and absorption of the epiphysis of the proximal humerus may occur, resulting in a stress fracture from sudden internal rotation and/or possibly an episode of avascularity.

Follow-through stage

The final stage starts with ball release and is characterized by forearm rotation into pronation. This may cause rotational and shearing forces on the lateral side of the elbow and compression on the posterior elbow.

Soft tissue injuries around the shoulder are most frequent in adults and affect the muscles, ligaments and capsular structures. The most common injuries include: bicipital tendinitis, subluxation of the long head of the biceps, chronic tendinitis, acromial bursitis and rotator cuff injuries due to impingement (see page 174).

Elbow injuries in children

Unique bony problems of the elbow are seen in children and adolescents. The pathology of these problems corresponds to each stage in the development of the elbow; that is, prior to the appearance of all the secondary centres of ossification in children, prior to fusion of the ossification centres in adolescents, and prior to the completion of bony growth in young adults. The majority of injuries are due to overuse resulting from an increase in frequency, rapidity and duration of throwing. Elbow injuries can be divided into three distinct areas:

Medial injuries   The medial side of the elbow is subjected to distraction forces which may cause injury to the medial epicondyle and the medial soft tissues, including the capsular structures and the ulnar nerve. In children, ossification of the medial epicondyle may be disturbed by enlargement of the epicondyle or by osteochondritic changes. In adolescents, avulsion fractures of the medial epicondyle may occur. The epicondyle may occasionally displace in the joint causing mechanical derangement. After fusion of the medial epicondyle, muscular injuries are more frequent and may cause the development of osteophytes.

Lateral injuries   On the lateral side of the elbow, bony disturbance from repetitive compression and shearing forces may occur during childhood at both the head of the radius and the capitellum. Injury to the lateral aspect may affect the entire epiphysis with enlargements and fragmentation throughout. During adolescence, the periphery of the ossification centre is affected more with subchondral necrosis and avulsion fractures damaging the articular cartilage and forming loose bodies. The capitellum and sometimes the head of the radius are affected by lesions.

Injuries to the lateral side of the elbow often result in permanent impairment.

Posterior injuries   In children, stress fractures and non-union of the olecranon epiphysis may occur as well as ectopic bone formation around the olecranon tip and loose body formation at a later date.

Elbow injuries in adults

These can similarly be divided into medial, lateral and posterior areas.

Medial injuries   These include medial epicondylitis, injury to the common flexors (myositis or acute rupture), compression of the hypertrophied pronator teres by the overlying fascia, chronic elongation and/or rupture of the medial collateral ligament with or without spur formation and development of traction osteophytes medially. Ulnar neuropathy is also frequent.

Lateral injuries   These involve the formation of loose bodies and post-traumatic hypertrophic arthritis. As this area is subjected to compression rather than traction, soft tissue injuries are less common.

Posterior injuries   Loose bodies may again result from traction injuries, such as overpull of the triceps or compression of the tip of the olecranon in the olecranon fossa. Posterior elbow injuries occur with sudden extension and hyperextension of the elbow. Older pitchers may develop flexion deformities that limit full extension. In these cases, an injury thought to be due to compression of the olecranon into the olecranon fossa may actually be an avulsion injury.

In summary, the various throwing injuries can be related to the various stages of the throwing mechanism. An understanding of this mechanism as well as the stages of the skeletal maturation in the youthful athlete, are important in diagnosing and treating throwing injuries.

Rupture of the supraspinatus tendon

Rupture of the supraspinatus tendon occurs typically in older athletes, who, after a long period of inactivity, have resumed training and competition in sports such as team handball, soccer, American football, tennis, badminton, cricket, table tennis, throwing sports and skiing. This injury is quite common in young athletes who partake in throwing and racket sports as well as wrestling and weight-lifting.

The shoulder joint is surrounded by a rotator cuff comprising four tendons. The supraspinatus, infraspinatus and teres minor muscles are attached to the upper posterior part of the humerus; the latter two rotate

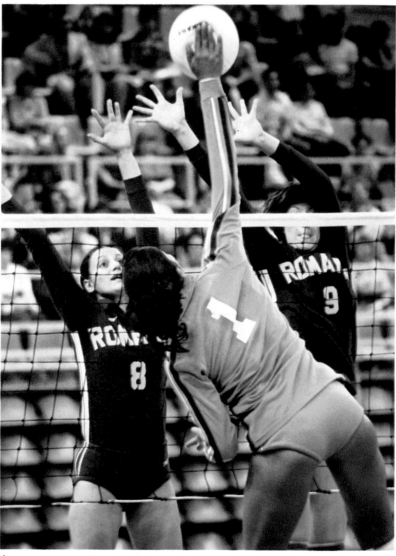

Arm movements above the horizontal plane may cause injuries to tendons and muscles in the shoulder region. *Photo: EPU.*

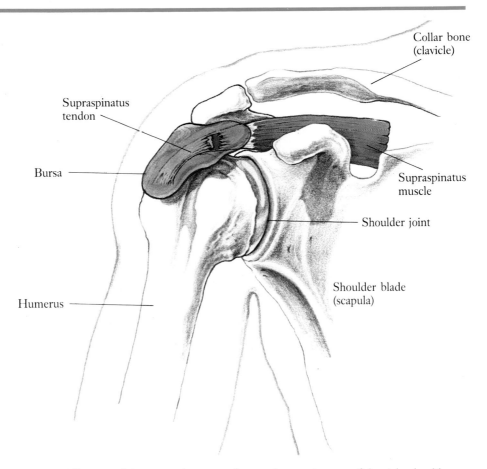

Rupture of the supraspinatus tendon on the anterior part of the right shoulder.

the arm outwards, while the subscapularis muscle which is attached to the front of the upper part of the humerus rotates it inwards. It is the tendons of these muscles which form the rotator cuff and strengthen the shoulder joint capsule behind, above and in front. On abduction of the shoulder joint the supraspinatus tendon glides into the space roofed by the acromion and the coraco-acromial ligament. If abduction is combined with extreme outward (external) rotation, the tendon instead glides towards the ligament and may impinge upon it. The infraspinatus, teres minor and subscapularis tendons act in a downwards direction and stabilize the head of the humerus against the socket of the scapula during abduction.

In 75 per cent of cases, the source of shoulder pain is found in the rotator cuff, and usually the supraspinatus tendon. The supraspinatus, together with the deltoid, raises the arm to initiate abduction. With a total rupture, the athlete has to drop the shoulder so the arm swings outwards due to gravity; then the deltoid takes over. The weakest point of the supraspinatus tendon is the part which forms a cuff over the joint less that $\frac{1}{2}$ in (1 cm) from the attachment of the tendon to the humerus. It is at this point that ruptures most often occur. They may be either partial or total.

In the vulnerable area is a network of capillaries in which typical degenerative changes, which diminish blood flow, are often apparent even in athletes of thirty to thirty-five years of age. When the arm is abducted to an angle of 80–120° to the body, and during static work in this position, the blood vessels are compressed; this further impairs the blood flow, reduces tissue oxygen supply and increases the risk of injury.

Causes
— Any force that rotates the arm inwards against a resistance or which prevents the arm from turning outwards, as may occur, for example, during team handball, American football or wrestling.
— Falling directly on to the shoulder or on to an outstretched arm.
— Lifting or throwing heavy objects.

Symptoms and diagnosis
— Intense pain is felt when the injury occurs. The pain returns on exertion, may increase during the next 24 hours and can then extend towards the upper arm. A diagnosis of rupture of the supraspinatus tendon is supported by the fact that the athlete has fallen on to his shoulder or has lifted or thrown a heavy object.
— Pain occurs when the arm is rotated outwards or is raised upwards and outwards. When the tendon is only partially torn, the arm can be lifted outwards to an angle of 60–80° to the body with little or no pain. The pain increases as the arm is lifted at an angle of 80–120° and then decreases again (see photograph below). Between these angles the arm is also weaker. When the tendon has sustained a *total rupture* the arm can be held at an angle of more than 120° to the body, but when it is lowered further it suddenly 'drops'. This is an important diagnostic sign.

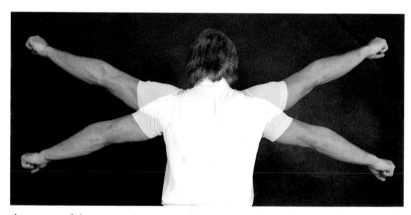

A rupture of the supraspinatus muscle causes muscle weakness in the range of movement of the injured arm. Pain will increase when the arm is lifted above an angle of 80–120° to the body.

— Muscular movements of the arm on the injured side are impaired due to pain and weakness.
— Local tenderness is felt over the tendon or its attachment.
— Arthroscopy and/or contrast X-ray of the shoulder joint may confirm the diagnosis.

Treatment	The *athlete* should:
	— treat the shoulder by cooling at the scene of the injury;
	— rest;
	— consult a doctor if the symptoms persist.

The *doctor* may:
— operate in cases of a total tendon rupture in young athletes;
— if the tendon rupture is partial, prescribe rest and immobilize the arm with a bandage for a short time;
— prescribe mobility training (see page 419) and other rehabilitative exercise.

Healing and complications
— After the bandage has been removed, conditioning exercises such as running can be resumed. Lifting and throwing exercises, however, should be avoided from for 8–12 weeks, depending on the degree of severity of the injury.
— A neglected supraspinatus tendon rupture can cause permanent disability due to impaired function, but can sometimes be surgically repaired at a later date.

Inflammation of the supraspinatus tendon or its attachment (supraspinatus tendinitis)

Inflammation of the supraspinatus tendon or its attachment is a common injury caused by overuse in contact sports and also amongst throwers, weight-lifters, racket players, wrestlers and others; it is one of the most frequent causes of shoulder pain.

Causes
— Prolonged and repeated use of the shoulder muscles with the arm at or above shoulder level.
— Repeated outward rotation of the upper arm.
— Incomplete healing after supraspinatus tendon rupture.

Symptoms
— Pain during movements of the shoulder joint, particularly when the arm is rotated outwards or lifted upwards and outwards at an angle of between 80° and 120° to the body. The photograph opposite shows a possible mechanism for the occurrence of pain under these circumstances.
— Tenderness felt when direct pressure is applied to the front of the upper part of the shoulder.
— Weakness when executing arm movements upwards and outwards (abduction) at an angle of 80–120° to the body.

Treatment
The *athlete* should:
— rest, but maintain mobility, until there is no pain when a load is applied;

— apply local heat and use a heat retainer;
— consult a doctor if the pain is severe or persistent.

The *doctor* may:
— prescribe analgesic and anti-inflammatory medication;
— administer a steroid injection when there is local tenderness in the tendon's attachment to bone;
— advise mobility training without load (see page 419), followed by strength training with increasing load;
— operate in cases of persistent pain and impaired function due to inflammation caused by partial supraspinatus tendon rupture.

Healing and complications
— If there are no complications the injured athlete can often resume his sporting activity after 1–3 weeks.
— Supraspinatus tendinitis, if neglected, can become prolonged or chronic, in which case it can be very difficult to treat. It may necessitate the injured athlete taking a long break from his sporting activity or even giving it up completely.

Subacromial bursitis

The bursa in the shoulder is located between the supraspinatus muscle and the acromion process of the scapula, and in its inflated state is about the size of a golf-ball. It is commonly affected by inflammation.

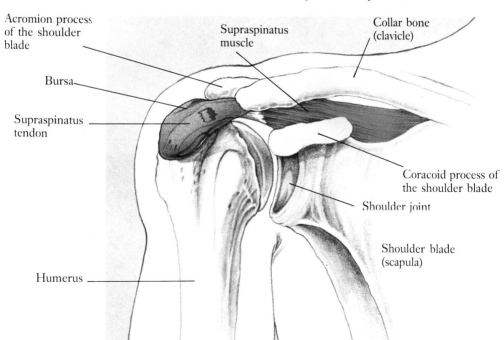

A. The arm and shoulder blade in a resting position showing rupture and inflammation of the supraspinatus tendon attached to the supraspinatus fossa. The adjacent bursa is shown.

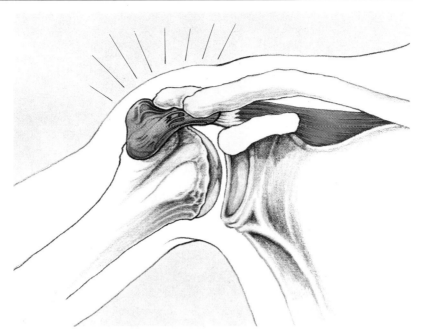

B. When the arm is lifted upwards and outwards (abduction) at an angle of 70–80° to the body, the bursa and the injured tendon may be trapped against the lower edge of the shoulder blade and against the coraco-acromial ligament, causing pain. The condition is called trapping or impingement syndrome.

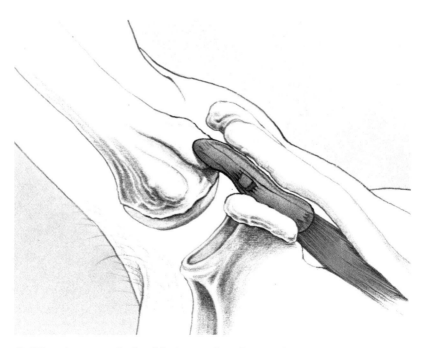

C. When the arm is further lifted upwards and outwards at an angle greater than 120°, the bursa and the injured tendon slide under the acromion process of the shoulder blade. This releases the pressure, and therefore the pain, on the tendon.

Causes	— A fall or a blow to the shoulder or a supraspinatus tendon rupture can cause bleeding into the bursa resulting in inflammation. — Repetitive movements can cause bursitis which, in turn, causes accumulation of fluid in the bursa. The effusion causes tension in the tissues and pain in the anterior (front) and upper part of the shoulder. — Inflammation in an adjacent tendon can easily spread to include the bursa.
Symptoms and diagnosis	— Pain in the anterior, upper part of the shoulder. — Pain which begins when the arm is lifted upwards and outwards (abduction) and the shoulder joint rotated (see diagrams on pages 190–1). — Tenderness on palpation. — Sometimes the bursa feels 'spongy' on palpation. — Examination using an arthroscope and/or bursography.
Treatment	The *athlete* should: — rest until the pain has resolved; — apply local heat and use a heat retainer. The *doctor* may: — aspirate the bursa when bleeding or effusion is accompanied by pain; — prescribe analgesic and anti-inflammatory medication; — advise mobility exercises (see page 95); — in cases of chronic inflammation, administer a steroid injection and advise rest; — use transarthroscopic surgery if necessary; — remove the bursa by surgery in some chronic cases, including resection of the coraco-acromial ligament (see below).
Healing	When bursitis is treated promptly, symptoms usually resolve in 2–3 weeks after which sporting activity can be resumed.

Impingement syndrome ('swimmer's shoulder')

'Impingement' can be defined as a trapping of soft tissues leading to painful inflammation.

Athletes including tennis players, swimmers, throwers and weight-lifters, who make repetitive movements of the arms in or above the horizontal plane, can develop this painful condition of the shoulder. It is caused by the trapping of the soft tissues between the head of the humerus and the vault formed by the acromion process of the scapula and the coraco-acromial ligament. The space between the ligament and the process is small and can be restricted further if the ligament is thickened or calcified. The anterior (front) edge of the acromion process can become irregular with bony outgrowths, especially in elderly people. The coraco-acromial ligament shows degenerative changes in the form of bone formations or calcification which render it inelastic. In the limited space between the two lie the tendons of the supraspinatus, infraspinatus, teres minor and subscapularis muscles, the long tendon of the biceps, and the bursa which overlies the supraspinatus tendon.

When the upper arm is moved forwards and upwards (its usual functional position) to an angle of 90° to the body and is then rotated inwards, the soft tissues are compressed against the sharp edge of the coraco-acromial ligament. During movements the tendons and the bursa rub against the ligament, and this mechanical irritation gives rise to painful inflammation. As inflammation is accompanied by swelling, the space is even further reduced, and the condition becomes progressively worse.

Repeated loading causes thickening of the soft tissues and leads to a chronic inflammatory reaction. It is often the vulnerable areas of the supraspinatus and biceps tendons which are involved in this process.

Symptoms and diagnosis
— When the arm is lifted above the horizontal plane, pain similar to that of supraspinatus tendinitis is felt (see page 189). The pain is particularly pronounced when the arms are raised upwards and outwards at an angle of 80–120° to the body, with maximum pain at an angle of 90°.
— Trapping of soft tissues can occur in 'swimmer's shoulder' when the forward and inward movements of the arms in the crawl and butterfly strokes trigger pain.
— The 'impingement sign' is seen. This means that the injured person feels intense pain, often sufficient to cause a grimace, when his arm is lifted vigorously forwards and upwards by the examiner.
— Tenderness is felt over the upper aspect of the head of the humerus and, if the biceps tendon is also inflamed, at the anterior aspect of the shoulder joint where the tendon lies.
— Impaired mobility can occur when the pain is prolonged.
— In the chronic condition the tissues thicken and become inelastic. The pain takes on a nagging quality and can occur even at rest and often at night. Tennis players who develop the condition may be inhibited during serving because they are afraid of triggering pain.

Preventive measures
— Proper warm-up exercises followed by flexibility training.
— Strength training.

Treatment
The *athlete* should:
— carry out active movements of the shoulder joint;
— keep up his conditioning exercises;
— apply local heat and use a heat retainer;
— resume his sports training gradually when the pain has resolved.

The *doctor* may:
— give instructions on active mobility training;
— prescribe anti-inflammatory medication;
— treat with ultrasound;
— use steroid injections selectively (when local steroids are justified, the injection should be followed by 2 weeks' rest);
— operate in chronic cases to remove the coraco-acromial ligament and

create more space for the soft tissues. In the elderly, more extensive measures may be necessary. After surgery, early mobilization is recommended, and training should comprise pendular exercises, active exercises with rotation and lifting, and strength training.

Inflammation of the subscapularis tendon

The subscapularis muscle, which originates on the inner surface of the scapula, runs anterior to the shoulder joint and is inserted high into the anterior (front) aspect of the head of the humerus, is the most important inward rotator of the upper arm. Its tendon can be affected by partial or total ruptures. A partial rupture, which is commonest, heals with inflammation. A total rupture is uncommon but can occur in conjunction with dislocation of the shoulder joint.

It is principally throwers, for example baseball pitchers and quarter-back players in American football, as well as overhead players in racket sports who suffer from injury and inflammation of the subscapularis tendon. Typical movements are also carried out by javelin throwers, team handball players, wrestlers, weight-lifters and goal keepers. First, the arm is raised outwards to an angle of about 90° to the body, with simultaneous straightening of the elbow joint in the horizontal plane and extreme outward rotation of the shoulder joint. During the 'throw' itself the arm is brought forwards with a simultaneous inward rotation of the shoulder joint. Tennis players make a similar movement when serving, smashing and volleying, but they keep the elbow joint bent until it is extended at the moment of impact. About 25 per cent of top-level tennis players examined had indications of overuse of the subscapularis tendon.

Symptoms and diagnosis
— Pain on moving the shoulder joint, particularly when the arm is held above the horizontal plane and is turned inwards.
— Pain initiated by rotating the arm inwards against resistance.
— Tenderness when direct pressure is applied against the tendon and the tendon attachment anterior to the shoulder.
— Impaired power of the arm during movements involving inward rotation.

Treatment
The *athlete* should:
— start active mobility training;
— rest until no pain is felt under load;
— apply local heat and use a heat retainer;
— see a doctor if pain is severe.

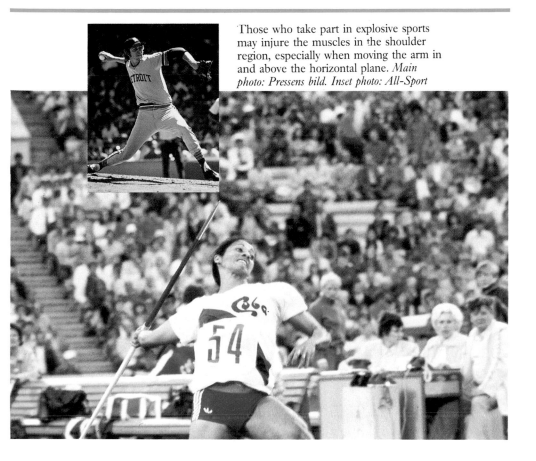

Those who take part in explosive sports may injure the muscles in the shoulder region, especially when moving the arm in and above the horizontal plane. *Main photo: Pressens bild. Inset photo: All-Sport*

The *doctor* may:
— advise active flexibility training (see pages 95);
— prescribe anti-inflammatory medication;
— arrange physiotherapy with flexibility training and heat treatment;
— administer a steroid injection, followed by 2 weeks' rest from movements under load, when symptoms are chronic.

Healing and complications

With appropriate treatment, the injured athlete can, in most cases, resume his training after 1–3 weeks. As soon as signs of inflammation in the subscapularis tendon appear, he should rest from sporting activity as the injury might otherwise easily become chronic and force him to interrupt his training for several months or give up his sport completely.

Dislocation of the long tendon of the biceps muscle

On the anterior aspect of the humerus, between the attachments of the supraspinatus (greater tuberosity) and the subscapularis muscles (lesser tuberosity), is a ligament which retains the long biceps tendon in the groove in which it glides (see diagram on page 174). If this ligament stretches or tears or if the groove is shallow, the biceps tendon may become partially or totally dislocated. Normally dislocation takes place inwards, giving the tendon a straighter course to run on contraction. It can also dislocate laterally in abduction and outwards rotation. Apart from its other functions, the long biceps tendon plays some part in inwards rotation of the shoulder joint.

Symptoms and diagnosis
— Bending movements of the elbow and abduction of the shoulder may cause pain extending up to the shoulder.
— Abduction of the humerus at the shoulder joint can cause pain over its anterior aspect.
— The fingers can feel the biceps tendon slipping in and out of its groove.

Treatment
The *athlete* should:
— rest;
— apply local heat and use a heat retainer.

The *doctor* may:
— prescribe anti-inflammatory medication;
— immobilize in acute cases;
— perform arthroscopy or X-ray by contrast medium;
— operate if the tendon is completely dislocated or causes persistent problems.

This injury can result in inflammation of the tendon and its sheath. Symptoms and treatment of this condition are given on page 37.

Calcific tendinitis

The degenerative changes which occur in tendons as part of the ageing process can, in combination with exertion, cause chronic inflammation with deposits of calcium in the supraspinatus tendon at an early age of thirty to thirty-five years. The calcium deposits can rupture into the bursa overlying the supraspinatus tendon, bringing about a temporary improvement of the condition but causing bursitis. Alternatively, the deposits can disappear spontaneously 2–3 weeks after formation or simply remain without causing any symptoms.

Symptoms and diagnosis
— Intense pain begins suddenly in the anterior upper part of the shoulder. It can be so severe that it prevents sleep, and is relieved by holding the arm still against the body.

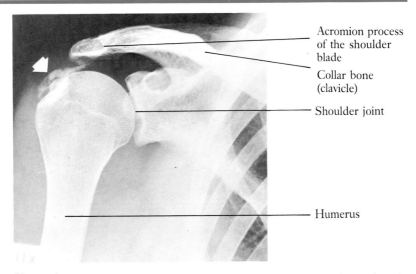

Acromion process of the shoulder blade

Collar bone (clavicle)

Shoulder joint

Humerus

X-ray of a shoulder showing calcification. The arrow indicates a calcium deposit just above the joint head at the bursa (compare with diagram on page 190).

— Because of the intense pain, a doctor is often consulted immediately. He will detect a distinct tenderness over the anterior upper part of the shoulder; an X-ray confirms the diagnosis.

Treatment   The *athlete* should:
— keep the shoulder joint in motion so that it does not stiffen;
— take a pain-relieving preparation.

The *doctor* may:
— puncture and aspirate the calcium deposit;
— administer a local anaesthetic and steroid injection;
— prescribe an analgesic preparation;
— advise flexibility exercises (see page 95);
— operate in order to remove the calcium deposit.

Rupture and inflammation of the deltoid muscle

Ruptures of the deltoid muscle, though infrequent, do occur in team handball and volleyball players, American footballers, weight-lifters, wrestlers and other athletes. The muscle is damaged in most cases by direct impact, but sometimes by overuse. The rupture affects only a small part of the muscle making it difficult to raise the arm upwards and outwards (abduction). Local tenderness is felt over the region of the rupture, and the treatment is rest.

197

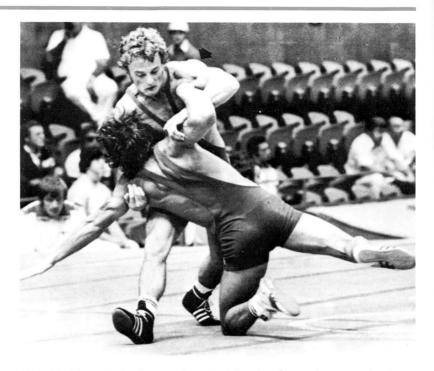

The deltoid muscle (at the arrow) can be injured under maximum exertion in strength sports.

Overuse injuries can affect the deltoid attachment to the humerus, particularly in young athletes who repeatedly raise the arm upwards and outwards under a heavy load. Overuse of the posterior part of the deltoid muscle occurs in, for example, butterfly-stroke swimmers because of their vigorous backward arm movements. Overuse of the anterior part of the muscle is not uncommon in certain contact sports when players use their outstretched arms to try to prevent someone holding the ball from passing them or in rugby tackles. The treatment for these overuse injuries is, as a rule, rest and heat.

Nerve injuries in the shoulder region

Nerve damage in the shoulder region is uncommon but should nevertheless be considered. It occurs mainly after injuries caused by impact and external pressure but also as a result of overuse.

Injuries to the suprascapular nerve

The suprascapular nerve supplies the supraspinatus and infraspinatus muscles and runs in a groove on the upper edge of the scapula, held in place by a ligament.

The suprascapular nerve can be damaged at the time of forward or backward dislocation of the shoulder joint which stretches the nerve over the edge of the scapula. During sports, the nerve can be damaged by a direct blow to the scapula, by external pressure (for example from a backpack) or by repetitive, one-sided motions of the shoulder which cause tension in the nerve leading to swelling and entrapment.

Symptoms and diagnosis
— Pain which radiates out towards the upper posterior part of the shoulder.
— Weakness in the supraspinatus and infraspinatus muscles, manifested by impaired abduction of the shoulder joint to an angle of 80–120°.
— Decreased volume (atrophy) of the supraspinatus and infraspinatus muscles. This change can be very pronounced and readily noticeable.

Treatment
— active rest;
— flexibility training and, if there is no pain, strength training;
— local steroid injection;
— if the complaints persist, surgery may be performed to cut the enclosing ligament and free the nerve.

Injuries to the axillary nerve

The axillary nerve supplies the deltoid and teres minor muscle and runs close to the shoulder joint. Damage to this nerve usually occurs as a complication following dislocation of the shoulder, but also sometimes in fractures of the upper part of the humerus. The symptoms include radiating pain and impaired sensation over the side of the upper arm, together with weakness (due to paralysis of the deltoid muscle) when the arm is abducted.

Since the course of the axillary nerve takes it around the upper part of the humerus close to the bone, a hard blow in this area can sometimes affect it, but the symptoms are usually transitory.

Injuries to the long thoracic nerve

The long thoracic nerve supplies the serratus anterior muscle which holds the scapula in position. An isolated injury to this nerve can occur during violent shoulder movements carried out with great force, for example during weight-lifting. Backstroke swimmers may sustain similar damage as their arm movements are a combination of outward rotation and forward and upward lifting.

When the long thoracic nerve is damaged, there is usually a dull ache which disappears spontaneously.

The ability to lift the arm is impaired and, at the same time, 'winging' of the scapula is seen, the bone protruding backwards on the damaged side. One way of revealing the injury is to ask the athlete to perform press-ups (push-ups) against a wall when the scapula will protrude posteriorly. The treatment consists of anti-inflammatory medication and gradually increased strength training.

Rupture of the pectoral (pectoralis major) muscle

The pectoral muscle has its origin in the anterior chest wall and its insertion in the anterior surface of the upper part of the humerus. Its function is to draw the upper arm in towards the chest and rotate it inwards. When it is subjected to a heavy load, the pectoral muscle can tear, and a total rupture can be induced by strength training (especially bench press training), heavy weight-lifting and other strength sports such as wrestling, shot putting, discus- and javelin-throwing. It is usually the insertion of the muscle into the humerus that is damaged.

Symptoms and diagnosis
— Pain at the insertion of the pectoral muscle into the humerus under heavy load.
— Swelling and bruising (secondary to bleeding) over the anterior aspect of the upper arm.
— Tenderness over the anterior aspect of the upper arm.
— Impaired strength when the upper arm is drawn inwards towards the chest (adducted) or is rotated inwards against resistance.
— Failure of the pectoral muscle to contract when the upper arm is pressed inwards against resistance. This can be felt by placing a hand over the muscle so that it covers both the damaged and healthy portions.
— A visible deformity or loss of definition of the muscle.

Treatment
The *athlete* should:
— apply emergency treatment according to the guidelines indicated on page 31 and page 64;
— carry out a gradually increased strength training programme when rupture is partial;
— consult a doctor.

The *doctor* may:
— operate in cases of total muscle rupture. After surgery, a supportive bandage should be worn for about 4 weeks.

Healing
After surgery a period of rest of 4–6 weeks is required, after which mobility and toning exercises can begin. Strength training, however, should not be resumed until at least 6–8 weeks after the injury and then only with a very light load.

Return to sport
In partial rupture, early strength training is initiated and sport is resumed when normal strength and pain-free normal range of movement is achieved.

Opposite top: The pectoralis major muscle. **Below left:** total rupture of the pectoralis major muscle at its insertion in the humerus. **Below right:** the pectoralis major muscle has been anchored to the humerus with bone sutures.

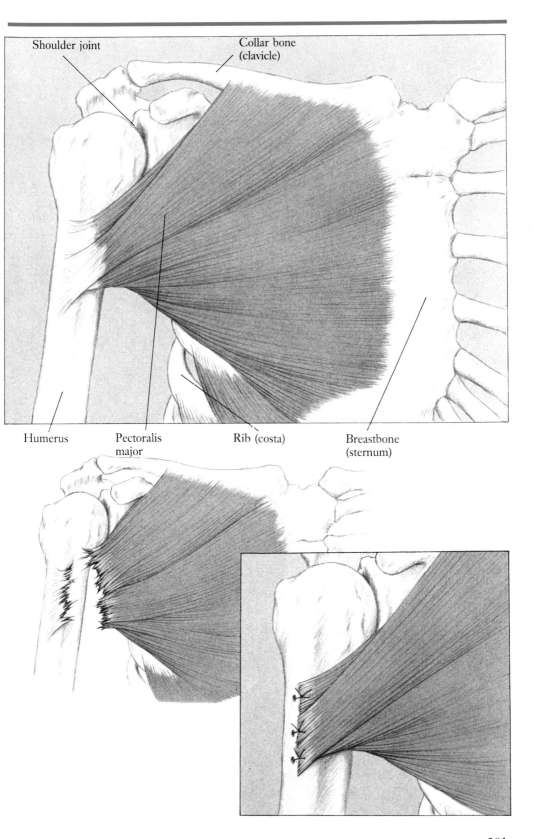

Shoulder joint

Collar bone
(clavicle)

Humerus

Pectoralis
major

Rib (costa)

Breastbone
(sternum)

Inflammation of the insertion of the pectoral muscle

The insertion of the pectoral muscle can be the site of local inflammation. The injury occurs particularly in gymnasts, tennis, badminton, squash and golf players, oarsmen, weight-lifters, swimmers and throwers. The immediate cause is often intensive strength training and acute overuse.

Symptoms and diagnosis
— Pain in the region of the insertion of the pectoral muscle into the humerus.
— Tenderness at a spot over the tendon attachment.
— Pain, and sometimes weakness, when the upper arm is drawn towards the chest (adducted) against resistance.

Treatment
The *athlete* should:
— rest the damaged area;
— apply local heat and use a heat retainer.

The *doctor* may:
— prescribe anti-inflammatory medication;
— give a local steroid injection and prescribe rest;
— initiate strength and flexibility training.

INJURIES OF THE UPPER ARM

The humerus articulates with the scapula at its upper end and with the radius and the ulna at its lower end. The biceps muscle, which flexes the elbow joint and rotates it outwards, lies in front of the humerus, while the triceps, which extends the elbow joint, lies behind.

Rupture of the long tendon of the biceps muscle

Ruptures of the long tendon of the biceps muscle are seen in gymnasts, tennis and badminton players, wrestlers, oarsmen, weight-lifters and javelin-throwers.

The long biceps tendon runs over the head of the humerus inside the shoulder joint and is inserted immediately above the articular cavity of the scapula. It is susceptible to degenerative changes, and ruptures occur most often in athletes over the age of forty to fifty years. In younger athletes this injury is relatively unusual.

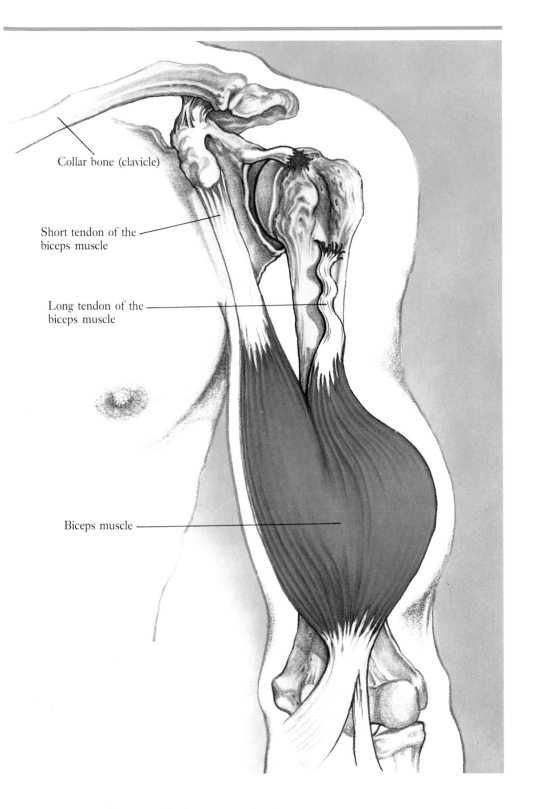

Collar bone (clavicle)

Short tendon of the
biceps muscle

Long tendon of the
biceps muscle

Biceps muscle

Rupture in the long tendon of the biceps muscle of the upper arm.

Symptoms and diagnosis	— Moderate pain over the anterior aspect of the shoulder joint. — Swelling (secondary to bleeding) over the anterior aspect of the upper arm. — Inability to contract the muscle against resistance in the acute stage. — Moderately impaired strength when the elbow joint is flexed and the forearm is rotated outwards. — Slow contraction of the biceps producing a more prominent swelling (see diagram on page 203) than that produced by a normal biceps in a healthy arm. The muscle fails to make its full contribution to flexing of the elbow joint.
Treatment	The *athlete* should: — consult a doctor for advice. The *doctor* may: — prescribe physiotherapy and mobility exercises (see page 419); — operate when a total rupture has affected a young, active athlete.
Healing	— If surgery is not considered necessary, mobility, strength and toning exercises can be started as soon as the pain begins to subside. — If surgery is carried out, immobilization is maintained for 4 weeks, after which mobility exercises and conditioning can be started. Strength training should not be resumed until a few weeks later. Contact sports should not be played until 4–6 weeks after the bandage has been removed.

Inflammation of the long tendon of the biceps

Inflammation of the long tendon of the biceps is a relatively common cause of shoulder pain. This tendon glides over the articular head of the humerus and leaves the joint through a special groove. When the tendon is inflamed, tenderness at the uppermost extremity is very noticeable (see diagram on page 174). The injury occurs in canoeists, oarsmen, weight-lifters, swimmers, javelin-throwers, fencers, wrestlers, golfers, and tennis, table tennis, badminton and squash players.

Symptoms and diagnosis	— Tenderness over the anterior aspect of the upper arm and shoulder when the elbow joint is flexed. — Pain over the anterior aspect of the shoulder can be brought on if the injured person turns his forearm outwards against resistance at the same time as the elbow joint is held flexed at a right angle. — Tendon creaking (crepitus) can be felt over the anterior aspect of the shoulder during flexion and extension of the elbow joint.
Treatment	The *athlete* should: — rest; — apply local heat and use a heat retainer. The *doctor* may: — prescribe anti-inflammatory medication;

Healing   The injured person can resume his sporting activity when symptoms have disappeared.

Rupture of the tendon of the triceps muscle

Falling on to the hand when the arm is flexed or forceful throwing can cause a rupture in the tendon of the triceps, and sometimes the tendon attachment can be torn away from the tip of the elbow.

Symptoms and diagnosis
— Pain in the tip of the elbow where a gap can be felt in the tendon.
— Impaired power in the arm or inability to straighten the arm at the elbow. An X-ray should be carried out to exclude bony injury.

Treatment
— In cases of minor ruptures no treatment, apart from rest, is necessary.
— Surgery should be carried out when young, active athletes have suffered a total rupture of the tendon or the tendon attachment.

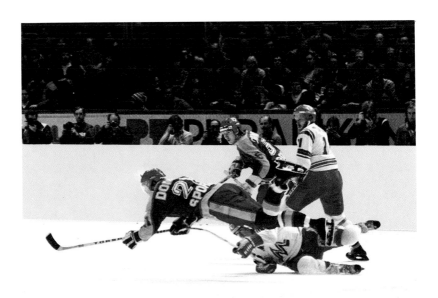

Falling forwards at speed can cause injuries to the triceps muscle. *Photo: Marie Hedberg/Reportagebild.*

Heterotopic bone formation ('Blocker's exostosis' or myositis ossificans)

After a blow to the arm, intramuscular haematoma can occur in the muscles. Pain, swelling and impaired muscle function are common. Swelling of the muscle may result in a compartment syndrome (see page 320). In spite of early treatment with ice, compression bandage and rest, the injury may be complicated with heterotopic bone formation. For treatment guidelines, see page 283.

Fractures

Fractures of the *upper part of the humerus* (see page 177) can be caused by falling on to an outstretched arm or on to the shoulder.

Fractures of the *mid-shaft of the humerus* can occur in riders, wrestlers and other athletes and are usually treated by strapping the arm to the body for 3–6 weeks. Surgery may occasionally be necessary. A rehabilitation period of 3–6 months is advisable before resumption of any sporting activity involving the use of the injured arm.

Stress fractures (see page 54) of the humerus can occasionally occur, for example, in javelin-throwers.

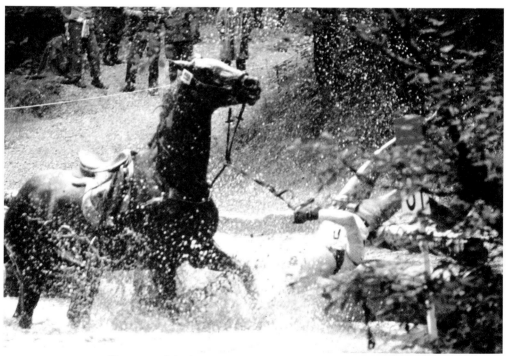

Fractures of the humerus can occur when falling. *Photo: Pressens bild.*

ELBOW INJURIES

The elbow joint not only allows the arm to flex but also permits the forearm to rotate inwards and outwards (pronation and supination). Good interaction between the skeleton, the ligaments and muscles surrounding the elbow joint is critical in coping with such basic parts of the daily routine as dressing, taking meals and attending to personal hygiene. Apart from interference with these activities, serious complications can occur in elbow injuries because of the close proximity to the joint of major blood vessels and nerves. Elbow injuries often occur during throwing. The mechanism of throwing is described on page 183.

'Tennis elbow' (lateral epicondylitis)

'Tennis elbow' has been known since the beginning of the nineteenth century. As the name implies, the injury is common among tennis players, but squash, badminton, table tennis, golf players and others can also be affected, as well as those who carry out repetitive, one-sided movements in their jobs (for example, electricians, carpenters) or leisure activities (for example, needlework).

'Tennis elbow' can be caused in tennis players by faulty stroke technique. Faulty backhand technique often causes lateral tennis elbow; faulty forehand technique may cause medial tennis elbow in the recreational player. A twisted serve may cause medial and posterior problems in competitive players. Recreational players often develop elbow problems as a result of hitting backhand balls by using wrist movements instead of hitting the strokes with a firm wrist and a movement of the whole arm and shoulder. Hitting a tennis ball which is travelling at a speed of 30 m/hour (50 km/hour) is theoretically equivalent to lifting a weight of 55 lb (25 kg). The forces that arise when the ball hits the racket have to be distributed over the player's body. It is therefore essential that the whole of the shoulder and the trunk, including the larger muscles, are used so that the forces and vibration can be dissipated as widely as possible. Recreational players may also play faulty strokes which give rise to torsional forces and vibration which then have to be distributed through the tissues.

'Tennis elbow' is a common complaint, and studies have shown that 45 per cent of the athletes who play tennis daily and 25 per cent of those who play once or twice a week have suffered from it. It is particularly common in athletes over forty years of age. The problems arise in the area of a small bony protuberance (the lateral epicondyle) on the outer (lateral) side of the elbow, which is the site of origin of the muscles which extend the fingers and the wrist (see diagram on page 208). The main muscles affected in 'tennis elbow' are the extensor carpi radialis brevis, the extensor digitorum communis, the carpi radialis longus and the extensor carpi ulnaris.

Because the extensor origin is small, the forces which develop in the muscles create a high load per unit area.

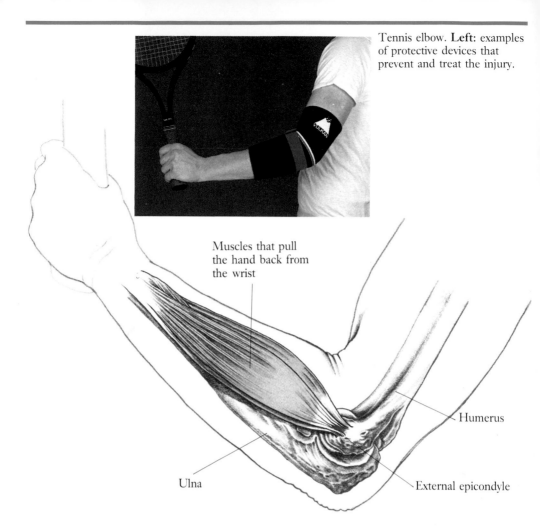

Tennis elbow. **Left:** examples of protective devices that prevent and treat the injury.

Muscles that pull the hand back from the wrist

Humerus

Ulna

External epicondyle

Symptoms and diagnosis

— Pain which mainly affects the outer aspect of the elbow, but can also radiate upwards along the upper arm and downwards along the outside of the forearm.

— Weakness in the wrist. This can cause difficulty in carrying out such simple movements as lifting a plate or a coffee-cup, opening a car door, wringing a wet dishcloth and shaking hands.

— A distinct tender point is elicited by pressure or percussion over the lateral epicondyle.

— Pain over the lateral epicondyle when the hand is bent backwards (dorsi-flexed) at the wrist against resistance (see photograph on page 209). This sign alone is sufficiently important to justify a diagnosis of 'tennis elbow'.

— Pain on the outer aspect of the elbow triggered by straightening the flexed fingers against resistance.

— The elbow can be X-rayed in order to exclude other diagnoses such as a loose body in the joint or a fracture. Other diagnoses that the doctor should consider are rheumatic disorders, trapping of a nerve (the deep branch of the radial nerve or the ulnar nerve) and radiating

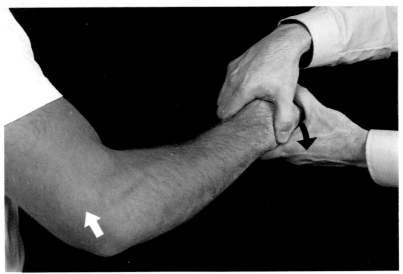

When bending the hand back from the wrist against resistance, pain is triggered over the epicondyle of the elbow (indicated by the white arrow).

pain caused by degenerative changes in the spine in the region of the 5th and 6th cervical vertebrae.

Preventive measures

— Correct playing and working techniques are the most important preventive measures.
— Sometimes a forearm brace or a heat retainer (see photograph on page 208) can be used as a means of dissipating the forces outwards before they reach the epicondyle.
— Asymmetrical training techniques should be avoided.

As far as the correct playing technique in tennis goes, the following points should be emphasized:

1. Good foot work so that the player approaches the ball correctly.
2. The ball should be hit correctly with the racket and at the right moment.
3. The shoulder and the whole of the body should take part in every stroke so that 'braking' does not occur when the ball is hit. The stroke should be followed through and the wrist should be firm.
4. The court surface should be slow in order to decrease the velocity of the ball. Fast surfaces such as grass or concrete cause the ball to hit the racket with increased force, resulting in increased load on the player's arm.
5. The balls should be light. Wet and dead balls become heavy.
6. The correct equipment should be used. The racket should be individually selected with regard to playing technique. A casual player should use a light racket, as a heavy racket causes greater load. The racket should be well-balanced and easy to manoeuvre as is necessary, for example, when making angled drop shots.
7. A tightly strung racket increases the impact and tension forces. The stringing of the racket should be individually adjusted and should not

be too taut. Anyone troubled by 'tennis elbow' should have the racket strung more loosely. Gut strings give more resilience and less vibration than nylon ones.

8. The size of the racket grip should be carefully chosen in order to suit the hand and be comfortable. A simple method of determining the appropriate size of grip is to measure the distance between the mid-

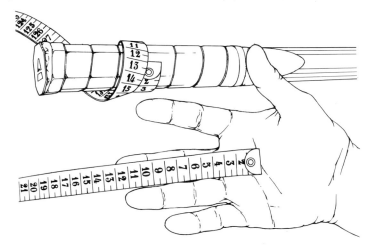

Measuring the right size racket grip. The distance between the mid-line of the palm and the tip of the middle finger is equal to the correct size of the grip.

line of the palm of hand and the tip of the middle finger (see diagram above). This distance should be equal to the grip's circumference.

9. A large 'sweet spot' (centre of percussion which is the mathematical point of the racket face where minimal torsion occurs on impact) is probably an advantage. Hits outside this spot will increase torsion and unwanted forces and vibrations.

Treatment

The *athlete* should:
— reduce pain and inflammation when the injury is in its acute stage by treating the injury with cooling for a couple of days (elevation and compression bandaging are not needed as swelling is not a problem);
— rest actively, that is, rest the injured area and avoid movements which trigger pain but continue with conditioning such as running, cycling or some similar activity;
— continue with tennis but avoid the strokes which cause pain;
— apply local heat and use a heat retainer after a couple of days when the injury is no longer in its acute stage;
— treat with ice massage, perhaps alternating with heat treatment;
— try taping the wrist to support the elbow joint under load;
— reduce the load on the extensors with the help of a brace which should be applied when the arm is relaxed and which should be kept in position until the rehabilitation period is over (see figure on page 122);
— improve strength, stamina and mobility by exercises when pain and inflammation are under control. When the athlete can tolerate the pain of a handshake, he or she can start the exercises. The training programme should follow the guidelines set out below:

1. Isometric training of the wrist extensors. The training is carried out with the wrist in three positions: first fully flexed, then in a neutral position and finally fully straightened. The joint should not be under load and the exercise should be carried out 30 times/day. The wrist extensors are flexed for 10 seconds at a time. When these exercises can be carried out without any pain, a load of 1 lb (0.5 kg) can be introduced.
2. Dynamic training. An elastic band is slipped over the ends of the fingers, and then an attempt is made to spread the fingers against its resistance. Another method is to extend (concentric) and flex (eccentric) the wrist with a load of 2–4 lb (1–2 kg) 20 times/day.
3. Flexibility training (static stretching) of the wrist. The joint is bent at an angle of 90° and the opposite hand is used to provide counter-pressure. The elbow of the injured arm should be held completely extended and the forearm should be rotated inwards (pronated). The bent wrist is stretched to its outer range and is held there for 4–6 seconds. After 2 seconds rest it is subjected to stretching for another 6–8 seconds. The exercise is repeated 15 times/day.
4. Training of strength and mobility in shoulder and arm (see page 419).

Increased training with a load can be introduced when the pain is under control, that is, when the patient can bear the pain that occurs when shaking hands.

The *doctor* may:
— prescribe anti-inflammatory medication;
— prescribe ultrasound treatment, high-voltage galvanic stimulation or and transcutaneous nerve stimulation;
— in persistent cases and if pain interferes with the exercises programme, administer local steroid injections. The injection should be given subperiostally to the extensor brevis origin. These injections have a early and beneficial effect. During the initial 24–48 hours, increased pain may be experienced.

A cortisone injection should be followed by 1–2 weeks' rest and should not be repeated more than 2–3 times. If, in spite of this treatment, the symptoms still persist, surgery should be considered. The results of such operations are usually good.

Healing   A genuine 'tennis elbow' often heals spontaneously and the prognosis is generally good. The symptoms can, however, persist for anything from a couple of weeks to a couple of years, especially if the athlete continues to load his arm. Strenuous activity can be resumed when the arm is fully mobile, has regained normal strength and is pain-free. After surgery, an interval of 8–10 weeks should elapse before tennis playing is resumed.

'Thrower's elbow' or 'golfer's elbow' (medial epicondylitis)

'Thrower's elbow' or 'golfer's elbow' is similar to 'tennis elbow', but the symptoms are located over the inner (medial) epicondyle of the elbow. A right-handed golf player may well suffer from 'tennis elbow' in the leading left elbow and 'golfer's elbow' in the following right elbow. 'Thrower's elbow' is commonest in javelin throwers, but also occurs in cricket and baseball bowlers.

Top-level tennis players may develop medial epicondylitis despite good playing techniques, and it is usually caused by the serving action during which the wrist is bent at the same time as the forearm is turned inwards. Those who hit an exaggerated 'top spin' and in so doing rotate the forearm vigorously inwards (excessive pronation) can also be affected.

The flexor muscles that are principally responsible for these movements have their origins at the medial epicondyle of the elbow.

Symptoms
The symptoms are similar to those of 'tennis elbow' (see the previous section) but are located on the inner aspect of the elbow. There is pronounced tenderness when the medial epicondyle is subjected to pressure, and flexing the hand downwards (palmar flexion) at the wrist joint against resistance causes pain.

Treatment
The treatment is the same for this injury as for 'tennis elbow'. Rehabilitation, however, can sometimes take a little longer after surgery.

'Thrower's elbow' in growing individuals ('little league elbow') (see page 183 for the mechanism of throwing)

When a ball is thrown in baseball, for example, the wrist and the fingers are vigorously pronated. The muscles which are responsible for this movement are all located in the inner (medial) compartment of the forearm. The force of the throw is transmitted up through the arm to the weakest part of the muscle group which is the medial epicondyle from which the muscles originate. In growing adolescents these muscle origins are attached to a growth area (the epiphysis) which is considerably weaker than the adjacent bone, and problems are caused by the increased traction on the epiphyseal junction.

Symptoms and diagnosis
— Pain in the elbow, which often starts gradually. If the pain appears suddenly the epiphysis may have been torn off, which sometimes necessitates surgery. The pain can be induced when the elbow joint is flexed.
— Stiffness in the elbow.

— Local tenderness directly over the medial epicondyle.

— Both the elbows should be X-rayed. A fissure in the growth zone (epiphysis) can be seen if it is present.

Treatment

The *athlete* should:
— rest;
— give up throwing movements completely until the pain has resolved (usually after 8–9 weeks);
— continue with conditioning and general strength training.

The *doctor* may:
— prescribe rest and sometimes immobilize the elbow. If there is a fissure in the growth zone (epiphysis), a cast may be used;
— operate if displacement is significant. Neither steroid injections nor anti-inflammatory medication should be given to growing adolescents.

Healing

If the growth zone (epiphysis) has been injured, throwing training can be resumed at the earliest 8 weeks after the injury occurred. Prior to that, careful rehabilitation should aim to maintain muscle function.

Entrapment of the radial, ulnar and median nerves

Entrapment of the radial nerve

The deep-seated branch which arises from the radial nerve just below the elbow in the outer part of the medial compartment of the forearm can be trapped where it passes through a narrow channel in the supinator muscle which rotates the forearm outwards (supinates). The symptoms may be similar to those which occur in 'tennis elbow'.

Symptoms and diagnosis

— Tenderness may be present below and slightly in front of the lateral epicondyle.
— Pain is felt and strength impaired when the wrist joint is extended and the forearm is supinated.

Treatment

The *athlete* should:
— rest.

The *doctor* may:
— prescribe anti-inflammatory medication;
— operate to free the nerve and enlarge the channel in which it runs. Surgery usually gives good results.

Entrapment of the ulnar nerve

If the medial aspect of the elbow is accidentally hit, pain can be felt which radiates to the fourth and fifth fingers of the hand. The ulnar nerve runs along the medial edge of the elbow just behind the epicondyle to which the flexor muscles of the wrist are attached. In throwing or racket sports the nerve can be stretched or slid out of its groove with subsequent mechanical irritation.

Symptoms and diagnosis
— Pain arising from the medial aspect of the elbow occurring, for example, after long tennis or golf matches, or throwing the javelin.
— Pain may increase and radiate to the fourth and fifth fingers of the hand.
— Numbness and impaired sensation may be present in the little finger and half the ring-finger.
— Tenderness may occur over the nerve on the medial-dorsal side of the elbow.
— In serious cases even tapping the ulnar nerve lightly can cause pain extending right down to the ring-finger.

Treatment
The *athlete* should:
— rest the arm.

The *doctor* may:
— prescribe anti-inflammatory medication;
— operate if the injury persists in order to free the nerve or move it to a position in which it is subjected to less tension. Surgery usually gives good results.

Entrapment of the median nerve (pronator teres syndrome)

The median nerve runs in front of the elbow joint and past the pronator muscle. Entrapment of this nerve is a rare condition in sport.

Symptoms and diagnosis
— Pain and tenderness in the middle anterior aspect of the elbow.
— Numbness in the second, third and radial half of the fourth finger.
— Pain elicited by pronation of the lower arm against resistence.
— Weakness present in palmar flexion of the hand.

Treatment
The *athlete* should:
— rest;
— use heat;

The *doctor* may:
— prescribe anti-inflammatory medication;
— immobilize for a short time;
— operate in chronic cases.

Bursitis ('student's elbow')

Just below the tip of the elbow (olecranon) there is a bursa into which bleeding can occur following an accidental blow to the area or a fall on to the elbow. In many sports, including orienteering, wrestling, volleyball, basketball, soccer, rugby and team handball, this injury is common as the participants wear no elbow guards, and in others, such as ice hockey, where the guards which are worn may provide incomplete protection.

After bleeding into the bursa, and also after prolonged loading of the elbow, the bursa can become inflamed and swollen. The condition is often called 'student's elbow' since it was popularly supposed to have affected students who used to rest their elbows on the desk while supporting their heads in their hands during studying.

Symptoms and diagnosis

— Pain at rest and during movement.
— Swelling and tenderness over the tip of the elbow after *acute bleeding into the bursa* following a violent impact. Sometimes the skin is broken.
— Small blood clots form in the bursa and cause irritation of the surrounding tissues. This results in inflammation and effusion of fluid.
— When there is *inflammation of the bursa*, or when it has been subjected to prolonged pressure it becomes distended with fluid and the overlying

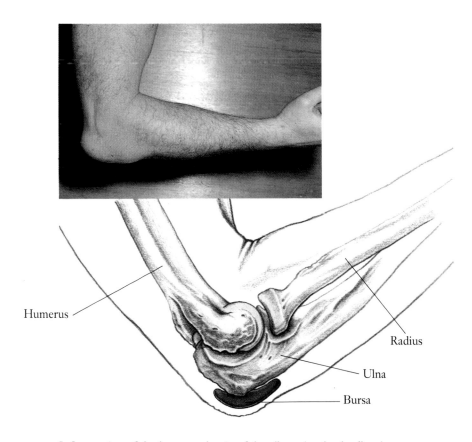

Inflammation of the bursa at the tip of the elbow, 'student's elbow'.

skin becomes red and tender. The swelling can extend to the forearm.
— Limitation of mobility in the elbow joint.

Preventive measures

Elbow guards of a type which protect the tip of the elbow (olecranon) (see page 117) should be used, especially by goalkeepers in team handball and soccer.

Treatment

The *athlete* should:
— rest until symptoms have resolved.

The *doctor* may:
— puncture the bursa and aspirate or drain out blood or fluid;
— apply a bandage to be kept in position for 4–7 days;
— administer a local steroid injection when inflammation is persistent;
— remove the bursa by surgery if it has been affected by repeated inflammation, especially when loose bodies are present.

Healing

After an episode of mild inflammation of a bursa in the elbow, the athlete can return to training one week after medical treatment has started. A severe bursitis can force rest for a long period of time.

Dislocation

Dislocation of the elbow joint occurs mainly in contact sports, such as football, rugby and ice hockey, but also in riders, cyclists, wrestlers, skiers and squash players amongst others. A common cause of this injury is falling on to the hand with a bent elbow. A similar injury can occur if the elbow is overstretched in a fall.

A backward (posterior) dislocation of the elbow joint is most commonly seen and may be combined with a fracture. Dislocations always involve injuries to surrounding soft tissues, such as the medial and lateral collateral ligaments, so that even when the injured joint is realigned promptly it can take some time for complete healing to take place.

Symptoms and diagnosis

— Intense pain, swelling, tenderness and limitation of mobility.
— Deformity of the elbow joint.
— An X-ray confirms the diagnosis.
— Stability testing of the collateral ligaments at 20° flexion.

Treatment

The *doctor* may:
— after having checked nerve function and circulation, replace the joint to its normal position and test it for stability; the sooner this is done, the easier the manipulation;
— X-ray the joint after it has been restored to its correct position;
— immobilize the elbow joint in a brace which is kept on for 2–5 weeks depending on the extent of the injury. Mobility training (see page 424) can be started thereafter;
— operate if there are extensive ligament injuries and instability in the joint.

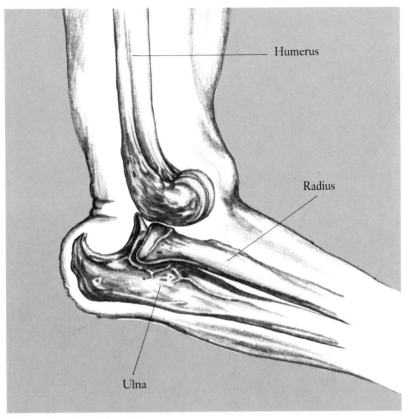

Humerus

Radius

Ulna

Dislocation of the elbow joint.

Healing and complications

When the plaster cast brace has been removed the injured athlete can resume conditioning exercises such as running. Not until 8–10 weeks after the occurrence of the injury, when the ligaments have healed and full mobility is restored, should he return to his usual sport.

Nerve and circulatory injuries may occur and give permanent symptoms in the forearm and hand.

If a dislocated elbow is treated inadequately, the result may be incomplete healing of the ligaments and joint capsule, and a susceptibility to recurrent dislocation.

Loose bodies in the elbow joint (osteochondritis dissecans)

In throwing movements, the elbow joint is exposed to considerable loads, especially during forward movement when the arm relaxes and there is major deceleration. This can cause the convex upper articular surface of the radius in the forearm to come into violent contact with, and even to injure, the outer portion of the articular surface of the humerus at the elbow. Cartilage from the articular surface, together with a fragment of the underlying bone, may become detached and form a loose body in the joint.

Symptoms and diagnosis
— Pain in the upper outer aspect of the elbow, triggered mainly by throwing movements.
— Difficulties in straightening and bending the elbow joint.
— A locking of the joint during elbow movements. The loose body prevents completion of the intended movement, and such an occurrence is always painful. Muscle cramp and swelling follow.
— Swelling around the elbow.
— Tenderness, mainly on the outer aspect of the elbow joint.
— Both elbow joints should be X-rayed, especially when the injured person is young and therefore still growing. On the X-ray of the injured elbow joint the osteochondritis, the defect or loose bodies (calcifications) can be seen.
— Arthroscopy confirms the diagnosis.

Treatment
— Rest.
— When the complaints are persistent surgery should be performed, possibly by arthroscopy.
— In the early stages, immobilization can be of value to secure healing in young athletes.

Healing
As a rule, the injured athlete can resume his sporting activity 2–3 months after surgery.

Fracture of the lower end of the humerus (supra-condylar fracture)

Children often sustain fractures of the lower part of the humerus because of falls from gymnasium apparatus and in riding or cycling falls.

Symptoms and diagnosis
— Intense pain during arm movements.
— Tenderness on pressure.
— Swelling and bruising.
— Contour changes.

Treatment
The injured person should be taken to a doctor as quickly as possible. Fractures of the lower part of the humerus very often require hospital treatment, especially in children or adolescents, as the important nerves and blood vessels situated near the broken ends of the bone can be affected by the resultant bleeding and are vulnerable to damage. Pulse and sensation below the injury should be checked.
— The *doctor* will attempt to realign the fractured bones, and if this is not possible, surgery may be necessary.

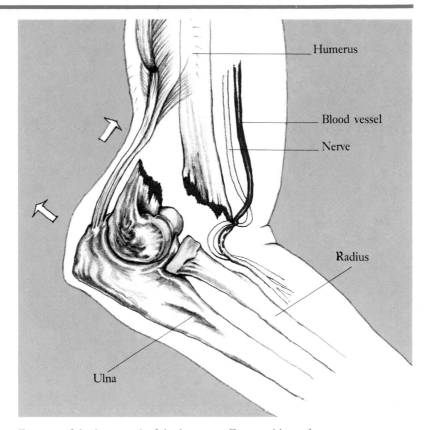

Humerus

Blood vessel

Nerve

Radius

Ulna

Fracture of the lower end of the humerus. Fractured bone fragments may press against and possibly damage blood vessels and nerves.

Healing

Mobility exercises (see page 424) are started at an early stage if the injury is less serious. After 8–10 weeks, when full mobility of the arm has been regained, sporting activity can be resumed.

Fracture of the head of the radius

The radius is comparatively thick and strong at the wrist, but considerably smaller in circumference and more fragile at the elbow. When the arm is stretched out to break a fall, the forces imposed are distributed through the forearm to the upper part of the radius. The radial head, which forms part of the elbow joint, can be fractured with the possibility of chronic problems.

Symptoms and diagnosis

— Instant pain when the injury occurs. This increases as the joint becomes swollen due to bleeding.
— Limitation of movement which increases with the swelling. The elbow is usually held flexed at an angle of 90°.
— An X-ray confirms the diagnosis.

Treatment	The *doctor* may:

The *doctor* may:
— aspirate the blood from the injured joint with a syringe if severe swelling is causing pain;
— apply a brace which is worn for 1–2 weeks (after that the arm muscles should be strengthened by training);
— operate if the radius is badly fragmented.

Healing

A properly reduced (set) fracture of the radial head heals in 6–8 weeks. Conditioning can be carried out through the rehabilitation period.

Fracture of the tip of the elbow (olecranon fracture)

A fracture of the tip of the elbow (the olecranon process) can be caused by a fall on to a bent elbow during contact sports or, for example, in speedway racing. The symptoms are swelling and tenderness over the elbow and an inability to straighten the joint. Surgery is often required as the triceps tendon pulls the fractured surfaces away from each other. It is 2–3 months before sporting activity can be resumed after an injury of this nature.

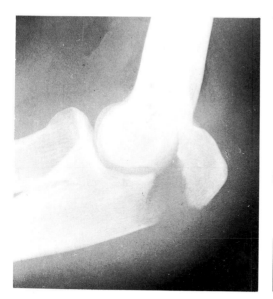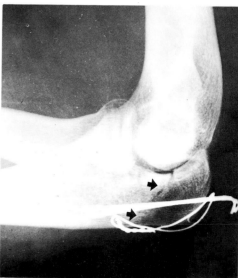

X-rays of fractures to the tip of the elbow. In the right-hand picture the displaced fragment has been fixed with a pin and steel wire (cerclage).

FOREARM INJURIES

The bones of the forearm are the radius and the ulna, which work in conjunction with each other.

Inflamation of tendons, tendon sheaths and muscles

As a result of external pressure or repetitive one-sided movements, the extensor and flexor muscles of the forearm and their tendons and tendon sheaths can become inflamed. The injury occurs mainly in oarsmen and canoeists at the start of their intensive training periods at the beginning of the season, but tennis, squash, table tennis and badminton players, skiers and others can also be affected.

Symptoms and diagnosis
— Pain when the hands are flexed and extended.
— Local swelling and tenderness over the affected muscle and tendon.
— Tendon creaking (crepitus) felt over the affected tendons on the back of the hand and the forearm when movements are made with the fingers and wrist (see diagram below).

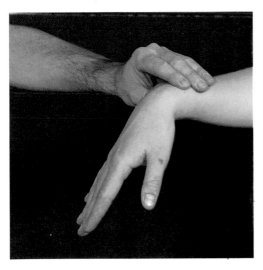 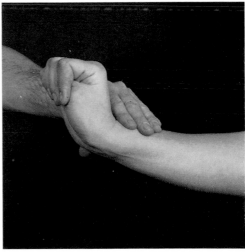

Preventive measures
— Gradually-increased training and load.
— Varied training avoiding one-sided movements.
— Correct technique.
— Correct equipment.

Treatment
The *athlete* should:
— rest. The injury often heals spontaneously, though it can take a considerable time to do so.

The *doctor* may:
— treat with a plaster cast for 1–4 weeks;
— prescribe anti-inflammatory medication.

Fractures of the forearm

Fractures of the forearm can occur after a fall or a direct blow and usually involve both the radius and the ulna. Fractures of the ulna alone can occur when parrying a blow with the forearm.

A fracture of the ulna can be combined with a dislocation of its articulation at the elbow joint (Monteggia's fracture). The elbow should therefore be examined and X-rayed when a fracture of the ulna occurs.

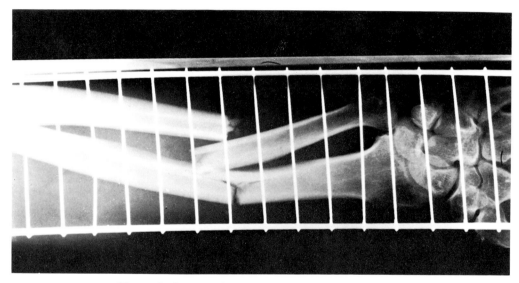

X-ray of a fracture of both the radius and the ulna. The striped background is a splint lying underneath the arm.

Treatment

It is important that the two bones, the ulna and the radius, are restored to their precise anatomical positions. Immobilization in plaster cast for 6–10 weeks is advisable, and surgery is frequently indicated, especially in cases of displacement.

When the plaster cast is removed the arm should be strengthened by training for 6–10 weeks before the injured athlete can return to sporting activity.

WRIST INJURIES

Fractures of the wrist (the distal radius and ulna)

A fracture of the distal radius (Colles' fracture) is the commonest of all fractures. It usually occurs as a result of a fall headlong on to the extended arm, forcing the hand backwards and upwards. A less common injury is the Smith's fracture where the mechanism is a forward flexion (palmar flexion) of the wrist. The injury is not uncommon amongst ice hockey, soccer, rugby and team handball players, riders, wrestlers, Alpine skiers and others.

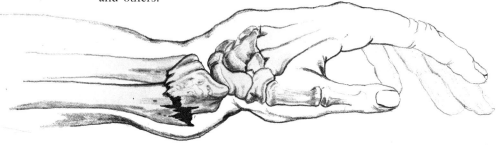

A side view of a fractured wrist.

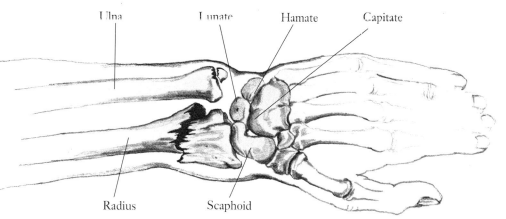

Ulna   Lunate   Hamate   Capitate

Radius   Scaphoid

A fractured wrist seen from above. Sometimes only one bone is injured.

Symptoms and diagnosis

— 'Dinner fork' deformity (see diagram above) of the wrist in Colles' fracture. The position is caused by the fractured fragment of the lower radius being driven backwards (dorsiflexed) in relation to the forearm. In Smith's fracture a forward (palmar flexion) dislocation of the distal radius is present.
— Swelling and tenderness in the wrist.
— Pain on wrist movements.
— In milder cases, swelling and displacement may be minor. The injury may then be mistaken for a sprain, but when this is so the wrist should be X-rayed to reveal any bony injury.

Treatment	The *doctor* may: — restore the fractured ends of the bone to their correct position; — apply a plaster cast (usually a splint or brace which can be removed after 4–5 weeks if the fracture is uncomplicated). The wrist is later strengthened by training; — operate in cases of more serious fractures.
Healing	Conditioning can often be maintained during the plaster period. Other forms of sporting activity involving the wrist can be resumed after 8–12 weeks.

Weakness in the wrist

Women aged about twenty and of slender build sometimes complain of pains in the wrist which occur on exertion (but often disappear at rest) and which radiate along the upper side of the forearm. On examination, a degree of hypermobility and laxity of the wrist may be noticed, but often no significant abnormality can be found. Sometimes a small swelling, or ganglion, can be found on the back of the hand. This should not prevent training, but a support bandage should be applied round the wrist and strength training carried out in parallel with the usual training. The symptoms often disappear in time.

Fractures of the scaphoid

A fracture of the scaphoid bone in the wrist can occur as the result of a fall with the wrist bent backwards on an extended arm. The injury is particularly common in contact sports such as soccer, American football, rugby, ice hockey and team handball but can also occur in skiers and others.

The blood flow to the scaphoid is easily compromised, especially in fractures of its middle portion which tend to heal badly. Athletes often find it difficult to accept the prolonged treatment that is needed for this injury to heal.

Symptoms and diagnosis	— Moderate pain with tenderness and swelling in the scaphoid region, that is, in the hollow formed at the base of the thumb when it is extended towards the wrist. — Moderately impaired power during hand movements. — The injury is often disregarded and is looked upon as a sprain because of the apparent triviality of immediate symptoms; — X-ray and bone scan (examination with radioisotopes).
Treatment	The *athlete* should: — consult a doctor for an X-ray in the case of any hand injury that could involve a fracture of the scaphoid. The *doctor* may: — apply a plaster cast when there is a suspected fracture even if the early

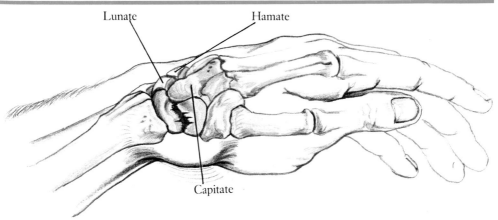

Lunate   Hamate

Capitate

Fracture of the scaphoid.

X-ray does not show one. A further X-ray should be taken 2–3 weeks later as it can take a long time for the bony changes to be revealed; a bone scan can, in some cases, be carried out earlier;
— when a fracture is present, apply a plaster cast which for the first 4–6 weeks should cover the elbow joint (preventing pronation and supination but allowing extension and flexion), the wrist and the thumb as far as the base of the nail. Such extensive immobilization is necessary if movements in the fracture area are to be prevented effectively. After 4–6 weeks the elbow can be left free. Immobilization of the wrist should continue for at least 3 months after which another X-ray

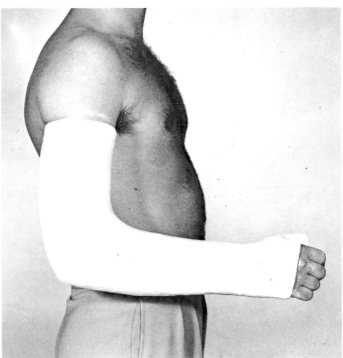

A plaster cast applied to a fracture of the scaphoid. The plaster extends over the top of the thumb joint.

225

examination is carried out. If the fracture is then healed, the plaster can be removed.

Healing and complications

— It is not unusual for the injured athlete not to consult a doctor and for the early symptoms to disappear. In these circumstances, healing may fail to occur and a false joint can be formed. This may ultimately cause degenerative changes in the wrist with discomfort, pain during movement, stiffness and impaired function.
— Premature cessation of treatment or even adequate treatment can be followed by formation of a false joint which should be operated on.
— Athletes can, in spite of a fracture of the scaphoid, continue with acceptable conditioning.

Pressure on the median nerve ('the carpal tunnel syndrome')

One of the nerves which supplies the hand, the median nerve, crosses the middle of the palmar aspect of the wrist in a narrow channel, the carpal tunnel. Acute or chronic inflammation of the tendons and tendon sheaths, an incompletely healed fracture of the wrist or an infection in the hand can reduce the space in this tunnel so that the nerve is subjected to pressure. This causes a persistent dull ache, with radiating pain and numbness in the thumb, index finger, middle finger and half the ring-finger. The symptoms generally get worse at night and the sensation is

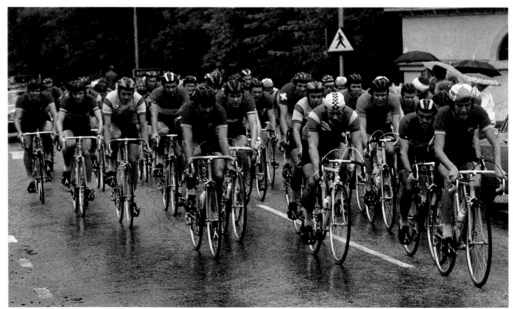

The position of the hand when cycling may increase pressure against the ulnar nerve in the palm.

often described as one of the hand having 'gone to sleep'. Shaking the hand and exercising the fingers brings relief in the short-term. When the condition is persistent, sensation in the hand is diminished and muscular atrophy occurs. The treatment in the first instance is rest, anti-inflammatory medication and sometimes diuretics ('water tablets') and splinting. Surgery is sometimes necessary, and is generally successful.

Pressure on the ulnar nerve (ulnar neuritis)

The ulnar nerve can be subjected to pressure, particularly at the level of the elbow but also where it crosses the wrist on the inner aspect of the hand. The pressure is caused by friction or impingement of the local tissues against the nerve, as can happen, for example, during cycling, and this causes mechanical irritation. The symptoms of ulnar neuritis are muscular weakness on attempting to spread the fingers and pain and numbness in the little finger and half the ring-finger. The initial treatment is rest and anti-inflammatory medication, but, if this fails, surgery gives good results.

Dislocations around the wrist

Dislocations around the wrist are not common in sports, but are important to recognize when they occur because a good recovery depends on early and correct diagnosis and treatment.

The lunate (see page 225) can dislocate both posteriorly (in a dorsal direction) and anteriorly (in a palmar direction).

Posterior dislocation of the lunate

This occurs in forced dorsiflexion by falling or impacting on to the dorsiflexed hand.

Symptoms and diagnosis
— A changed contour of the dorsal aspect of the wrist.
— Swelling and tenderness over the dorsal aspect of the wrist.
— Painful and restricted movements.
— X-ray shows the dislocated lunate.

Treatment
The *athlete* should:
— cool down, compress and elevate the wrist;
— call a doctor as soon as possible.

The *doctor* may
— verify the diagnosis by X-ray;
— reduce the dislocated lunate;
— immobilize in a plaster cast for 3–4 weeks;

— operate when closed reduction is impossible or in late unrecognized cases;

Anterior dislocation of the lunate

This occurs in forced palmarflexion when falling on to an outstretched hand.

Symptoms and diagnosis
— 'Shortened' hand.
— Changed contour of the palmar aspect of the wrist.
— Swelling and tenderness over the palmar aspect of the wrist.
— Painful and restricted movement of the wrist.
— X-ray shows the anterior dislocation of the lunate.

Treatment
The *athlete* should:
— cool down, compress and elevate;
— call a doctor as soon as possible.

The *doctor* may:
— verify the diagnosis;
— reduce the dislocated lunate;
— immobilize in a plaster cast for 3–4 weeks;
— operate if closed reduction is impossible;

Complications
— The injury may compress the median nerve.
— Avascular necrosis may occur.

Perilunar dislocation

This means a dorsal dislocation of the capitate (see page 225) in relation to the lunate, which may sometimes be dislocated anteriorly at the same time. It may occur in association with a dislocation or fracture of the scaphoid and is caused by forced dorsiflexion or axial compression of the wrist.

Symptoms and diagnosis
— Changed contour on the dorsal aspect of the wrist.
— Swelling and tenderness.
— Painful and restricted movements.
— X-rays show the posterior dislocation of the capitate.

Treatment
The *athlete* should:
— cool down, compress and elevate;
— call a doctor as soon as possible.

The *doctor* may:
— verify the diagnosis by X-ray;
— reduce the dislocated capitate and, if necessary, the lunate;
— immobilize in plaster for 3–6 weeks;
— operate when closed reduction is impossible.

Separation between the scaphoid and lunate

This may occur in forced dorsiflexion of the wrist. Ligamentous disruption between the scaphoid and lunate will cause the two bones to separate.

Symptoms and diagnosis
— Pain on movement.
— Swelling of the wrist, tenderness over the lunate and scaphoid.
— X-ray shows an increased joint span between the scaphoid and the lunate.

Treatment
The *athlete* should:
— cool down, compress and elevate the wrist;
— call a doctor.

The *doctor* may:
— verify the diagnosis by X-ray;
— reduce the displacement, and suture the ligament and joint capsule;
— immobilize in a plaster cast for 3–4 weeks.

Malacia of the lunate (Kienböck's disease)

This injury may occur as a result of repeated trauma or impacts. The circulation of the lunate is disturbed, and the bone softens and becomes devascularized.

Symptoms and diagnosis
— Painful and restricted movements.
— Tenderness over the lunate.
— Weakness of the hand.
— Decreased size and sclerosis of the lunate on X-ray (increased bone density).

Treatment
The *athlete* should:
— rest the wrist;
— call a doctor.

The *doctor* may:
— verify the diagnosis by X-ray or bone scan;
— immobilize in the acute stage;
— resort to surgery in chronic cases.

Fracture of the hook of the hamate

The hook of the hamate projects anteriorly on the lateral side of the palm. A compression fracture of the hook of the hamate is a rare injury, but it may occur in racket sports, baseball, ice hockey and bicycling if the handle of the racket, bat, club or stick is compressed on to the hook of the hamate.

Symptoms and diagnosis
— Pain and tenderness on the lateral aspect of the palm.
— Poor power grip.
— Numbness of the little finger due to irritation of the ulnar nerve.
— X-ray with a carpal tunnel view is necessary to verify the diagnosis.

Treatment
The *athlete* should:
— rest and cool down the injury;
— call a doctor.

The *doctor* may:
— verify the diagnosis with X-ray;
— immobilize in a short plaster cast that includes the little finger until healed 4–6 weeks in general;
— operate and remove the hook in some dislocated fractures or when nonunion is present.

Complications
— This fracture is easily overlooked. Untreated fractures lead to nonunion, but this may even occur in adequately treated fractures.
— Ulnar neuritis.
— Flexor tendinitis and/or rupture.

The athlete can usually return to sport with some protection after 6–8 weeks.

HAND AND FINGER INJURIES

Fractures of the metacarpal bones

Fractures of the metacarpal (hand) bones are particularly common among handball players but also occur among volleyball, ice hockey, basketball, soccer and American football players, cricketers and others. Such fractures can be caused by forcible extension of the fingers, (as, for example, during shooting in team handball when the hand in question hits the covering arm of the defence player) or as a result of a direct blow. Even a blow to the end of the bones, as in boxing and ice hockey, can result in fractures of the metacarpal shafts.

Symptoms and diagnosis
— Tenderness, swelling and pain in the hand.
— The injury should be X-rayed.

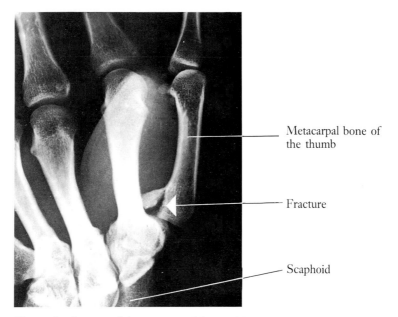

Metacarpal bone of the thumb

Fracture

Scaphoid

X-ray of a fracture of the metacarpal bone of the thumb. The fracture involves the joint surface and is a fracture dislocation ('Bennett's fracture').

Treatment — A fracture of the metacarpal bone of the thumb which impinges upon its articular surface (a Bennett's fracture) should be treated surgically in most cases. Inadequate treatment can result in permanently impaired function as the thumb becomes weak and loses its ability to grasp.
— Fractures of the metacarpal bones of the other fingers do not need surgery if the bone ends are well aligned. In most cases, treatment with a firm bandage, for example a plaster cast, for 3–4 weeks is quite sufficient.

Healing The injured athlete can return to playing handball and similar sports 6–8 weeks after the occurrence of the injury.

Rupture of the ulnar collateral ligament of the thumb
(Stener's lesion, skier's thumb, game keeper's thumb)

Around 10 per cent of all injuries in Alpine skiing involve the ulnar collateral ligament complex of the thumb making this the second most common injury sustained by skiers. Its incidence in skiing has been estimated to be between 50,000–200,000 per year.

Injury will result if the skier falls on to an outstretched arm. In so-doing, the pole forces the thumb upwards (abduction) and backwards (extension) putting stress on the metacarpo-phalangeal joint. This often results in an injury to the ulnar collateral ligament or a fracture or dislocation of the first metacarpal bone. To prevent this injury, skiers should use poles without straps or avoid using the straps already attached to the poles.

This injury is not uncommon in cross-country skiing. In this sport, however, the strap is grasped between the palm of the hand and the pole grip so injury will occur when carrying out a forceful pole-plant; it also occurs in ice hockey when a player's stick gets trapped, forcing the thumb backwards, or when the thumb is trapped by an opponent in team handball.

Symptoms and diagnosis
— Pain in the thumb web on movement.
— Tenderness when pressure is applied to the thumb web.
— Bleeding which causes bruising and swelling.
— Instability in the joint when the thumb is tested in abduction (movement away from the palm) at an angle of 20–30°. The critical degree of laxity, that is, the degree at which total rupture occurs, ranges from 20–45°. In total rupture the ligament is displaced to such an extent

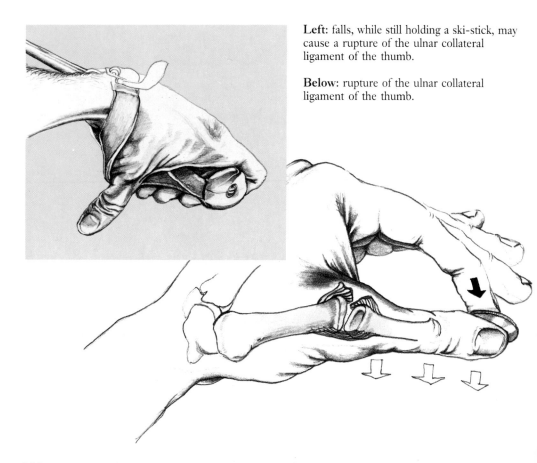

Left: falls, while still holding a ski-stick, may cause a rupture of the ulnar collateral ligament of the thumb.

Below: rupture of the ulnar collateral ligament of the thumb.

that the ulnar extension of the adductor aponeurosis becomes lodged between the ruptured end of the ligament and its attachment to the base of the first phalanx (finger bone). In this case, surgery is necessary. The ligament may, however, be totally ruptured and displaced without this complication.

— Arthrography may help to show displacement when deciding if surgery is necessary.

Treatment

The *athlete* should:
— cool the injury with ice packs, apply compression and keep the thumb elevated;
— consult a doctor.

The *doctor* may:
— carry out a thorough stability examination;
— mobilize a partial rupture to preserve joint mobility as soon as possible;
— apply a cast for 5–6 weeks — this does not guarantee the ligament will heal completely in its correct position;
— operate if there is instability in the joint and if clinical examination and arthrography show ligament displacement with interposition of the adductor aponeurosis. Compare stability with the same joint on the uninjured side.

Healing and complications

— Injured athletes can return to sporting activity 4–6 weeks after the completion of cast treatment and a strength training programme.
— If this injury is inadequately treated, there is a risk of permanent instability, resulting in weak grasp and osteoarthrosis. Surgery on a neglected injury can often be effective.

Rupture of the attachment of the long extensor tendon of the finger ('mallet finger')

The extensor tendon of a finger is attached to the end of its terminal phalanx (bone in the finger-tip) and can rupture when, for example, a ball unexpectedly hits the finger-tip and forces the finger to flex. A small bone fragment may be torn loose (avulsion) together with the tendon and will show up on X-rays.

Symptoms

— Slight tenderness between the nail and the first joint of the finger.
— The finger-tip is slightly bent, and the first (distal) joint cannot be actively extended.

Treatment

The *doctor* may:
— treat with a splint which keeps the first (distal) finger joint overextended for about 6 weeks (see diagram on page 234);
— operate when a bone fragment has been torn away.

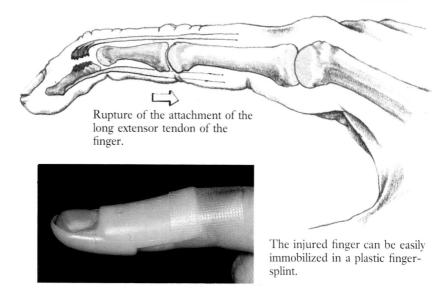

Rupture of the attachment of the long extensor tendon of the finger.

The injured finger can be easily immobilized in a plastic finger-splint.

Healing and complications

Ruptures of the attachment of the long extensor tendon of the finger heal in 6 weeks. If the injury is not treated, the injured person will have a permanent 'mallet finger' deformity.

Ligament injuries to fingers

Ligament injuries to the fingers are common, and the collateral ligaments of the fingers are often damaged in sports such as team handball, volleyball, basketball and rugby.

Symptoms and diagnosis
— Pain and distinct tenderness in the injured area.
— Impaired mobility.
— Instability can be present if the tear is complete.

Treatment
— Ligament injuries can be treated by bandaging or taping the injured finger to an adjacent finger for support. Active flexion and extension exercises of the injured finger can then start without any lateral load. The bandage is worn for about 2 weeks.
— Major ligament injuries are treated with a plaster cast. As a rule, surgery is not needed except for injuries to the ligaments of the thumb.
— Residual effects with slight swelling and stiffness of the injured finger can continue for a long time (6–9 months) after the injury has occurred.

Dislocation of finger joints

Dislocation of finger joints is a common injury which often affects team handball, basketball and volleyball players, and cricketers. In 80 per cent of cases it is the little finger or the thumb that is damaged. In cases of lateral dislocation, it is the ligaments on the side of the joint opposite the direction of the dislocation which are damaged. In cases of posterior dislocation (that is, dislocation upwards and backwards) both lateral ligaments are damaged, at least partially, as well as the anterior capsular ligaments.

Symptoms
— Pain, tenderness and impaired function.
— Deformity of the joint outline.

Treatment
The *doctor* may:
— reduce the joint back into its normal position;
— tape the digit to the adjacent finger or, in severe injury, immobilize by applying a plaster cast which is worn for 2–3 weeks;
— X-ray the joint as a bone fragment may have been torn loose.

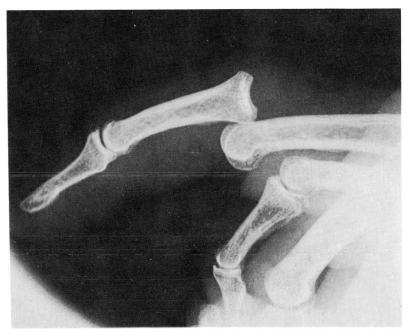

X-ray of a dislocated finger joint.

The sooner the joint can be restored to its normal position after the injury has occurred, the easier the procedure. If manipulation is carried out within a few minutes, severe pain is not generally experienced. Protected early return to sport is usually possible.

Fractures of fingers

Fractures of finger bones are not particularly common but sometimes occur in team handball, volleyball, basketball, soccer and other sports. Such fractures may be treated with a plaster cast for 2–4 weeks if they do not affect the joints. Sporting activity can be resumed 2–3 weeks after the plaster has been removed, but general conditioning can be carried out during rehabilitation.

Finger fractures which affect the joint surfaces and those with severe displacement sometimes need surgical treatment. A plaster cast is subsequently applied and kept in position for 3–5 weeks. After a further 3 weeks the injured athlete can resume his sporting activity.

Infections

Open wounds of the fingers or palms of the hands must be cleaned particularly carefully. If they are neglected, bacterial infection can easily arise and prolonged treatment can then be necessary. Anyone who has a red, swollen and tender finger-tip, for example, should see a doctor as soon as possible, for an infection in a finger can spread to the palm of the hand via the tendon sheaths, in which case emergency surgery may become necessary.

Infected wounds, especially on hands and fingers must never be neglected since the consequences can be catastrophic.

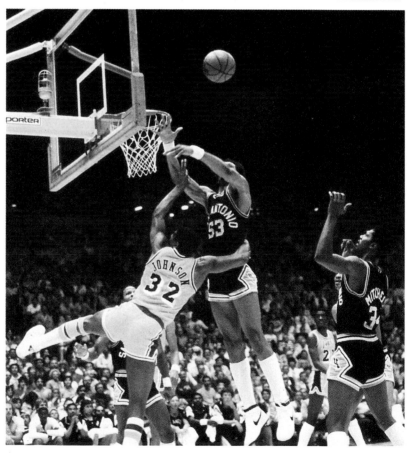

Finger injuries can occur when playing ball games, such as basketball. *Photo: All-Sport/Tony Duffy*.

BACK INJURIES

The spine is composed of seven cervical (neck) vertebrae, twelve thoracic (chest) vertebrae and five lumbar (lower back) vertebrae, plus the sacral and coccygeal vertebrae. Each vertebra consists of a body from which an arch of bone arises. On each arch there are articular processes which allow limited mobility between adjacent vertebrae. Between the vertebral bodies are flexible plates of fibrocartilage, the discs, which facilitate movements of the spine and act as shock absorbers. Intervertebral discs have no blood or lymph supply and only a limited nerve supply.

The spinal column has a supportive, a protective and a locomotive function. The neck region is very mobile and the lowerback region is fairly mobile with most movement between the fifth lumbar vertebra and the first sacral vertebra. The chest region, on the other hand, is less mobile because the ribs are attached to their constituent vertebrae. The regions of the spine which have most mobility generally give rise to most problems.

There is one anterior and one posterior longitudinal system of ligaments along the spine. In addition there are smaller ligaments around the joints and between the vertebrae and their spinous processes. These ligaments are responsible for the passive stability of the back. Active stability is contributed by the muscles of the back and the abdomen and is of great importance. These muscles can be divided into an anterior group, which includes the psoas musculature, and posterior deep and superficial groups.

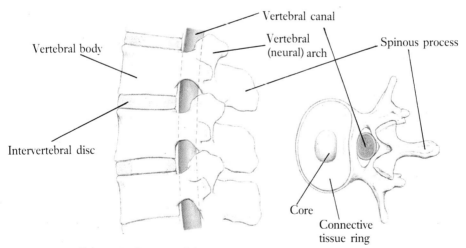

Schematic diagram of the anatomy of the spine.

The spine is exposed to a heavy load when the body is bent forwards or turned, and the activity of the muscles of the back increases noticeably when the body is bent forwards at an angle of 30°. The same muscles have to work harder when the body is in the sitting rather than the standing position and this exposes the discs to increased pressure. In general, injudicious flexing of the spine, side bending, excessive twisting or loading asymmetrically should be avoided. During lifting, the load should be placed as near to the body as possible.

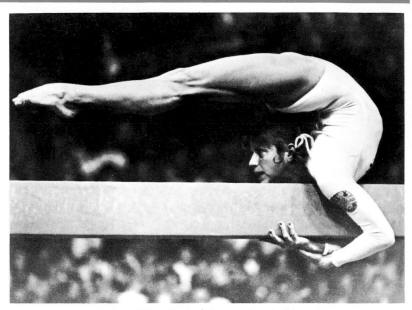

Extreme load on the back (Olga Korbut, Soviet Union). *Photo: Reportagebild.*

Back problems in general

Back problems affect 80 per cent of all people at some time in their life. There is no specific category of subjects who suffer back pain more frequently than others — labourers are affected as often as clerks, men as often as women. Important contributory factors are hard physical work, lifting, static working postures and vibration. In spite of the fact that the heaviest industrial tasks are now carried out by machines, the number of people seeking advice for back pain does not seem to have decreased. Of all sufferers, 70 per cent return to work within a week and 90 per cent within 3 months, regardless of the treatment they receive.

Diagnosis in general

Diagnosis of back problems depends on expert evaluation of pain, physical examination results, back function, constitutional factors and X-ray findings. With regard to pain, its location, intensity, duration and quality should be considered as well as factors which precipitate or relieve it. The function of the back should be studied with regard to its range and pattern of movements, posture, muscle tone and control, and constitutional factors should be evaluated. Changes in the shape of the spine, for example an exaggerated S-shaped curve (scoliosis), can, like the overall physique, be of importance.

A number of skeletal changes such as slipping of one vertebra on another, stress fractures, bony outgrowths along the edges of the vertebral bodies, and degenerative joint changes, can be identified by ordinary X-ray examination, while a slipped disc can be seen with the help of a contrast medium. Computerized serial X-rays (tomography) can give additional information about the various tissues which make up the spinal column.

X-ray should be performed in maximal flexion, extension or any other position which evokes pain. Instability or other causes of pain can then be revealed.

The injured person's social situation and psychological mood can be important when a history of back problems is given and should be evaluated by enquiring into family circumstances, education, working conditions and so forth.

Injuries to the neck

The cervical portion of the spine comprises seven vertebrae which are connected by joints and ligaments and between which there are discs. The two uppermost vertebrae in the neck bear the brunt of turning (rotatory) movements, while flexion and extension occur most conspicuously between the fourth, fifth and sixth vertebrae.

The injuries which may affect this area include fractures and dislocations with ligament damage. Degenerative changes can affect the discs and give rise to bony outgrowths (osteophytes) along the edges of the vertebral bodies which can result in pressure on nerves and thus pain. Injuries and diseases of the cervical spine can cause discomfort and pain which not only affects the neck but can radiate to the back of the head, and to the shoulders, arms and hands.

Injuries to the cervical spine resulting from accidents

Blows to the head and cervical region can cause fractures of the cervical vertebral column and also dislocations with simultaneous injuries to the joint capsules, ligaments and discs. The injuries can be either stable or unstable.

The commonest causes of injury are bending backwards (extension) or forwards (flexion), rotating too violently, or hitting the head so that the impact is transmitted to the cervical region (axial compression).

Bending forwards can cause a compression fracture at the front, and ligament injuries at the back, of a vertebral body. Sometimes fractures of the joint processes and injuries to the joint capsule can also occur, and ligament injuries may be present without any visible injury to the skeleton. After an injury associated with flexion it is essential to decide, with the help of X-rays, whether the injury is stable or unstable.

Extension (bending backwards) produces similar injuries with disc and ligament damage at the front and compression damage at the back of the vertebral bodies.

A twisting impact can occur in isolation or in combination with flexion or extension. As a result of twisting, unilateral damage to joint processes and ligaments can occur with a resultant dislocation.

A fracture and/or ligament injury of the cervical spine can occur as a result of a violent collision with an opponent or with surrounding objects, for example the goal posts, and can be serious. Within the cervical vertebral column, in the vertebral canal, runs the spinal cord, which, together with its nerve roots, can be subjected to pressure and damaged by bone and ligament injuries.

Another important cause of cervical spine injury is the 'whiplash' which involves the neck being rapidly extended then flexed. This can happen for example, in road traffic accidents when one vehicle is run into by another from behind. Ligament, bone and muscle injuries, which may result in chronic pain, can occur and anyone who has suffered a whiplash injury should be X-rayed.

Symptoms and diagnosis
— Pain in the cervical region, especially during movements.
— Radiating pain with numbness in the arms.
— Impaired sensation in the skin below the level of the injury.
— Muscle weakness or paralysis below the level of injury.

Treatment
The *trainer* should:
— arrange transport of the injured athlete to hospital for examination;
— delegate further handling to expert staff if available.

The injured athlete needs to be carefully placed on a stretcher in such a way that his head and body are lifted simultaneously and the position of the cervical vertebrae is not disturbed. Clothing, cushions or similar supports are placed on each side of the neck during the journey to hospital, to splint the neck and prevent further injury.

The *doctor* may:
— carry out a careful examination of the nervous system and X-ray the cervical vertebral column in order to assess its stability. Depending on the severity of the injury the treatment may consist of a neck collar, traction, Halo-west or surgery.

Pain radiating from the neck (cervical brachialgia, cervical rhizopathy)

Pains in the cervical region can be caused by disc degeneration and osteophyte formation. The changes affect nerve roots which can produce waves of pain. Even a temporary strain or trapping of a nerve can produce similar symptoms.

It is usual to distinguish between pain which is confined to the nape of the neck and back of the head (see page 241) and that which radiates into the arms with either a widespread (cervical brachialgia) or clearly defined (cervical rhizopathy) distribution.

Symptoms and diagnosis
— Pain radiating from the nape of the neck into the shoulder, arm and/or fingers. The pain is usually deep and widespread (brachialgia), but it can have clearly defined limits with intense sharp pain following the distribution of the affected nerves (rhizopathy). The pain is felt more acutely during neck movements than during shoulder movements.
— Pain radiating up the neck and into the back of the head can cause headaches, insomnia and sometimes dizziness.
— Numbness and weakness in the arm and fingers. There may be areas of complete anaesthesia.
— An X-ray examination should be carried out, especially if pain is caused by movement. The examination should elicit those positions which provoke the pain in order to detect any abnormal mobility.

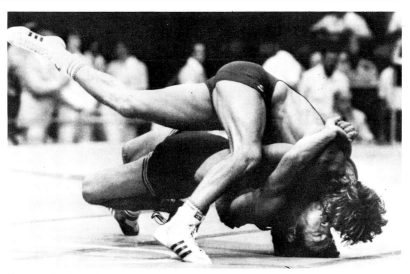
Extreme load on the neck region of the back.

Treatment
— Rest.
— Neck collar and a heat retainer.
— Analgesic and anti-inflammatory medication.
— Physiotherapy with traction.

Pain in the neck (cervicalgia) and wry-neck (torticollis)

Pain which is located in the neck and does not radiate out into the arms is called cervicalgia (see lumbago, page 246).

Wry-neck is a painful condition which can occur in young athletes after violent turning movements of the neck, for example when diving and also when heading or jumping in soccer. It is probable that the nerve roots arising from the cervical spinal cord are affected by, for example, a momentary compression or stretching, causing a reflex spasm in the neck muscles.

Symptoms and diagnosis
— Vice-like pain felt in the neck and in the angle between the nape of the neck and the shoulder, never extending below the shoulder joint. The pain is triggered by neck movements. The musculature is tender and tense.
— Painful twisting of the head to one side.
— Impaired mobility of the back of the neck.

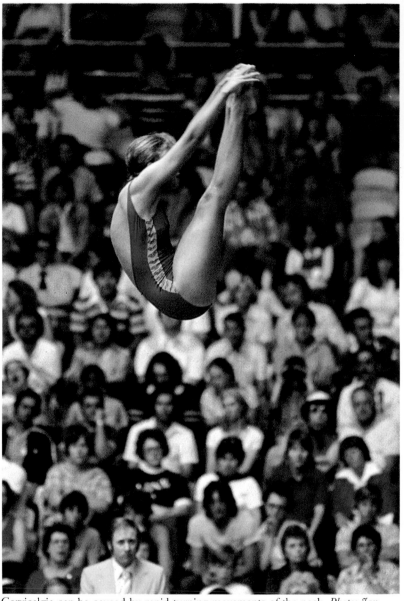

Cervicalgia can be caused by rapid turning movements of the neck. *Photo: Jan Düsing/Pressens bild.*

Treatment
— Local heat treatment and a heat retainer.
— Muscle relaxants.
— Analgesic medication.
— Rest.
— Traction.
— Neck collar.

The condition often improves within a week. If this is not the case a doctor should be consulted.

Injuries to the thoracic and lumbar spine

Fractures of thoracic and lumbar vertebrae

Fractures of vertebrae in the thoracic and lumbar regions are uncommon in sports but can occur in riders, Alpine skiers, ski jumpers and contact sports.

Symptoms and diagnosis
— Severe pain at the site of the fracture.
— Pain on any back movement.
— If pain radiates into the legs it must be assumed that the spinal cord or its nerve roots have been affected.
— Loss of sensation and paralysis are signs of a serious injury.

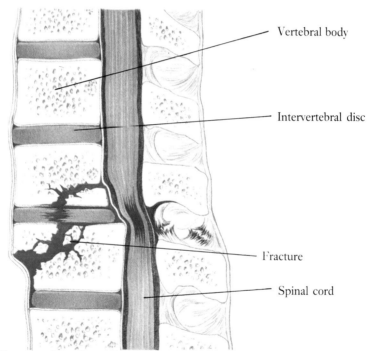

Fracture of vertebrae with displacement and pressure on the spinal cord.

Treatment
— The injured person is taken to hospital for a neurological examination and an X-ray and assessment of the stability of the vertebral column.
— When thoracic and lumbar vertebrae have been damaged during sporting activity, compression of the damaged vertebral body is usually only moderate and heals after a period of rest.
— In extreme cases, severe compression of the vertebrae may occur, and injury may also be caused to the spinal cord and nerve roots. These injuries are treated with bed rest, perhaps with a corset or other immobilization, for 2–3 months, or with surgery.

Fractures of the transverse processes of the lumbar vertebrae

Fractures of the transverse processes of the vertebrae can occur as a result of a direct violent impact to the side of the vertebral column or as a result of a tearing mechanism in cases of muscle injury, especially in the lumbar region.

Symptoms and diagnosis
— Tenderness over the transverse processes at the side of the vertebral column.
— Pain on movement, especially when the back is bent sideways.
— An X-ray examination confirms the diagnosis.

Treatment
— Rest until the pain has resolved. The injury is benign and heals in 6–8 weeks.

Muscle ruptures in the back

Ruptures of the back muscles occur in weightlifters, javelin and discus throwers, pole-vaulters, football, handball, basketball and volleyball players, wrestlers, boxers and many others. The injury usually consists of minor ruptures of the fasciculi and is most often located in the long back extensors and the large flat back muscles (dorsal).

Symptoms
— Piercing pain on flexion, extension and rotation.
— Local tenderness over the area of rupture.

Treatment
The *athlete* should:
— begin controlled muscle training after a few days;
— rest actively for 3–8 weeks or until there is no pain on exertion;
— apply local heat and use a heat retainer, though not until 2–3 days after the injury has occurred.

The *doctor* may:
— give analgesic and (perhaps) anti-inflammatory medication.

Healing
If training and competition are resumed before the injury has healed completely there is a risk of renewed bleeding and delayed healing.

Inflammation of muscle attachments

The muscle attachments around the spinous processes of the thoracic and lumbar spine can, like the attachments of the muscles to the sacrum and the hip bone, become inflamed as a result of overuse. Such injuries are commonest among cross-country skiers, javelin, discus and hammer throwers, weightlifters and in racket sports.

Symptoms
— Pain during exertion.
— Aching after exertion.
— Tenderness on pressure over the spinous processes.
— Pain in the attachment of the muscle in question which is triggered by its contraction.

244

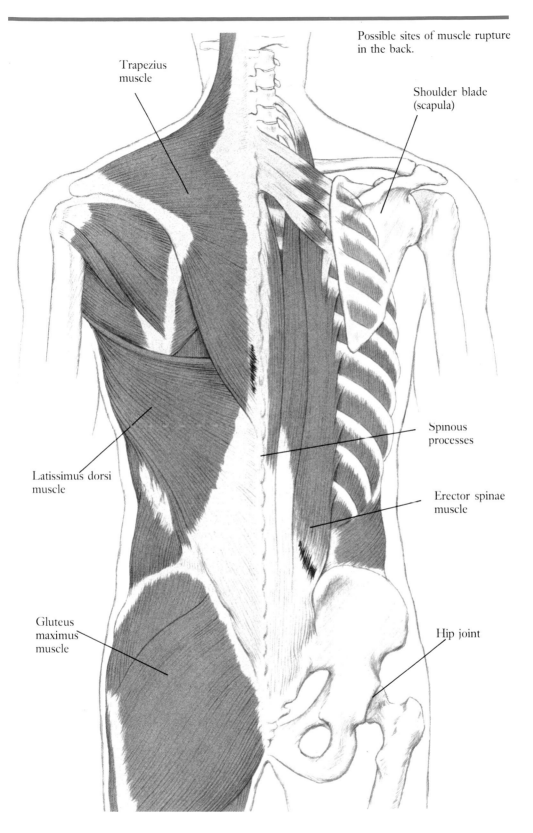

Trapezius
muscle

Possible sites of muscle rupture
in the back.

Shoulder blade
(scapula)

Latissimus dorsi
muscle

Spinous
processes

Erector spinae
muscle

Gluteus
maximus
muscle

Hip joint

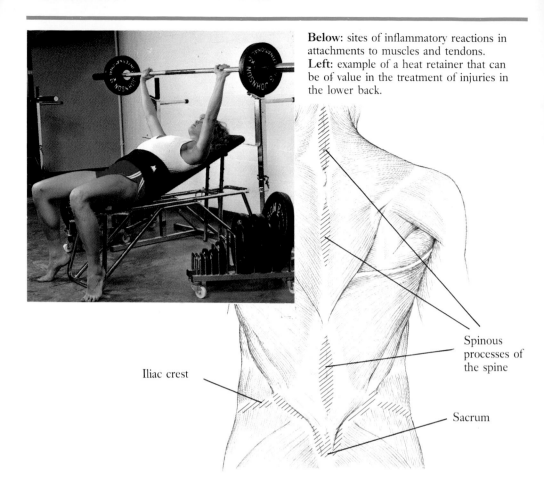

Below: sites of inflammatory reactions in attachments to muscles and tendons.
Left: example of a heat retainer that can be of value in the treatment of injuries in the lower back.

Iliac crest

Spinous processes of the spine

Sacrum

Treatment	The *athlete* should: — rest until there is no pain on exertion; — apply local heat and use a heat retainer. The *doctor* may: — prescribe anti-inflammatory medication; — administer local steroid injections followed by 2 weeks' rest if complaints are persistent.
Healing	The inflammation often heals after a few weeks.

Lumbago (low back pain)

Low back pain can occur in connection with most sports, and its precise cause is unknown. Acute lumbago mainly affects those between thirty to forty years of age. After the age of fifty years the complaint is rare.

Symptoms and diagnosis	— The symptoms often appear after lifting a heavy object or turning rapidly, but they can also occur without previous exertion.

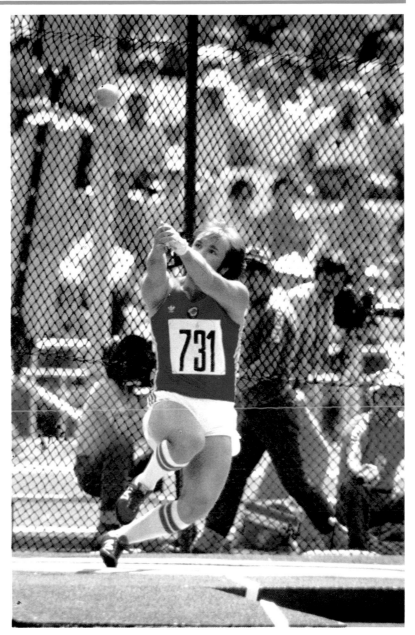

Muscle attachments of the back may become inflamed when subjected to repeated load, for example in throwing sports. *Photo: Pressens bild.*

— The pain is usually located in the lower back and does not radiate down into the legs.
— Stiffness occurs in the back.
— The posture may appear asymmetrical with the back bent to one side as a result of muscle spasm that prevents the movements of the back which trigger pain.

Treatment

The *athlete* should:
— spend 1–3 days (or as long as it takes for the pain to subside) in bed, adopting the position that causes the least possible pain;
— apply local heat, for example with a heat retainer and hot baths;
— avoid body movements which involve flexing or turning the spine.

The *doctor* may:
— give ergonomic advice;
— prescribe analgesic drugs in order to break the pain cycle which arises from reflex muscle spasm impairing circulation and thus causing muscle pain which in turn precipitates more reflex spasm and so on. Peripheral muscle relaxants can sometimes be of value;
— recommend rest several times daily in a psoas position (see photograph on page 251) and give other advice about having good support when in the sitting position and avoiding positions and movements that cause pain. When the patient is lying on his side he should get up by using his arms to support his weight. Similarly, when rising from a chair, he should do the same with the help of the chair arms;
— prescribe a course of physiotherapy, for example, the Swedish back school, when symptoms are recurrent;
— prescribe traction or manipulation in chronic cases;
— prescribe a corset or body belt which gives temporary support and can be worn when the patient carries out activities that usually trigger the problem. A corset can be of value in the acute stage of lumbago but should be used for the shortest possible time if muscle atrophy is to be prevented;
— X-ray the lumbar region if the pain has been present for more than 2 months or if symptoms are recurrent. A raised erythrocyte sedimentation rate (ESR) may be a sign of infection, tumour or joint inflammation;
— prescribe preventive and rehabilitative training (see page 429) as early as possible. Jogging has been shown to be beneficial.

Healing time and complications

Lumbago is often benign and as a rule the symptoms disappear spontaneously within 1–3 weeks. In certain individuals, however, symptoms may be prolonged.

> People with back complaints should lead physically active lives. Their activities, however, should be tailored to suit the symptoms in question.

Sciatica, slipped disc (herniated disc)

Pain which radiates from the back down one or other leg is known as sciatica. It is often exacerbated by exertion, coughing, sneezing or straining. One of its commonest causes is a slipped disc which exerts pressure on one of the roots of the sciatic nerve, and it can also be triggered by a temporary local trapping or straining of the nerve or its roots. Rarer causes include tumours, bony deposits and infections which can affect the sciatic nerve throughout its course.

The intervertebral discs between the vertebral bodies are composed of a connective tissue ring and a core of a pulpy, semi-fluid substance. Slipped discs often show signs of changes due to age (disc degeneration), which can occur even in relatively young individuals. Cracks form in the connective tissue ring of a disc, allowing the pulpy substance to seep through and cause pressure on the adjacent nerve roots (see diagram below). The prime cause of a slipped disc is bending forwards and to the side to lift a heavy object. Athletes who suffer slipped discs have often had previous attacks of acute lumbago. Depending on where the slipped disc is located in relation to the nerve root, different syndromes occur:

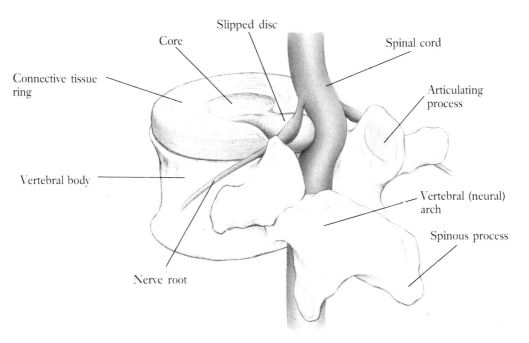

Slipped disc causing pressure on a nerve root.

— *L 4 syndrome* when the nerve root adjacent to the disc between the third and the fourth lumbar vertebrae is damaged;
— *L 5 syndrome* when the nerve root adjacent to the disc between the fourth and fifth lumbar vertebrae is affected;
— *S 1 syndrome* when the nerve root adjacent to the disc between the fifth lumbar vertebra and the first sacral vertebra is affected.

Symptoms As a rule, the S 1 syndrome affects people up to about thirty-five to forty years of age, while the L 5 syndrome is commoner in older individuals. The different syndromes each show the characteristic pain radiation patterns (see diagram on page 250) and affect sensation, reflexes and muscle power.

A combination of lumbago and sciatica occurs in which pain is felt mainly in the lumbar region but radiates into one leg and increases on exertion. There may be numbness in the area of distribution of the nerve,

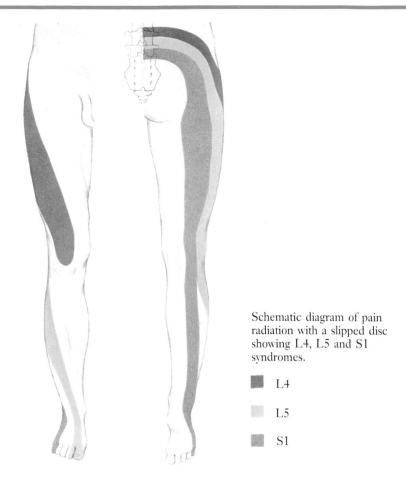

Schematic diagram of pain radiation with a slipped disc showing L4, L5 and S1 syndromes.

■ L4

■ L5

■ S1

weakness in the leg and diminution of the reflexes. The pain can be triggered by coughing or straining and can be so severe that the lumbar region becomes locked into a position of lateral flexion (scoliosis).

Diagnosis

— The diagnosis is confirmed by the history of the pain which is typical.
— Examination of the spine may reveal a scoliosis caused by strong muscular contraction in the lumbar region.
— Mobility is impaired and the musculature is tender and tense.
— Lasègue's sign is seen; that is, with the patient lying on his back, the extended leg is raised by another person. At some point the patient experiences pain radiating down the leg.
— Neurological examination of the nervous system reveals diminished reflexes, weakness or paralysis, and impaired sensation.
— In serious cases, disturbance of the nerve supply to the bladder results in difficulty in passing water. If this occurs, a doctor should be consulted immediately.
— A diagnosis of slipped disc is confirmed by X-raying using a contrast medium (myelography).

Treatment

The *athlete* should:
— rest in bed in the appropriate position (psoas position, see photograph

250

below). As rest causes rapid wasting of the back muscles, special training exercises should be started as soon as possible;

— apply local heat and use a heat retainer.

The *doctor* may:

— advise continued rest and limitation of activity for 8–12 weeks;
— prescribe analgesics, anti-inflammatory medication and muscle relaxants;
— start gentle traction treatment under the supervision of a physiotherapist when the condition has passed its acute stage;
— prescribe transcutaneous nerve stimulation (TNS, see page 171);
— perform emergency surgery in cases of bladder function impairment;

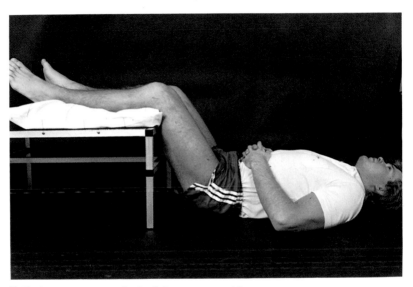

Relieving pressure on the back in a psoas position.

— operate when acute pain persists in spite of analgesic drugs, when paralysis occurs and/or when a disabling postural defect resulting from reflex muscle spasm fails to correct itself or deteriorates further. A new procedure involves injecting an enzyme called chymopapain into the disc. The enzyme dissolves the centre (nucleus) of the disc and relieves pressure on the nerve roots. In cases without urgent complications, frequent re-examinations should be carried out, and usually a 'wait-and-see' policy is adopted for 3–6 months. Before surgery on a slipped disc, X-ray examination with a contrast medium (myelography) is carried out so that the doctor can identify and locate the slipped disc. CAT scans can also be helpful.

Healing and complications

— Most individuals who suffer from a slipped disc recover gradually with rest alone.
— Hospital treatment after surgery for a slipped disc lasts for 4–8 days

or sometimes longer followed by 4–8 weeks convalescence. Not until 3–4 months later can a return be made to active sport or heavy work.
— The results of surgery in these cases are good. Of those who are operated on, 95 per cent make a complete recovery and can return to their original jobs.

Narrowing of the vertebral canal (spinal stenosis)

The vertebral column can be affected by narrowing as a result of causes other than a slipped disc, including wear of the facet joints and osteophyte formation. This condition, which is not common, mainly affects those over sixty years of age and especially middle-aged former wrestlers and weightlifters who have sustained strenuous loads to the back.

Symptoms and diagnosis
— The symptoms are often indeterminate, with just a vague aching discomfort.
— Pain starts in the back, especially when it is straightened from the flexed position.
— Pain is felt in the legs after walking a short distance. The pain recedes at rest, especially if the patient is sitting down, but returns after further brief exertion.
— X-ray examination, myelography or computerized tomography confirm the diagnosis.
— Other possible causes of the pain, for example arteriosclerosis, have to be eliminated.

Treatment
The *doctor* may:
— prescribe physiotherapy;
— prescribe a corset;
— operate in exceptional cases and remove the causes of the narrowing. It is, however, a major operation and there is the risk of relapse.

Wear in the intervertebral joints between the vertebral arches (facet joint syndrome)

The joints between the vertebral arches are called intervertebral facet joints. They are oriented in such a way that they reduce the rotation capability of the vertebrae. If there were no facet joints the discs would wear out more quickly as a result of rotatory movement in the spine.

When the discs are affected, with age, by degenerative changes, a decreased compression and displacement of the vertebrae occur, and the possibility of disc compression is increased. This in turn can lead to increased load on the joints causing osteoarthritis. The cartilage of the articular surface is destroyed, and the resulting osteophytes then press on the nerves so that radiating pain is experienced without a disc having slipped.

Symptoms and diagnosis
— Facet joint syndrome affects those of forty years of age and over and manifests itself as a sudden pain in the lumbar region.

— Rest makes the pain worse, but it is helped by movement and training, a feature which distinguishes this type of osteoarthritis from others.
— Stiffness and limited range of movement in the back.
— Tenderness beside or along the spinous processes and pain when straightening the back.
— Pain in the back and buttock when lifting the extended leg.
— An X-ray confirms the diagnosis.

Treatment

The *doctor* may:
— prescribe physiotherapy;
— prescribe analgesic medication;
— inject local anaesthetic into the area of the affected joint (this is carried out in an operating theatre under X-ray control);
— operate to divide the nerve which supplies the facet joint;
— prescribe lumbar heat retainer.

'Weak back'

Some people have a 'weak back' which means that they show symptoms such as fatigue, stiffness and weakness accompanied by aching during or after slight loading of the back.

Treatment

The *athlete* should:
— improve his technique or change his working posture in order to relieve the symptoms;
— improve his back muscles by comprehensive training (see page 429) which should be included in all training programmes.

The *doctor* may:
— prescribe physiotherapy with a back muscle programme, give advice on lifting technique, and so on.

Scheuermann's disease (Roundback)

Scheuermann's disease is a hereditary back disease which produces progressive rounding of the back (kyphosis) and which can sometimes hinder sporting activity. The complaint mainly affects adolescent boys, and usually three to five thoracic vertebrae are involved and become wedge-shaped.

Symptoms and diagnosis

— Slight fatigue in the thoracic region on exertion after the affected person has, for example, been sitting in school for a whole day.
— Weakness and pain in connection with strenuous back exercise or loading the back.
— The complaints are often pursued by parents, coach or trainer when they notice that the shape of the back changes in the individual affected.
— Increased breathing capacity in swimmers, for example.
— An X-ray examination confirms the diagnosis.

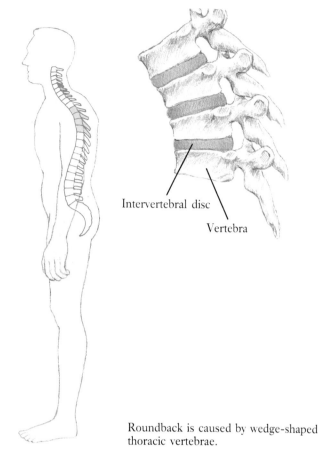

Intervertebral disc

Vertebra

Roundback is caused by wedge-shaped thoracic vertebrae.

Treatment	— Adolescents who have long-standing back complaints of this type can be X-rayed so that infectious diseases and tumours of the vertebral column can be ruled out as causes of the complaints. — In cases of weakness of the back, physiotherapy and muscle strength training can be prescribed and may be of help.
Healing and complications	The disease progresses relatively slowly until the skeleton has stopped growing. In cases of exceptionally rapid progression, a corset, brace or support is prescribed. — The disease seldom causes any further symptoms once the growth of the skeleton has ceased. — Individuals who suffer this back deformity have, as adults, a lower rate of absenteeism from work because of back problems than other people.

Lateral curvature of the spine (scoliosis)

Lateral curvature to the left or right of part of the spine can render the vertebral column S-shaped. The cause of this complaint, which affects growing children, is unknown. It is often discovered by the PT teacher, coach or parents and should lead to a visit to the doctor.

Scoliosis occurs in about 5 per cent of all children in a normal population, but a mild form is more common than that among athletes who pursue asymmetrical training, for example tennis players and javelin-throwers. Javelin-throwers who have been training for more than 8 years can develop a type of scoliosis which appears to cause them no problems in the short term. The explanation might be found in the mechanism of javelin-throwing: — during the throw the body is bent towards the throwing arm and is twisted at the same time as the back becomes more lordotic (sway-backed). Repeated training with throwing movements results in the upper back muscles on the throwing-arm side of the body becoming more highly developed than those of the other side.

Symptoms Scoliosis hardly ever causes discomfort or pain and does not preclude suitable physical activity. The most important sign is the curvature of the spine which is established by X-ray. Severe scoliosis can cause complications involving the heart and lungs in middle life.

Treatment — All children and young people with scoliosis should be examined by an orthopaedic specialist.
— In mild cases the patient should be kept under observation while in more severe cases a corset or surgery may be needed.

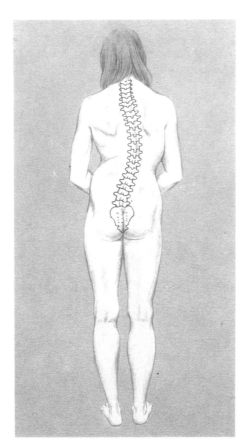

Scoliosis. This illustration shows the vertebral column with lateral curvature.

Defective vertebral arches (spondylolysis) and forward slipping of vertebrae (spondylolisthesis)

A defect in a vertebral arch is called spondylolysis. The defect can be congenital or may have been caused by injury or overloading resulting in stress fracture. Spondylolysis creates the necessary conditions for one vertebra to be able to slip forwards in relation to that below it. Once this has occurred the condition is called spondylolisthesis. The younger the individual in whom the arch defect occurs, the greater the risk of the vertebral body slipping forwards. The risk of slippage is very small in individuals over the age of twenty-five years.

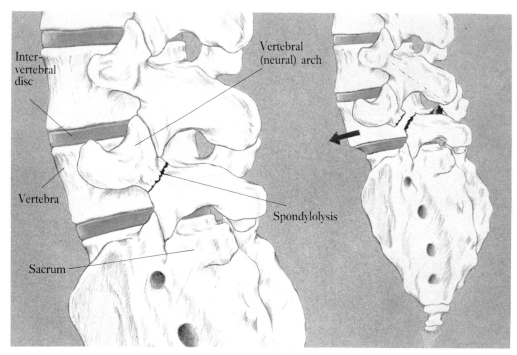

Left: spondylolysis (defective vertebral arch). **Right:** spondylolysis with spondylolisthesis (slippage of vertebra).

The problems which arise are determined partly by the speed with which the slippage takes place and partly by its extent. Spondylolysis can in itself cause problems including pain in the back and sciatica. These are precipitated by a local effect on the nerves due to changes around the defect without any slippage having occurred. The symptoms of spondylolisthesis begin as the vertebral body slips forwards and begins to exert traction and compression on the nerve roots. In growing adolescents the symptoms often appear after physical exertion.

Spondylolisthesis occurs in only about 3–7 per cent of the population, and it is usually the fifth lumbar vertebra that is involved. In sports in which the back is exposed to heavy shear loads, for example gymnastics, diving, javelin-throwing, wrestling, weightlifting and golf, a comparatively larger proportion of participants is affected. The injury occurs above all in growing adolescents during sports involving frequent bending of the spine to extreme extended positions, for example, in gymnastics and linemen in American football.

Symptoms and diagnosis

— Fatigue accompanied by aching in the lumbar region in young people, most frequently after physical exertion.
— Sometimes sciatic symptoms develop in both legs, in which case Lasègue's sign is often seen on both right and left. Sometimes a notch can be felt in the spine during examination.
— X-ray examination in a position that triggers the pain confirms the diagnosis.

Treatment

The *athlete* should:
— rest until symptoms have resolved;
— consult a doctor for an opinion;
— in most instances, continue training, provided that the back is protected from overexertion, sciatic symptoms are absent and the symptoms do not become worse. Exercises such as sit-ups, weightlifting and other forms of strength training which stress the back should be avoided. Young people below sixteen to eighteen years of age should avoid extreme movements in the lumbar region.

The *doctor* may:
— prescribe rest when the injury is in its acute stage;
— prescribe physiotherapy with a back muscle programme, give advice on lifting technique, and so on;
— prescribe a cloth corset and a lumbar heat retainer;
— recommend a change of sport;
— operate in exceptional cases when other treatment has not been successful;
— keep growing adolescents who have had this condition under observation with annual X-ray examinations.

Rheumatoid spondylitis (Bechterew's disease, pelvospondylitis ossificans, spondylarthritis ankylopoietica)

Bechterew's disease mainly affects the sacro-iliac joint, the joints between the vertebral arches and the anterior long ligament of the spine, which may gradually ossify. It usually afflicts young and middle-aged men and should be suspected in cases of chronic, but not severe, pain in the lumbar region.

Bechterew's disease is always associated with other disorders. Of the men who suffer from Bechterew's disease, about 75 per cent have chronic inflammation of the prostate gland (chronic prostatitis), 20 per cent have intestinal inflammation and 5 per cent psoriasis. In women Bechterew's disease is connected with an intestinal disease in 80 per cent of cases, with recurrent urinary tract infection in 15 per cent and with psoriasis in 5 per cent.

Symptoms and diagnosis	— Stiffness and pain in the morning.
	— Aching in the small of the back that disturbs the night's sleep.
	— Pain which radiates out towards the groin and down into the legs.
	— Other joints can also be affected, for example, hip, shoulder and toe joints. Increasing kyphosis may appear.
	— Recurrent eye inflammations (iritis).
	— X-ray examinations of the sacro-iliac joint can show irregularities in the joint. When the thoracic and lumbar regions are X-rayed early ossification of the anterior long ligament can be identified as well as an increase in the angularity of the shape of the vertebrae.
	— The erythrocyte sedimentation rate (ESR) is somewhat raised, and special blood tests may confirm the diagnosis, as can examination with radioactive isotypes.

Treatment

The *athlete* should:
— relieve stress on the affected joints;
— avoid rapid twisting movements and also cold and draughts;
— use a heat retainer;
— consult a doctor.

The *doctor* may:
— prescribe Bechterew exercises, a special type of physiotherapy which aims to counteract incorrect posture and increase mobility in back, shoulders and hips;
— prescribe anti-inflammatory medication;
— treat other associated diseases.

Healing and complications

Active mobility training should be commenced at an early stage, but the disease from which the patient suffers in addition to Bechterew's disease should be treated before he or she returns to training and competition. In the early stages and during symptom-free periods, sporting activities can be carried on without any major limitations, though a doctor should be consulted. During active exacerbation sporting activity is limited.

HIP JOINT AND GROIN INJURIES

Pain in the hip joint and the groin

The symptoms of injuries to the hip joint and groin can be vague and non-specific, and the doctor must therefore consider a variety of diagnostic possibilities. Disorders of the hip joint and groin are considered together because pain from the former can often radiate to the latter.

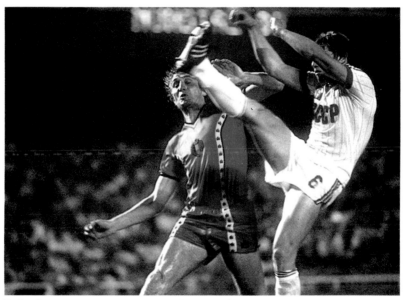

Risk of injuries to the groin. *Photo: Pressens bild.*

Hip disorders are caused mainly by injuries to the articular cartilage, while pain in the groin can be caused by inflammation resulting from overexertion or overloading of muscles, tendons and tendon attachments. The underlying cause of the inflammatory changes is thought to be microscopic ruptures which lead to minor tissue damage and an inflammatory reaction associated with symptoms typical of overuse injuries. Pain in the groin can also result from partial or total ruptures of muscles or tendons.

Other conditions which can cause problems in the hip and groin region are various fractures, bursitis, herniae, inflammation and infection of abdominal organs and genitalia, entrapment of various nerves including the sciatic nerve, tumours and general articular changes.

259

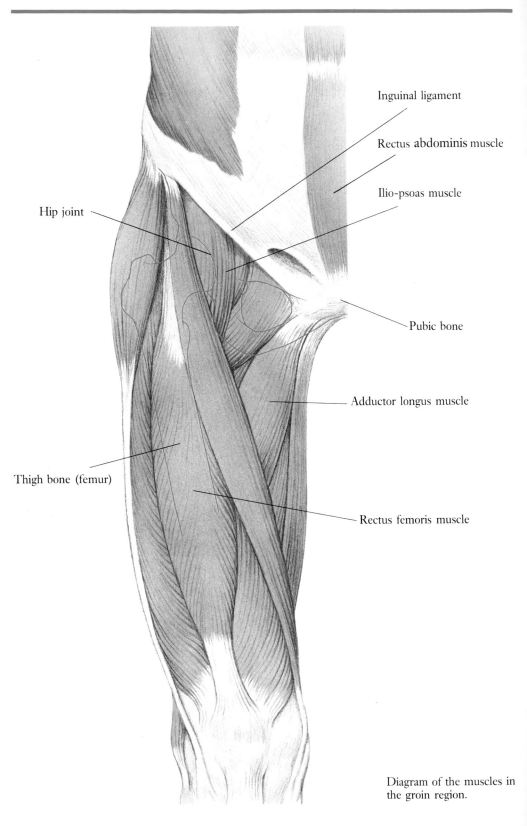

Inguinal ligament

Rectus abdominis muscle

Ilio-psoas muscle

Hip joint

Pubic bone

Adductor longus muscle

Thigh bone (femur)

Rectus femoris muscle

Diagram of the muscles in
the groin region.

During sporting activities, one of four muscle groups is generally involved in injuries to the hip and groin region. These are:
— the adductor longus muscle; the muscle that moves one leg inwards towards the other (adduction);
— the ilio-psoas muscle; the muscle that flexes the hip joint;
— the rectus femoris muscle; the thigh muscle which flexes the hip joint and extends the knee joint;
— the rectus abdominis muscle and other abdominal muscles.

In cases of injuries to hip and groin an early diagnosis is essential so that treatment can be commenced as soon as possible. If they are neglected they can cause very prolonged complaints or become chronic in which case they can be very difficult to treat.

Inflammation of the adductor muscles

The muscles that draw the leg inwards, that is, adduct at the hip joint, are primarily the adductor longus, the adductor magnus, the adductor brevis and the pectineus muscles. The gracilis muscle and the lower fibres of the gluteus maximus also work as adductors. However, it is usually the adductor longus that is damaged during sporting activity.

The adductor longus muscle arises from the pubic bone and is inserted into the back of the mid-shaft of the femur. Overloading can be caused by sideways kicks in soccer, hard track training and drawing the free leg inwards when skating. It is also common among team handball and ice hockey players, skiers, weightlifters, hurdlers and high-jumpers. The symptoms may begin insidiously, perhaps at a training camp or during other intensive training periods.

Symptoms and diagnosis

— Pain can often be located in the origin of the muscle and may radiate downwards into the groin. The pain often decreases after initial exertion and can disappear completely, only to return after training with even greater intensity. There is a risk that athletes will enter a cycle of pain (see page 41) in which case the condition is difficult to treat.
— Tenderness at one particular point on the pubic bone over the origin of the muscle. This tenderness is distinct.
— The pain can be triggered by adducting (pressing) the legs in towards each other against resistance (see photograph on page 262).
— Functional impairment is common. Sometimes the athlete cannot run but can manage to bicycle. The athlete should not participate in explosive sports.
— An X-ray examination sometimes shows calcification around the origin of the muscle on the pubic bone (see diagram on page 264).

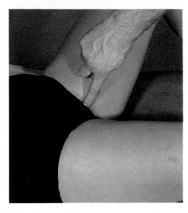 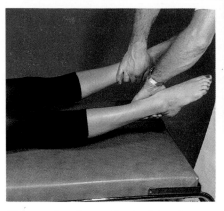

Tenderness in one area over the origin of the muscle in the pubic bone.

Pain can be triggered in the injured area by pressing the leg inwards against resistance.

The distance between the origins of the adductor longus and the rectus abdominis muscles is small, and inflammatory changes probably affect both muscles simultaneously.

Preventive measures

Preventive training with specially designed strength and flexibility exercises (see page 434) is essential and should be included in every training progamme as an integral part of the warm-up. The coach should be well aware of the training level of the different athletes and should, if possible, vary the training individually with this in mind. Athletes who undergo good basic fitness training are injured less often than others, and this is true especially with regard to muscle injuries.

Treatment

The *athlete* should:
— rest as soon as pain in the groin is felt. The condition will then resolve relatively quickly without any other treatment. This, of course, is based on the assumption that the injured athlete does not return to training and competition until there is no tenderness or pain when making movements with the leg under load;
— apply local heat and use a heat retainer;
— use general heat-treatment in the form of hot baths;
— maintain basic fitness by cycling (preferably on an exercise bicycle) or swimming, using a crawl stroke, but only if these activities can be carried out without pain.

The *doctor* may:
— prescribe anti-inflammatory medication;
— prescribe a special programme of muscle training. This should prefer- ably take place under the supervision of a physiotherapist. Below is a suggested outline of a training and rehabilitation programme for anyone who has injured the adductor longus muscle (see opposite).
   1. Warm-up: a light dynamic training programme, such as using an exercise bicycle, for 5–10 minutes.

2. Static training without loading the adductor muscle at different joint angles up to the pain threshold.
3. Dynamic training without resistance.
4. Isometric training, gradually increasing the external load.
5. Static stretching according to the method described on page 96.
6. Dynamic training with gradually increasing load.
7. Technique-specific co-ordination training.
8. Sport-specific training.
— administer a steroid injection around the muscle attachment or tendon attachment in question, and also prescribe 2 weeks' rest after the injection (the injection should only be given when there is distinct tenderness over the attachment into the bone);
— prescribe local heat treatment;
— operate in cases of delayed resolution.

Healing and complications

The exercises and movements which caused the inflammatory condition in the adductor muscle should not be resumed until the pain and tenderness have disappeared. If the affected athlete rests immediately pain begins, the condition will heal quite quickly (in 1–2 weeks), but if training is resumed too early treatment can be much more difficult. If the condition is not treated there is a risk that it will become prolonged or chronic.

Rupture of the adductor muscles

Ruptures of the adductor longus can be partial or total. Complete ruptures are usually located at the muscle's insertion into the femur, but can also occur at its origin in the pubic bone. Partial ruptures usually occur in the muscle itself or in its pubic origin. A rupture of the adductor longus muscle can occur when the muscles of the adductor group are tense and overused, for example in soccer, when the ball and an opponent's foot are kicked with the inside of the foot at the same time, or when a fast start, a gliding tackle or a sudden turn is made.

Symptoms and diagnosis

— Sudden momentary stabbing pain in the groin region is experienced. When attempts are made to restart activity, the pain returns.
— Local bleeding which can cause swelling and bruising. These do not, however, necessarily show themselves until a few days after the injury has occurred.
— If the muscle cannot contract there is reason to suspect a total rupture.
— When the rupture is in the belly of the muscle a defect can be felt at the site of injury, and the muscle is also most tender here.
— If there is bony tenderness an X-ray should be carried out.
— A clinical examination should be performed when the muscle is in a relaxed as well as in a contracted state.
— An X-ray should always be taken in athletes with groin pain. If a tumour is present, as in total rupture, a soft tissue X ray could be performed.

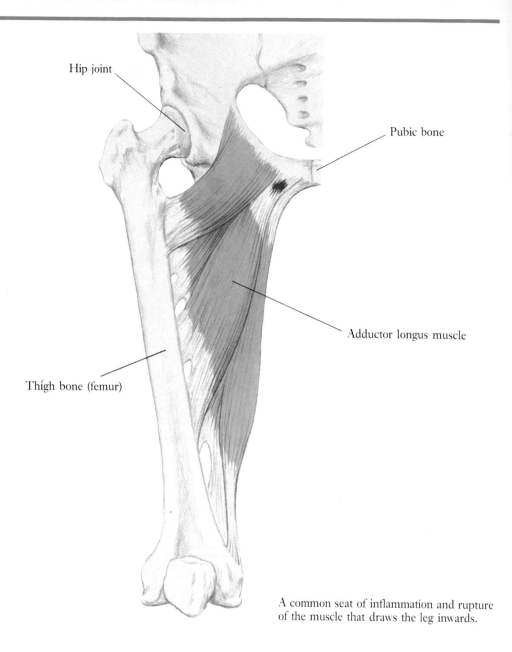

Hip joint

Pubic bone

Adductor longus muscle

Thigh bone (femur)

A common seat of inflammation and rupture of the muscle that draws the leg inwards.

Treatment

The *athlete* should:
— treat the injury immediately with cooling, compression bandaging and elevation (see page 68);
— rest and sometimes crutches.

The *doctor* may:
— operate in cases of a total rupture;
— in cases of a partial rupture take the steps described on page 262. A partial rupture will heal with scar tissue and a subsequent inflammatory reaction after the acute stage.

Healing and complications	During the rehabilitation period the injured athlete should continue muscle training (see page 434), cycling, light jogging, swimming and gradually increased conditioning. Not until the athlete is completely free from discomfort when the injured muscle group is subjected to a load can regular training be resumed. Its intensity should at first be limited and then increased gradually. Matches and competition should not be participated in until recovery from the injury is complete, and the athlete is fully trained and has been tested under competition conditions.

Total rupture of the adductor longus muscle can occur without any extensive problems. It can, however, cause the affected individual to suspect that he has a tumour as the belly of the muscle increases in size due to compensatory growth (see page 35).

Inflammation of the ilio-psoas muscle

The ilio-psoas muscle is by far the strongest flexor of the hip joint. It arises from the lumbar vertebrae (psoas) and the inner aspect of the hip bone (ilium) and is inserted into the inner aspect of the femoral shaft (lesser trochanter). Load on the muscle essentially means load on the insertion.

Inflammation of the ilio-psoas muscle can occur during strength training with weights and simultaneous knee-bending, sit-ups, rowing, ploughing through the snow for conditioning, running uphill, intensive shooting practice in football, badminton, long-jump and high-jump, hurdling and steeplechasing.

Beneath the ilio-psoas muscle tendon lies a bursa which can become the location of inflammation, either in isolation or simultaneously with the tendon of the ilio-psoas muscle. These conditions can be difficult to distinguish, and in the following section they will therefore be treated together.

Symptoms and diagnosis	— As a result of this injury the athlete can enter a cycle of pain similar to that described on page 261 under the heading 'Inflammation of the adductor muscles'.
	— Tenderness at the insertion of the tendon into the femur may be present but can be difficult to demonstrate in a muscular individual.
	— Pain in the groin may occur on flexing the hip joint against resistance.
	— When the bursa as well as the tendon of the ilio-psoas muscle is inflamed, a sensation of tension and swelling can arise in the groin. In spite of the fact that the bursa is distended with fluid, it can still be difficult to feel in a muscular individual.
Treatment	The *athlete* should:
	— rest until the pain has resolved;
	— apply local heat and use a heat retainer.

The *doctor* may:
— prescribe anti-inflammatory medication;
— prescribe a muscle training programme according to the principles on page 91;
— administer a steroid injection into the muscle insertion to be followed by 2 weeks' rest;
— aspirate the bursa to confirm a diagnosis of 'suspected bursitis'. This may be difficult to perform and should therefore be done under X-ray control. After the bursa has been drained 1 ml of a steroid preparation can be injected into it.

Healing and complications

When there are signs of inflammation in the groin muscles the athlete should rest immediately otherwise the condition can easily become prolonged and chronic.

Rupture of the ilio-psoas muscle

Rupture of the ilio-psoas muscle is rare, but when it occurs it is usually located in the tendon or the tendon insertion at the lesser trochanter (see diagram on page 267).

Symptoms and diagnosis

— Pain appears suddenly like a stab in the groin and returns as soon as the injured athlete tries to flex the hip joint.
— When rupture is partial, deep pain is felt at the ilio-psoas insertion into the inner aspect of the femur when the hip joint is flexed against resistance.
— Swelling and local tenderness may be present at the tendon insertion.
— A definite weakness in flexion of the hip joint is apparent in cases of total rupture.
— Sometimes a bone fragment may be torn away, so an X-ray examination should be carried out, particularly when the injury has occurred in a growing individual.

Treatment

— A partial rupture of the muscle should be treated as described on page 263 under the heading 'Rupture of the adductor muscles'.
— Cases of total rupture of the ilio-psoas muscle require surgery.

Inflammation of the upper part of the rectus femoris muscle

The rectus femoris muscle arises above the articular cavity of the hip joint. The muscle flexes the hip and extends the knee joint. After intensive shooting practice in soccer, repeated fast starts, strength training and similar activities, pain can be felt just above the hip joint.

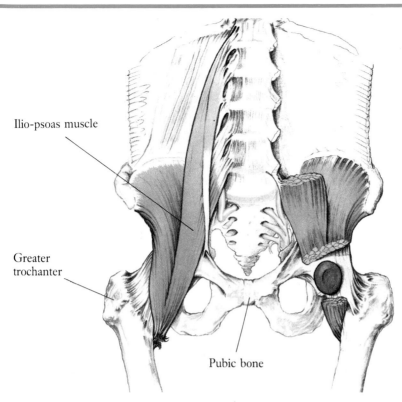

Ilio-psoas muscle

Greater trochanter

Pubic bone

Left of picture: partial rupture of the ilio-psoas muscle. **Right of picture:** inflammation of a bursa situated behind the ilio-psoas muscle; the muscle has been partly removed.

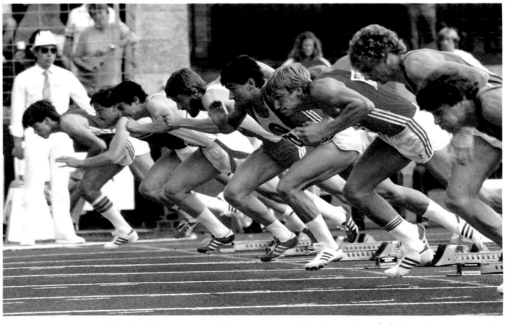

Injuries due to wear and tear can occur in the groin and thigh region as a result of repeated fast starts.

Symptoms and diagnosis	— Pain during and after exercise.
	— Pain which is triggered when the injured person flexes the hip joint or extends the knee joint against resistance (see photograph below).
	— Local tenderness at the origin of the muscle above and anterior to the hip joint (see photograph below).
Treatment	The treatment is in principle the same as that described on page 261 under the heading 'Inflammation of the adductor muscles'.

Rupture of the upper part of the rectus femoris muscle

Pain in the groin can be caused by a rupture in the origin or the upper third of the rectus femoris muscle. This rupture is usually partial, but total rupture may occur. The rupture can occur during shooting and tackling in football and also during fast starts in general (see diagram opposite).

Symptoms and diagnosis	— During vigorous flexing of the hip joint a sudden stabbing pain can be felt in the groin.
	— In cases of total rupture it is impossible to contract the muscle.
	— A defect and tenderness can often be felt in the belly of the muscle.
	— An X-ray examination should be carried out since a fragment of bone may have been torn away from the origin, especially in growing adolescents. At a later stage there may be residual calcification following bleeding.

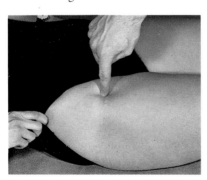

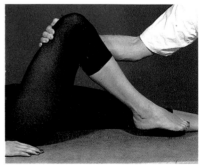

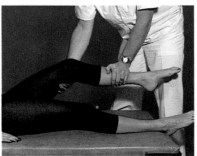

Above left: local tenderness around the origin of the muscle.

Above right: pain when bending the hip joint against resistance.

Left: pain when straightening the knee joint against resistance.

Treatment

— In cases of partial rupture, the same principles as described on page 263 can be used.

— In cases of total rupture, surgery is probably to be preferred, especially if the origin of the muscle has been torn away from the skeleton near the joint, taking with it a fragment of bone.

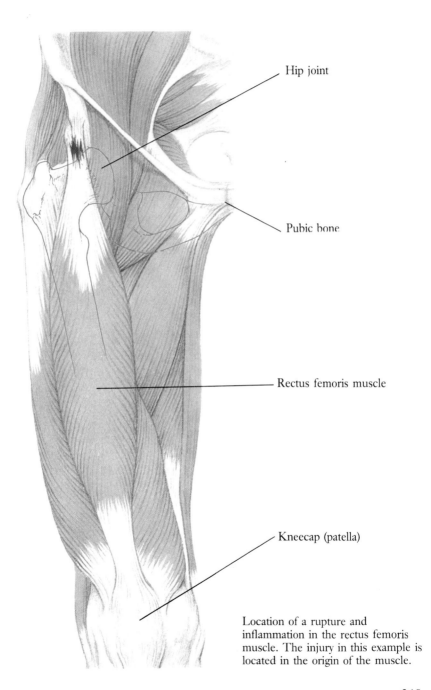

Hip joint

Pubic bone

Rectus femoris muscle

Kneecap (patella)

Location of a rupture and inflammation in the rectus femoris muscle. The injury in this example is located in the origin of the muscle.

Inflammation and ruptures of the abdominal muscles

In cases of ruptures and inflammation of the abdominal muscles it is usually the rectus abdominis muscle which is damaged, but the oblique and transverse muscles of the abdomen can also be affected. The rectus abdominis arises from the upper part of the pubic bone and the 5th, 6th and 7th costal cartilages. Inflammation and partial rupture of this muscle is located, as a rule, at its insertion to the pubic bone (see diagram below). Ruptures can also appear in the transverse muscles towards the sides of the abdomen and can cause confusion if, for instance, they are located over the appendix.

Ruptures of the abdominal muscles occur in weightlifters, throwers, gymnasts, rowers, wrestlers, pole-vaulters and others. Inflammation is often triggered by exertion, for example strength training, sit-ups, shooting practice in football and also serving and smashing in tennis and badminton.

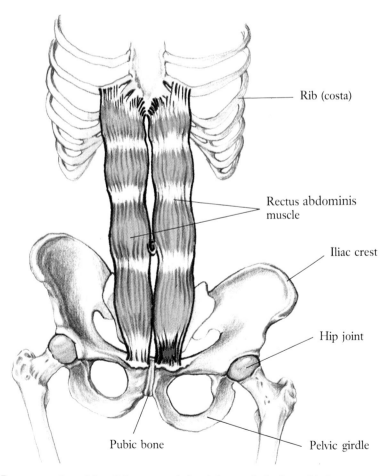

Rib (costa)

Rectus abdominis muscle

Iliac crest

Hip joint

Pubic bone

Pelvic girdle

Rupture at the origin of the rectus abdominis muscle in the pubic bone.

Symptoms and diagnosis

— On exertion of the abdominal muscles the athlete feels a sudden stabbing pain which indicates that a rupture has occurred.
— There may be tenderness over the area in which the rupture has occurred and/or inflammation (see photograph on page 268).
— There is impaired function affecting, for example, forceful forward thrust in walking and running.
— A rupture of the abdominal muscles can be difficult to distinguish from inflammation of the internal abdominal organs such as appendicitis. It is typical of a rupture that the tenderness and the pain are more pronounced when the abdominal muscles are contracted than when they are relaxed. The muscles can be flexed if the injured athlete lies flat and lifts his head and legs simultaneously into the air.
— In cases of inflammation of the abdominal muscles there is often tenderness and pain over the origin of the rectus abdominis muscle into the pubic bone. The symptoms are triggered when the injured athlete contracts the abdominal muscles as described above.

Treatment

The *athlete* should:
— rest until the symptoms have resolved;
— apply local heat and use a heat retainer.

The *doctor* may:
— prescribe anti-inflammatory medication;
— prescribe an exercise programme according to the guidelines on page 91;
— administer a local steroid injection followed by 2 weeks' rest when there are signs of inflammation of the tendon attachment;
— operate when there is prolonged pain.

Healing and complications

If the athelete rest immediately when there are signs of overuse of the abdominal muscles, healing takes only 1–2 weeks as a rule. In cases of muscle ruptures the healing time varies according to the extent of the injury. The injured athlete should not return to training and competition until healing is complete as new ruptures can otherwise ensue and the healing process can then be delayed considerably. Large muscle ruptures can lead to hernia formation in the abdominal wall.

Most athletes train their abdominal muscles by sit-ups. In order to prevent the ilio-psoas muscle being used during the rehabilitation period, the hip joint should be held bent so that this muscle does not contract. The best method of training the rectus abdominis muscle is half sit-ups, done slowly with bent knees.

Other causes of pain in the hip joint and the groin

Inflammation or ruptures of other groin muscles

There are a number of muscles which affect the groin region, including the pectineus, the sartorius, the tensor fascia lata and the gluteus medius, and these can also be damaged during sporting activity. When injuries are examined, the precise location of the pain must be sought. This, together with an assessment of muscle function, can elucidate the diagnosis.

Symptoms and treatment are in principle the same as those described on page 261 under the heading 'Inflammation of the adductor muscles'.

Hip joint changes

Pains in the groin may be referred from the hip joint and can be an early symptom of changes due to wear (osteoarthritis; see page 49), of rheumatoid arthritis (see page 51) or osteochondritis. Loose bodies can occur in the joint, formed, as they are in the knee, by a release of fragments of bone and cartilage (osteochondritis dissecans). In exceptional cases the edge (limbus) of cartilage which surrounds the joint cavity may have been displaced and driven into the joint. These conditions cause pain on exertion and loading, and also sometimes locking of the hip joint. Continuous and persistent aching discomfort is also often precipitated by exertion. Pain during movements of the hip joint, especially during extension, should motivate an X-ray examination. This should be carried out, with or without contrast medium, with the hip held in the position which triggers the pain. Arthroscopy may also be considered.

Dislocation of the hip joint

The hip joint is extremely stable under normal circumstances, but can be dislocated (usually backwards) by very violent impact. The injury is serious because the femoral head can be damaged permanently as a result of impairment of its circulation. Dislocations of the hip joint rarely occur without simultaneous skeletal injuries, and prolonged follow-up treatment is needed before a return to sporting activity can be made.

Fracture of the neck or upper shaft of the femur

Fractures of the neck of the femur and of the upper part of its shaft are comparatively common injuries in the elderly. The former, however, also occurs in younger individuals who have fallen directly on to the hip while skating or skiing, for example. It is typical of fractures of the neck of the femur that the injured leg is shortened and twisted outwards after the injury. These fractures are nearly always operated on, and healing and rehabilitation is a slow process.

Stress fracture of the neck of the femur

Stress fractures (see page 53) can occur in the neck of the femur in, for example, long distance runners as a result of prolonged and repeated load. Similar fractures can also affect the pubic bones.

(see page 53)

Symptoms and diagnosis

— Pain during loading of the hip joint and also aching in the joint after exertion.
— Pain in the hip joint on movement.
— When there is persistent pain in the hip region, X-rays should be carried out. If no signs of a stress fracture show up at the time, but the problems continue for another 3 weeks or so, the X-rays should be repeated.
— A specialized examination using radioactive isotopes (bone scan, scintigraphy) can be useful.

Treatment

— Rest the leg until the fracture has healed which as a rule takes 5–8 weeks, depending on the location of the fracture and the age of the injured athlete. Unloading with crutches may be necessary.

Hernia

Inguinal hernia
An inguinal hernia is a protrusion of the contents of the abdomen through the peritoneum resulting from a weakness of the muscles and connective tissue layers of the abdominal wall. Of all hernias, 80 per cent are inguinal (groin region), and appear as swellings at some point along the inner half of a line between the pubic tubercle and anterior superior iliac crest. They can be the cause of pain in the groin which is triggered by exertion or

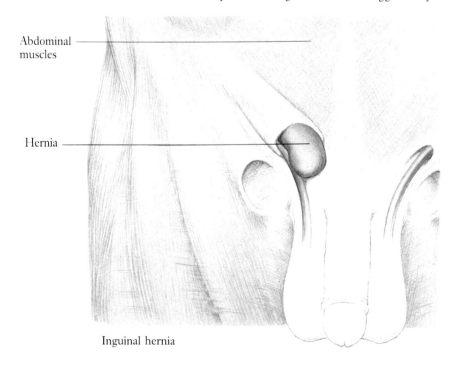

Abdominal muscles

Hernia

Inguinal hernia

even coughing, sneezing or straining. When the causes of vague pains in the groin are sought by a doctor he or she usually routinely checks for the presence of an inguinal hernia.

Hernias are treated by surgery, and the patient can often resume his toning exercises a few weeks after the operation, but should not return to strength training for at least 8–10 weeks.

Femoral hernia
Almost 10 per cent of all hernias are femoral hernias which protrude on the front of the upper thigh below the groin fold. Symptoms and treatment are similar to those of inguinal hernias (see above).

Abdominal hernia
Hernias within the abdomen can cause pain which radiates out towards the groin. Such hernias can be diagnosed by herniography which involves a contrast medium injected into the abdomen penetrating into the hernia and thereby revealing it. Soccer players can develop incipient hernias in the right half of the abdomen if the right leg is the one mainly used, and in the left if the player is 'left-footed'.

Hydrocele
A hydrocele is an accumulation of watery fluid around the testes. It does not as a rule cause any serious problems and is treated by draining the fluid. Large hydroceles may sometimes need surgical treatment.

Other conditions which can cause symptoms referred to the groin include tumours in the testes, inflammation of the tissues in the surrounding area, varicose veins in the scrotum and torsion of the testes.

Inflammation of internal organs

Appendicitis
Appendicitis is characterized by aching and pain in the lower right-hand side of the abdomen and mild fever. Nausea and vomiting often occur, and lifting the right leg exacerbates the pain. Symptoms like these which persist for more than a few hours should lead to urgent consultation with a doctor.

Prostatitis
Inflammation of the prostate gland can cause pain which radiates out towards the groin (see page 259). Difficulty in passing water is common and worse during cold weather. The condition should be investigated by a doctor and treated appropriately.

Urinary tract infection
Urinary tract infections are characterized by burning pains on urination and frequent, urgent passage of urine which may smell unpleasant. Such infections can cause pain which radiates out into the groin region (see page 259).

Urinary tract infections should be investigated by a doctor and treated with antibiotics active against the particular types of bacteria present in the urine.

Gynaecological disorders

Gynaecological disorders can cause pain which radiates to the groin. They include inflammatory conditions, venereal diseases, skin diseases and tumours.

Tumours

Tumours are not uncommon in the groin region and can cause pain and aching which at first may appear while playing soccer or performing some other physical activity. Other symptoms are similar to those caused by inflammation and ruptures of muscles and tendons, and when they are persistent investigation sometimes reveals a tumour as the cause. *If there is persistent pain in the groin region an X-ray examination should be carried out*, and the rectum should also be examined carefully.

Sciatica

Pain which radiates to the groin and down along the thigh may be caused by the L4 syndrome of sciatica (see page 248).

Pressure on nerves ('entrapment')

Nerves in the groin region can be subjected to pressure or load which is usually due to local anatomical conditions. The nerves in question are primarily the ilio-inguinal, the genito-femoral and the lateral cutaneous

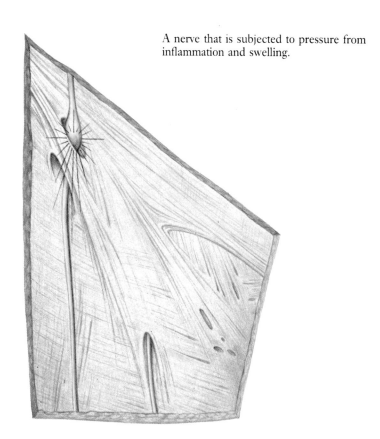

A nerve that is subjected to pressure from inflammation and swelling.

nerve of the thigh, which all supply skin areas around the groin folds, and also the anterior cutaneous nerve of the thigh and the obturator nerve.

The ilio-inguinal nerve supplies the skin just above the penis, the scrotum or the labia and the inside of the thigh and pain in these regions should lead to a suspicion of pressure on the nerve. The intensity and character of the pain varies. Increased sensitivity in the area can be demonstrated by scratching a needle lightly over the skin from a painless to a painful area, and the diagnosis can be confirmed by injecting local anaesthetic around the nerve. When pain is severe and persistent, surgery is sometimes resorted to.

The genito-femoral nerve supplies a skin area just below the groin fold and also parts of the external sexual organs, while the lateral cutaneous nerve of the thigh, as its name suggests, supplies the outside of the thigh. Symptoms and treatment in cases of pressure on these nerves are the same as those outlined above for pressure on the ilio-inguinal nerve.

Inflammation of the sacro-iliac joint

Inflammation of the sacro-iliac joint is not uncommon as an isolated condition among athletes who pursue winter sports, but can also be one aspect of a more generalized disease, such as a rheumatic joint disease or Bechterew's disease (see page 257).

Symptoms and diagnosis

— Vague symptoms include aching and stiffness in the lower part of the lumbar region. These are most pronounced in the morning and after periods of inactivity. They come and go, and long periods free from problems are typical.
— The aching can radiate out towards the back of the thigh, the hip joint or the groin. Changes in the sacro-iliac joint can occur, however, without the patient feeling any pain.
— Inflammation of the sacro-iliac joint can sometimes be combined with inflammation of other joints, for example, the knee and ankle.
— A raised erythrocyte sedimentation rate occurs along with other blood changes typical of inflammatory disorders.

Treatment

The *doctor* may:
— prescribe anti-inflammatory medication;
— prescribe physiotherapy;
— recommend a lumbar heat retainer.

Healing and complications

The symptoms are prolonged, but the condition is considerably more benign in women than in men.

Inflammation of the pubic bone (osteitis pubis)

Some athletes are afflicted by pain located in the anterior aspect (front) of the pubic bone. This may be combined with tenderness over the area where the right and left parts of the bone meet at the centre of the body (symphysis). X-ray changes indicative of inflammation of the bone in this area can sometimes be seen. When such changes are not apparent, examination with radioactive isotopes (bone scan, scintigraphy) can sometimes give positive results. The treatment consists of rest and prescription of anti-inflammatory medication.

It should be pointed out that X-ray changes resembling those seen in cases of osteitis pubis can sometimes be incidental findings which cause the athletes no problems whatever.

Inflammation and calcification of the greater trochanter

Some of the large muscle groups of the buttocks have their attachments to the greater trochanter of the femur in the upper, outer (lateral) part of the thigh. An irritant inflammatory condition can be initiated in the muscle attachment of the gluteal muscles in, for example, cross-country runners and orienteerers.

Symptoms and diagnosis

— Pain occurs over the upper part of the femur on the lateral aspect of the hip.
— Tenderness occurs on pressure over a small area around the greater trochanter.
— Pain is precipitated by pressing the leg outwards against resistance.
— X-ray examination sometimes reveals calcification in the area in question.

Treatment

The *athlete* should:
— rest until pain has resolved;
— apply local heat and use a heat retainer.

The *doctor* may:
— prescribe anti-inflammatory medication;
— initiate a muscle exercise programme according to the principles on page 91;
— administer a steroid injection combined with prescribed rest.

Bursitis of the hip (trochanteric bursitis)

Over the upper outer (lateral) part of the femur, beneath the fascia lata lies a superficial bursa, with a deeper one between the tendon of the gluteus medius muscle and the posterior surface of the greater trochanter. In cases of falls or blows affecting the hip, the superficial bursa can become the site of bleeding (haemobursa; see page 49). Minor bleeding resolves spontaneously, but a major bleed can sometimes result in clot

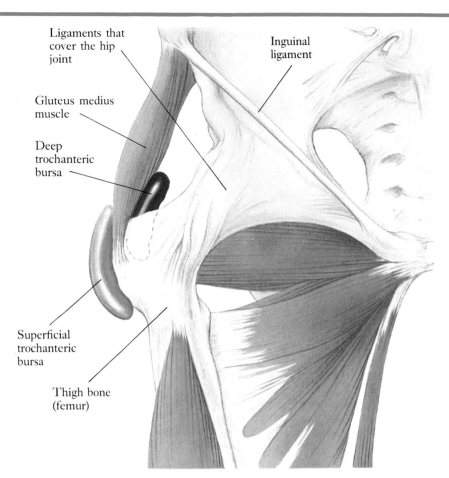

Ligaments that cover the hip joint

Inguinal ligament

Gluteus medius muscle

Deep trochanteric bursa

Superficial trochanteric bursa

Thigh bone (femur)

Inflammation of the superficial and deep bursae of the greater trochanter.

formation. Clots are gradually transformed into loose bodies or adhesions which give rise to inflammation and effusion of fluid.

Inflammation secondary to friction and overuse can affect either bursa and is a commoner cause of pain than a haemobursa. An excessive pronation of the foot (see page 354) can contribute to overuse in this region as can running on cambers.

Symptoms and diagnosis

— Pain which is particularly pronounced during running. When the leg is simultaneously adducted and rotated inwards with the knee joint straight, the pain increases.

— Intense pain is caused by the swelling which accompanies the onset of inflammation. Once this begins, it rarely resolves spontaneously so medical advice should always be sought.

— Local tenderness over the upper, lateral part of the thigh.

— Impaired function causing, for example, limping because of pain and discomfort.

— Pain which radiates down the thigh at night.

— Loose bodies and adhesions in the bursa can give rise to creaking sensations (crepitus) during hip movements and can sometimes be felt as small, mobile beads when the skin overlying the bursa is palpated.

— In order to confirm the diagnosis the doctor may ask the athlete to lie down on his healthy side and raise the leg on the tender side. As a result of this manoeuvre, the bursa is compressed resulting in severe pain. If the same movement is carried out against resistance the pain increases.

Treatment

The *athlete* should:
— rest the injured area;
— apply cooling to the area;
— run on even surfaces.

The *doctor* may:
— aspirate and drain the bursa in cases of bleeding or extensive effusion of fluid;
— prescribe orthotics if, for example, excessive foot pronation is present;
— prescribe anti-inflammatory medication;
— administer a local steroid injection and prescribe rest;
— in cases of prolonged problems operate in order to remove loose bodies and any adhesions in the bursa. Usually the bursa itself is also excised (see diagram opposite).

Hip complaints in children and adolescents

Perthes' disease

Perthes' disease, the precise cause of which is unknown, afflicts children between the ages of three and eleven years. The internal bone structure of the head of the femur degenerates and becomes deformed and flattened. The child complains of tiredness and pain in the groin and sometimes the knee, and a limp is present. The diagnosis is made by X-ray examination.

Depending on the severity of changes in the femoral head, the treatment varies from surgery to none at all. The healing process is prolonged.

Although Perthes' disease only affects the hip joint, pain is sometimes absent from that joint and felt only in the knee to which it is referred. Both joints should be X-rayed in cases of knee pain if Perthes' disease is not to be missed.

Slippage of the epiphysis at the neck of the femur

Slippage of the epiphysis (see page 406) at the neck of the femur (epiphysiolysis) occasionally affects boys between the ages of eleven and sixteen years. Pain begins in the groin region, but, as is usual in the case of hip disorders, is also felt in the knee. It can be triggered by sporting activity.

It is important that young people who complain of this type of symptom should be X-rayed to exclude the possibility of slipped epiphysis. The

Inflammation of the hip joint (synovitis)

Acute pains in the hip in children are usually caused by inflammation of the tissues surrounding the joint. The pain increases with time, and the child shows an aversion to making hip movements and sometimes has difficulty with walking. Inflammation of the hip joint is seen mainly in children below the age of ten years and is considered to be a benign condition which should be investigated by a specialist but which resolves spontaneously.

The hip disorders in children and adolescents described above should be distinguished from serious conditions such as bone infection (osteomyelitis), tuberculosis, rheumatic diseases and tumours.

Pain in knee and/or hip joints, and lameness in children and adolescents should prompt medical examination.

THIGH INJURIES

Rupture of the thigh muscles

Rupture of the muscles in the *front* of the thigh, the quadriceps muscles, can occur as a result of impact against contracted muscles, as during soccer when one player's knee hits another's thigh, or during a sudden, vigorous and explosive contraction of the muscles, in a fast start or rush. In cases of rupture caused by external impact, the muscles lying close to the bone are affected, while the more superficial muscles are affected, as a rule, by ruptures caused by overload (distraction ruptures see page 29).

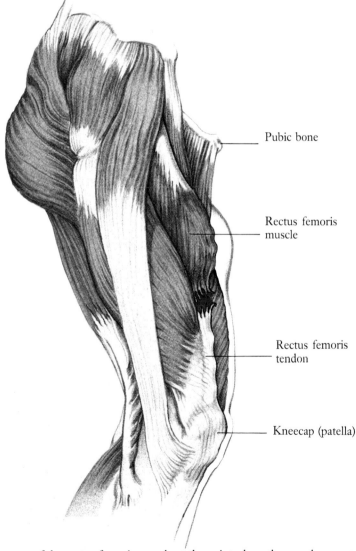

Pubic bone

Rectus femoris muscle

Rectus femoris tendon

Kneecap (patella)

Rupture of the rectus femoris muscle at the point where the muscle merges into a tendon.

Ruptures of the hamstring muscles (the biceps femoris, semimembranosus and semitendinosus muscles) usually occur as a result of overload and then forceful contraction of the flexors of the knee joint. Sprinters, middle-distance runners and players of contact sports are especially susceptible to this type of muscle injury, but long-jumpers, triple jumpers, badminton and tennis players, and others can be affected.

Symptoms and diagnosis — The athlete often notices a 'lash' or 'stab' of intense pain as the injury occurs. Similar pain recurs on exertion.

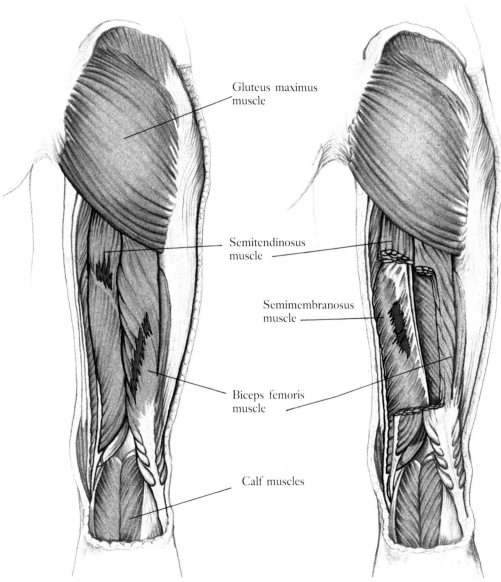

Gluteus maximus muscle

Semitendinosus muscle

Semimembranosus muscle

Biceps femoris muscle

Calf muscles

The injury on the left-hand side of the leg is a rupture of the semitendinosus muscle at the back of the thigh. The injury on the right-hand side of the leg is a rupture of the biceps femoris muscle.

Rupture of the semimembranosus muscle at the back of the thigh. The middle parts of the semitendinosus muscle and the biceps femoris have been removed to show the rupture.

- The muscle may go into spasm.
- There is intense tenderness over the injured area.
- Increasing swelling and bruising.
- Pain can be elicited by contracting the muscle against resistance.
- In cases of a total or major partial rupture a defect can be felt in the muscle.

Treatment
- Ruptures of the muscles of the thigh are treated according to the guidelines given on page 32.

Healing and complications
- The healing time varies between 2 and 12 weeks depending on the extent of the bleeding and whether the rupture is partial or total.
- Scar tissue in the muscles adds to the risk of a further haematoma or rupture occurring.
- Significant haematoma inappropriately treated can result in heterotopic bone formation (see below).

Heterotopic bone formation, myositis ossificans, 'charley-horse'

Bleeding, usually in association with tissue damage, can occur in the thigh muscles as the result of impact. This type of injury is especially common in the contact sports, for example, soccer, rugby, American football, team handball and ice hockey. A significant haematoma which is neglected can result in a healing condition called heterotopic bone formation or myositis ossificans. The scar tissue which forms calcifies and ossifies. The muscle function and mobility in the knee joint are impaired, and there is a risk of recurrent injury occurring in the same area.

Treatment
- Immediate treatment at the time of injury should be directed to restricting the bleeding according to the principles given on page 64.
- If myositis ossificans has occurred, rest is recommended.
- Careful static muscle contractions and active movements can sometimes be started when haemorrhage is under control. If there is an improvement in muscle function and mobility, gentle massage and alternate hot and cold baths can be tried and are often beneficial.
- For instructions on other aspects of treatment, see page 32.

Vague pains in the front, side or back of the thigh can be caused by sciatica (see page 248) or a stress fracture (see page 53).

KNEE INJURIES

The articular surfaces of the femur and the tibia in the knee joint are composed of cartilage. The anterior surface of the femur also articulates with the patella. The fibula, which provides attachment for ligaments and muscles, extends to the top of the lower leg but has no articulation with the knee joint.

The *passive stability* of the knee joint is maintained by the collateral ligaments, the cruciate ligaments and the menisci. The collateral ligaments stabilize the knee joint on the medial and lateral sides. The medial collateral ligament is composed of a superficial, long portion and a deeper, short portion which is attached to the medial meniscus. The lateral collateral ligament is not attached to the lateral meniscus. Antero-posterior stability is maintained by the anterior and the posterior cruciate ligaments respectively. These also contribute to maintaining the lateral stability and together they prevent hyperextension and hyperflexion. Hyperextension of the joint is also limited by the tight connective tissue capsule behind the knee joint.

The medial and lateral menisci, which are semilunar fibrocartilages, stabilize the knee joint during movements and load and also serve as shock absorbers between the tibia and the femur.

The *active stability* of the knee joint is maintained by contraction of the surrounding musculature. The main muscles that contribute to this stability are the extensors in the front of the thigh (the quadriceps muscle) and the flexors at the back of the thigh (the hamstring muscles).

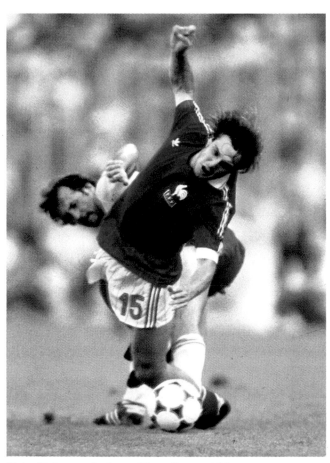

Risk of injury to the knee. *Photo: Pressens bild.*

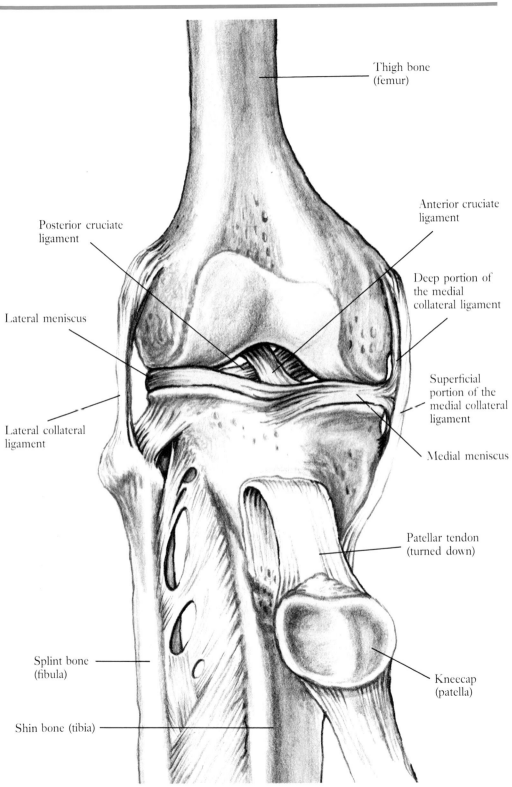

Thigh bone
(femur)

Anterior cruciate
ligament

Posterior cruciate
ligament

Deep portion of
the medial
collateral ligament

Lateral meniscus

Superficial
portion of the
medial collateral
ligament

Lateral collateral
ligament

Medial meniscus

Patellar tendon
(turned down)

Splint bone
(fibula)

Kneecap
(patella)

Shin bone (tibia)

Anatomical diagram of the right knee joint, seen from the front.

Ligament injuries in the knee joint

Ligament injuries in the knee joint should be treated as potentially serious since the passive stability of the joint is disturbed. They are as common as meniscus injuries and mainly affect athletes involved in contact sports such as football, ice hockey, team handball, basketball and rugby, as well as Alpine skiing.

The mechanism of injury
Ligament injuries in the knee joint occur mainly as the result of collisions with opponents in contact sports but also without body contact, in twisting and other movements that exceed the normal range of motion. The various ligaments of the knee joints cooperate in order to maintain the stability of the joint, and the stronger the stresses the joint is subjected to, the greater the degree to which the ligaments are engaged. Combination injuries are likely to occur as a result of violent impact, and the more violent the impact, the more serious and complicated the injuries. The following mechanisms are commonest:

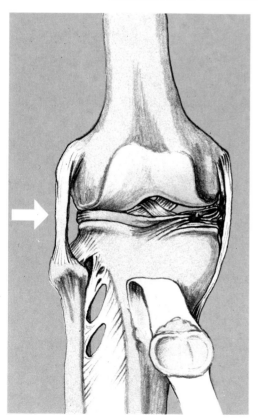

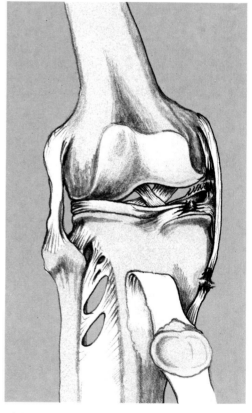

The stages in the development of injury caused by impact against the outer side of the knee joint. If the impact is moderate the deep portion of the medial collateral ligament ruptures first. The medial meniscus may also be injured.

If the impact is more violent, the superficial portion of the medial collateral ligament will rupture.

1. An impact which hits the knee joint from the lateral side or hits the fore-foot from the medial side;
2. An impact which hits the knee joint from the medial side or hits the fore-foot from the lateral side;
3. An impact which results in hyperextension or hyperflexion of the knee joint;
4. A twisting impact without body contact.

1. Impact against the lateral side of the knee joint

An impact against the lateral side of the knee joint which forces the joint inwards (in valgus) is considerably more common than an impact against the medical side of the knee joint which forces the joint outwards (in varus). The resulting mechanism of injury is similar whether there is an impact against the lateral side of the knee joint as described above or an impact against the medial side of the foot which forces it outwards in relation to the knee (see diagrams below). The latter situation can occur, for example, when two players kick the ball at the same time with the inside of their feet.

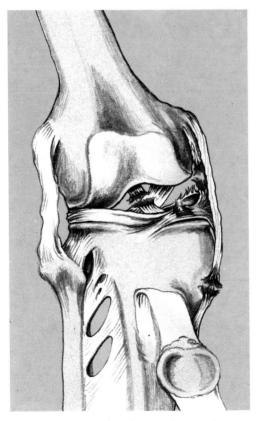 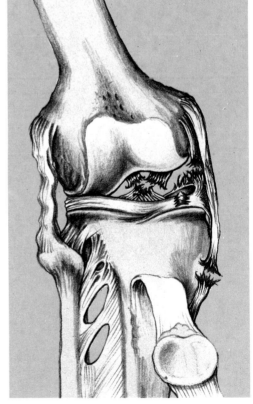

In an even more violent impact, the anterior cruciate ligament will rupture.

In an extremely violent impact, the posterior cruciate ligament can also rupture, resulting in damage to the medial meniscus and the medial collateral ligament as well as the anterior and posterior cruciate ligaments.

During sporting activities the lateral side of the knee is most often affected by impact when the foot is under load and the knee joint is slightly bent. The knee joint is then forced inwards and the tibia is rotated outwards in relation to the femur, possibly causing injuries to the medial meniscus or to the medial collateral ligament. Sometimes these two injuries are combined, probably because the two structures are attached to each other. The deep portion of the medial collateral ligament attached to the meniscus is short and tight, so that it takes the load before the superficial portion and ruptures first. In a more violent impact the anterior cruciate ligament is also loaded and subsequently tears. The result is a combination of damage to the medial collateral ligament, the anterior cruciate ligament, and possibly the medial meniscus, and an infusion into the joints.

In extremely violent impact against the lateral side of the knee joint, the posterior cruciate ligament ultimately tears, so that the structures affected include the medial collateral ligament, both anterior and posterior cruciate ligaments and possibly the medial meniscus. The overall result is medial as well as anteroposterior instability between the tibia and the femur (see below).

2. Impact against the medial side of the knee joint

In sports, the medial side of the knee is often subjected to impact when

The stages in the development of injury caused by impact against the inner side of the knee joint.

Right: if the impact is moderate, the lateral collateral ligament ruptures.

Opposite left: if the impact is more violent, the anterior cruciate ligament will also rupture.

Opposite right: in an extremely violent impact, the posterior cruciate ligament will also rupture resulting in damage to the lateral collateral ligament as well as the anterior and posterior cruciate ligaments.

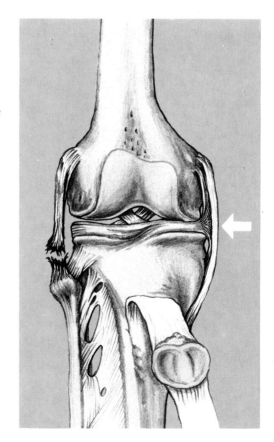

the joint is slightly bent and the foot is under load. The knee joint is then forced outwards and the tibia is twisted inwards in relation to the femur. At first the load is borne by the lateral collateral ligament which can tear as a result (see diagrams below). The probability of a meniscus injury occurring is less in this case than in the case of impact to the outside of the knee since the lateral collateral ligament is not attached to the adjacent meniscus. When impact is more violent, the anterior cruciate ligament is stretched and torn and the result is a combined injury involving the lateral collateral and anterior cruciate ligaments. A combined injury of this nature should be suspected if there is a simultaneous effusion due to bleeding in the knee joint (haemarthrosis).

When there is an extremely violent impact against the medial side of the knee, even the posterior cruciate ligament is stretched and torn, so that damage to the lateral collateral ligament is combined with injuries to both cruciate ligaments. The result is lateral as well as anteroposterior instability of the knee.

3. Impact causing hyperextension or hyperflexion

Impact on the knee joint from the front can cause hyperextension. Forced hyperextension can also occur without body contact. Falling on to a bent knee joint can cause hyperflexion. Isolated injuries which involve only the

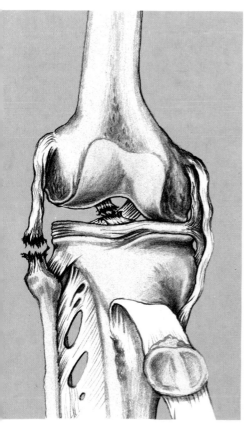 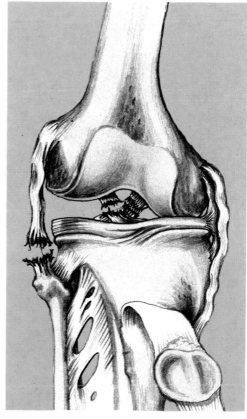

anterior or only the posterior cruciate ligament can result, but are rare. Injuries to the collateral and the cruciate ligaments are often combined with damage to the posterior joint capsule.

4. Twisting impact without body contact

Twisting impact without body contact takes place during a twisting turn with the foot fixed, for example, when the studs of the boot get stuck in the grass. This type of impact can cause both meniscus and ligament injuries in the knee. Anterior cruciate ligament injury can occur during forced internal rotation of the tibia relative to the femur.

Symptoms and diagnosis

— An important symptom of an acute knee ligament injury is pain which is extreme at the moment of impact but subsequently decreases. It recurs when the joint is moved or loaded.

— There is often local tenderness over an injured collateral ligament.

— When there is an effusion in the knee, the joint is swollen. It is important, particularly in cases of internal joint injury, to decide whether the effusion is caused by bleeding and this is done by joint aspiration under sterile conditions. There is usually a history of the effusion occuring rapidly after the injury.

— Instability in the joint is an important symptom which the injured person seldom notices while the injury is in its acute stage, but which often becomes apparent later, especially when the joint is loaded and exerted.

General examination of a knee ligament injury

The examination of an injured knee should always be carried out by a *doctor*. Knee injuries are common in sport, and it is important that they should be treated correctly. Information is therefore likely to be of interest to managers as well as athletes, and insight into the methods of examination of such injuries can increase the understanding of their handling by the medical profession. An adequate test is not possible unless the opposing muscles are relaxed.

1. *Analysis* of the injury mechanism. An idea of the magnitude of the energy and the direction of impact at the moment of injury is of value to the doctor and provides the basis for the assessment of the severity and type of injury.

2. *Inspection* of the injured area. There may be swelling around as well as within the joint. Bruising over or around the course of the collateral ligaments indicates bleeding and a ligament injury.

   In cases of effusion, swelling extends above the patella. The doctor can establish whether such an effusion is present by pressing with his hands against the areas above and below the patella at the same time as he presses the patella towards the femur with the thumb of one hand (see photograph opposite). When there is an effusion, the patella meets a spongy resistance that ceases when the articular surface of the patella is compressed against that of the femur. When the pressure on the patella is released, it can be seen to rise again because of the underlying fluid.

3. *Palpation.* The examining doctor palpates over the joint lines of the knee and over the entire course of the collateral ligaments and notes the location of tenderness. Even swelling caused by an effusion of blood (see above) spreading along the course of the ligaments can be felt during this part of the examination.

4. *Testing the range of movement.* The doctor checks whether there is any restriction of extension or flexion of the knee. Pain on movement or a decreased range of movement can be the sign of a meniscus injury.

5. *Stability examination.* Such an examination is essential in order to enable the doctor to decide whether a ligament injury is such that instability has resulted. An adequate test is not possible without being muscle-relaxed. Pain can sometimes make an adequate examination impossible.

a. *Testing of the collateral ligaments* is performed both when the knee joint is extended, and when it is flexed at an angle of 20–30°. In cases of medial instability the lower leg can be angled outwards (in valgus) and in lateral instability the knee joint can be angled inwards (in varus) at the knee joint in relation to the femur. The degree of instability is determined by comparison with the undamaged knee joint.

   If pain is too severe for this examination to be performed, it can be

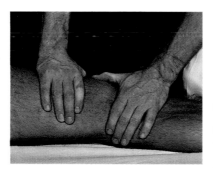

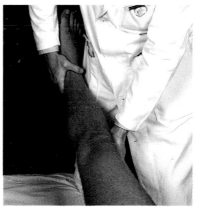

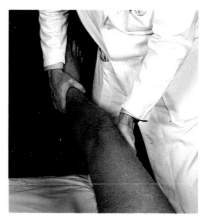

Above left: examination of an effusion in the knee joint. By moving his hands towards each other, the doctor will compress the fluid in the knee. Then, by pressing a thumb against the kneecap it will make it 'dance' against the bone underneath if an effusion is present.

Above right: stability examination of the ligaments of the knee joint when the leg is extended. If the knee joint wobbles, there is an injury to the lateral collateral ligament and also an injury to the posterior medial joint capsule and the anterior cruciate ligament.

Right: stability examination of the lateral collateral ligament of the knee joint, held bent at an angle of 20–30°.

reserved until a day or two after injury, or alternatively may be carried out under anaesthetic.

Moderate medial instability characterized by, for example, wobbling outwards of the lower leg when the knee joint is flexed at an angle of 20°, indicates an injury to the deep portion of the medial collateral ligament. If the wobbling is pronounced, both the deep and superficial parts of the ligament have probably sustained damage. If there is wobbling outwards when the knee joint is extended, there is, as a rule, also an injury to the anterior cruciate ligament and/or the posterior joint capsule as well as to the medial collateral ligament.

b. *Testing the anterior cruciate and medial collateral ligaments*
The *anterior drawer test* is carried out when injury to the cruciate or the collateral ligaments is suspected. The injured person lies supine with the knee joint bent at an angle of 90°. Excessive movement of the tibia

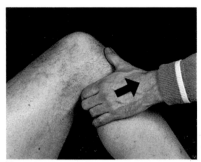

Examination of the anterior cruciate ligament by using an anterior drawer test on an uninjured knee.

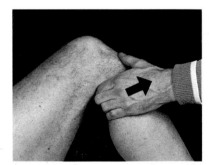

An anterior drawer test on a knee with an injured anterior cruciate ligament.

forwards in relation to the femur (the anterior drawer sign) indicates injury to the medial collateral ligament and/or the anterior cruciate ligament. The anterior cruciate ligament is examined by carrying out the drawer test with the lower leg rotated inwards while the medial collateral ligament is examined by a drawer test with the lower leg rotated outwards.

c. *Testing of the anterior cruciate ligament*
The anterior drawer test with the knee joint bent to an angle of 10–20°, *Lachman's test*, is used to examine the integrity of the anterior cruciate

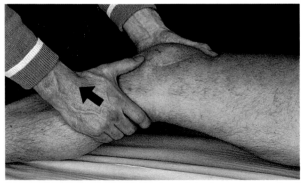

An anterior drawer test with the knee joint bent at an angle of 10–20°, Lachman's test.

ligament. The doctor holds down the patient's thigh on the lateral side with one hand and takes hold of the upper part of the lower leg on the medial side with the other hand. The lower leg is lifted forwards, and an anterior drawer sign can then be both seen and felt. A positive Lachman's test is a strong indication of a rupture in the anterior cruciate ligament.

The *flexion rotation drawer sign* is another stability test of the anterior cruciate ligament. The lower leg is held by the examiner and the knee is

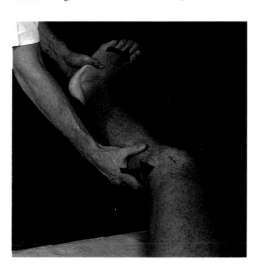

Stability examination of the anterior cruciate ligament – the pivot shift test.

passively flexed to about 20–30°; then the tibia subluxates forward (compare Lachman's test).

The '*pivot shift test*' and the '*jerk test*' are other methods that the doctor may use to decide whether there is an injury to the anterior cruciate ligament. He or she will rotate the foot on the injured side inwards with one hand and press the other hand against the lateral side of the upper part of the fibula.

In the 'pivot shift test' the examiner starts with the knee extended. The knee is pressed inwards (in valgus) during passive flexion and internal rotation of the lower leg. At 20–30° of flexion, a subluxation forward of

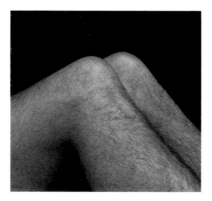
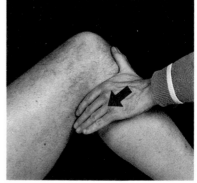

Left: on injury to the posterior cruciate ligament, lower leg of injured side is displaced backwards in relation to lower leg of uninjured side. **Right:** examination of the posterior cruciate ligament with a posterior drawer test.

the lateral tibial condyle can be seen. During further flexion to about 40–60°, the lateral condyle reduces and then the athlete experiences the 'giving way' phenomenon. The sequence of events for the 'jerk test' is reversed as the starting point is in flexion.

d. *Testing of the posterior cruciate ligaments*
The *posterior drawer sign*, that is, excessive backward movement of the tibia in relation to the femur, occurs in cases of injury to the posterior cruciate ligament. It is important that the doctor compares the contours of the healthy and injured knee joints in 90° flexion before performing the posterior drawer test. In cases of posterior cruciate ligament injury, it is not unusual for the lower leg on the injured side to be displaced backwards in relation to the lower leg on the healthy side. The forward pull of the lower leg to its normal position during the posterior drawer test can then be misinterpreted by the inexperienced examiner as a sign of an anterior cruciate ligament rupture.

6. *An X-ray examination* of the knee joint should be carried out to confirm or exclude a skeletal injury such as detachment of bone fragments at the points of insertion of the collateral or the cruciate ligaments. Arthrography (X-ray examination with contrast medium) is not necessary when the injury is in its acute stage.

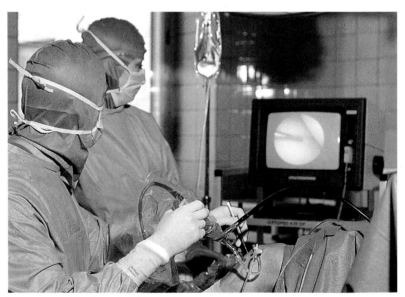

Inspection of the knee joint by arthroscopy.

7. *Aspiration of the knee joint* (withdrawal of fluid through a needle) can be performed in cases of extensive swelling in order to decide whether an effusion of blood is present. *When bleeding has occurred within the knee joint a serious injury inside the joint must be suspected.*

8. *Inspection of the joint by arthroscopy* means that the doctor examines the interior of the knee joint with a special instrument in order to obtain information about meniscus injuries, ligament injuries and injuries to the articular cartilage. The examination is performed under anaesthetic.

9. A *stability test of the knee joint under anaesthetic* is important if the diagnosis is uncertain and the patient is difficult to examine without anaesthesia. It should be carried out if pain is a limitation in the early stages of the injury. All the tests outlined here should be included.

Treatment of acute ligament injuries

The *athlete* should:
— start treatment as soon as possible according to the guidelines given on page 64;
— consult a doctor if there are symptoms such as pain during movement, limitation of movement, swelling of the knee joint, local tenderness along the course of the ligaments, or instability such as 'giving way'.

The *doctor* may:
— prescribe rest from sporting activity in cases of partial ligament injury, when there is no instabilty of the knee joint. Training of the muscles at the front and back of the thigh should start immediately. A support bandage or a plaster cast may sometimes be applied, and this treatment may be continued for some weeks;
— operate on unstable ligament injuries, especially combined instability, for example, collateral ligament injury together with anterior or posterior cruciate ligament injury. The ligament ends are sutured or reinserted into the exact anatomical postition. In cases of total rupture of the anterior or posterior cruciate ligaments, an augmentation is usually performed using, for example, a tendon or retinaculum. Post-operative management may vary from immobilization for 3–6 weeks to early protected movement or immediate continuous passive motion;
— immobilize in a plaster cast for some weeks followed by a movable cast for another 3 weeks in cases of total (grade III) isolated medial collateral ligament injury. This treatment can be used as an alternative to plaster immobilization or surgery. Total (grade III) rupture of the lateral collateral ligament usually requires surgical treatment for the best results;
— stress the importance of continuing training the thigh muscles in order to maintain their function. Such training should be carried out even when the leg is in plaster. After the plaster has been removed, training should be such that it increases the strength in the thigh muscles and the range of motion in the knee joint. A suggested training programme is described on page 444.

Treatment of old ligament injuries

It is not unusual for severe ligament injuries to be overlooked and for the patient to fail to consult a doctor during the acute stages. After a short period of rest, he or she then resumes training and competition. The knee is then often subjected to further trauma, or is found not to function satisfactorily. The indications of ligament instability and insufficiency are recognized by recurrent effusions or pain. These features get worse over the years when secondary restraints (ligament stabilizers) are insufficient.

The routine of the medical examination is basically the same in cases of old as in cases of acute ligament injuries, with an analysis of the mechanism of injury and stability tests. An X-ray examination with a contrast medium may be of value in assessing an old ligament injury. Arthroscopy will reveal the condition of the joint in detail.

Reconstruction of deficient collateral or cruciate ligaments is often a difficult task. The key to successful reconstruction is to stabilize all the deficient structures of the unstable knee. A new anterior cruciate ligament can be constructed inside the joint from a part of, for example, the patellar tendon, the semitendinosus tendon or the ilio-tibial band (intra-articular reconstruction). The function of the ligament can also be restored by using tissue taken from outside the joint, for example the ilio-tibial band (extra-articular reconstruction). A deficient collateral ligament can be stabilized by shortening. A deficient posterior cruciate ligament can be replaced by a free graft from the patellar tendon, the semitendinosus tendon or the ilio-tibial band. Treatment after surgery can include 6 weeks in plaster cast; in some cases this is replaced by an early range of motion training protected by a movable cast or brace, or by use of a continuous passive motion machine. The convalescence is more prolonged than that which follows an acute ligament injury and it often takes a year for a replaced ligament to regain the strength of the normal ligament. It is important that the injured athlete does not return to competitive sports too early and that there is satisfactory muscular strength in the leg.

Healing and complications

It is important that the injured athlete does not return to his usual training activity until the knee joint has attained almost full mobility, and the strength of the thigh musculature has returned. The period of physical fitness training after a ligament operation on the knee joint extends over the first 6–10 weeks after removal of the plaster. Only when the strength and function of the knee joint has been restored at leisure and the doctor in charge has been consulted should competitive sport be resumed.

After an operative reconstruction of ligaments of the knee joint the strength of these structures is reduced for up to one year. As a rule, competitive sports, particularly contact sports, should not be resumed before then. This is essential for the sake not only of the future functional capability of the knee joint but also of its renewed strength and mobility. With the introduction of artificial ligaments, the rehabilitation time may become shorter but clinical experience, so far, is too little.

Meniscus injuries

The menisci consist of a semilunar fibrocartilage, partly filling the space between the femoral and tibial articular surfaces. They stabilize the joint throughout its range of motion and contribute to the limitation of medial and lateral rotation as well as extension and flexion. They also serve as shock absorbers between the femur and tibia by increasing the contact area for weight-bearing. The menisci also take part in the lubrication of the joint.

Meniscus injuries occur in most sports but are commonest in contact sports. They often occur in combination with ligament injuries, particularly when the medial meniscus is involved. This is partly because the medial meniscus is attached to the medial collateral ligament and partly because tackles are often directed towards the lateral side of the knee, causing external rotation of the tibia. Injury to the medial meniscus is about five

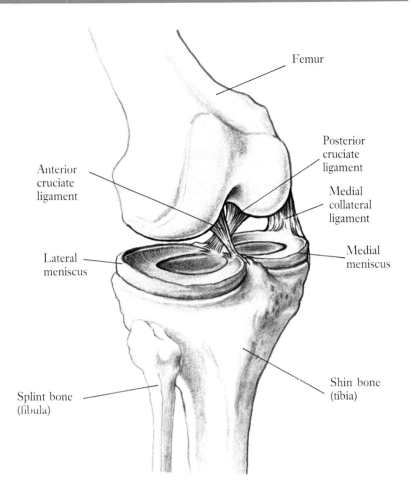

Anatomical diagram of the relationship between menisci, cruciate ligaments and medial collateral ligament. (Knee joint drawn diagonally from front, outer side).

times more common than injury to the lateral meniscus. Meniscal injuries are frequently caused by a twisting impact to the knee. In cases of outward (external) rotation of the foot and lower leg in relation to the femur, the medial meniscus is most vulnerable, while in cases of a corresponding inward (internal) rotation of the foot and lower leg the lateral meniscus is most easily injured. Meniscus injuries can also occur as a result of hyperextension and hyperflexion of the knee. In elderly individuals, a meniscus injury can occur during a normal body movement, such as deep knee bends, because of decreased strength due to degenerative changes.

When meniscus injuries have been caused by trauma the ruptures run vertically through the meniscal tissue (see diagram on page 298). In elderly people, horizontal ruptures are commoner.

Every suspected or confirmed meniscus injury should be subjected to a stability test by a doctor to exclude ligament deficiency.

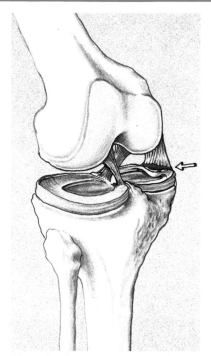

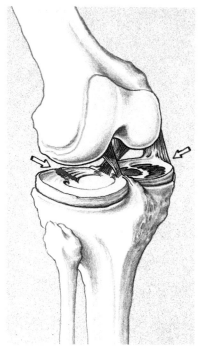

Example of a meniscus injury, showing detachment of the meniscus at its attachment to the medial collateral ligament.

Examples of meniscus injuries. **Right:** a longitudinal rupture. **Left:** a transverse rupture.

Medial meniscus injury

Symptoms and diagnosis

— Pain on the medial (inner) side of the knee joint during and after exertion.
— 'Locking', which means that the torn part of the meniscus is lodged in the joint thus blocking mobility so that a full extension or a full flexion is rendered impossible. The joint can lock momentarily of its own accord in certain positions.
— Pain which is located in the area of the medial joint line occurs during hyperextension and hyperflexion and also on turning the foot and lower leg outwards when the knee joint is flexed.
— Sometimes there is an effusion of fluid in the joint, especially after exertion.

The diagnosis of an internal meniscus injury is considered to be fairly certain if three or more of the following examination findings are present:
— tenderness at one point over the medial joint line;
— pain located in the area of the medial joint line during hyperextension of the knee joint;
— pain located in the area of the medial joint line during hyperflexion of the knee joint;
— pain during external rotation (outward turning) of the foot and the lower leg when the knee is flexed at different angles around 90°;
— weakened or atrophied quadriceps muscle.

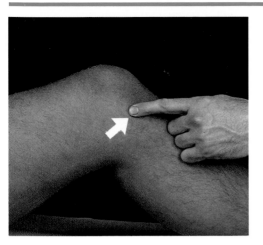

Injury to the medial meniscus; tenderness can occur over the inner synovial cavity (see arrow).

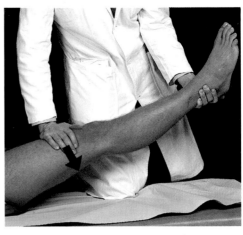

Injury to the lateral meniscus; pain can occur if the knee joint is over-extended.

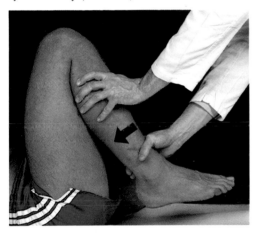

Injury to the medial or lateral meniscus; pain can occur in the knee joint during vigorous flexion of the joint.

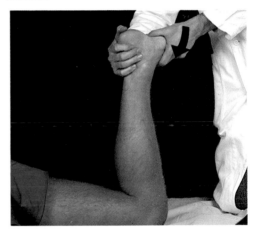

Injury to the medial meniscus; pain can occur when foot and lower leg are rotated externally with knee bent at 90°. Injury to the external meniscus; pain can occur when the foot and lower leg are rotated internally keeping knee bent at 90°.

Arthroscopy of the joint is the most certain way of confirming a diagnosis of meniscus injury. In doubtful cases an X-ray with contrast medium can also be helpful.

Lateral meniscus injury

Symptoms and diagnosis
— Pain which is located in the lateral aspect of the joint occurs in connection with exertion of the knee joint. In many cases the pain appears consistently after a specific amount of exertion.
— Locking phenomenon (see above).

— Pain located in the area of the lateral joint line occurs on hyperextension and hyperflexion of the knee and also on internal rotation of the foot and the lower leg in relation to the femur when the knee joint is flexed to 90°.
— Sometimes there is effusion of fluid in the joint.

The diagnosis of a lateral meniscus injury is considered to be fairly certain if three or more of the following findings are present on examination:
— tenderness at one point over the lateral joint line;
— pain located in the area of the lateral joint line during hyperextension of the knee joint;
— pain located in the area of the lateral joint line during hyperflexion of the knee joint;
— pain during internal rotation of the foot and the lower leg when the knee is flexed at different angles;
— weakened or atrophied quadriceps.

Arthroscopy confirms the diagnosis and an X-ray with contrast medium can be helpful.

Treatment

The *athlete* should:
— when he suspects a meniscus injury, carry out static quadriceps muscle exercises. It is important that anyone waiting for knee surgery should also train the thigh muscles daily according to the guidelines given on page 91. This prevents unnecessary weakening of the muscles, and enables rehabilitation to be shortened considerably.

The *doctor* may:
— operate by removing a portion or repair by suturing back the damaged part of the meniscus. In cases of acute locking the injury should be operated on as soon as possible. Certain types of meniscus injuries can be operated on successfully during arthroscopy. The doctor then makes small incisions in the joint through which various instruments are inserted. The damaged part of the meniscus is held with a pair of forceps and is cut loose with small scalpels (or scissors) which are inserted into the joint during arthroscopic observation. In this way, the operation scars as well as pain and swelling can be reduced in comparison with the usual 'open' meniscus surgery, and the knee joint regains its functional ability more quickly. In the long run, the end result is similar whichever method of operation is used;
— prescribe training of the quadriceps and hamstring muscles (see page 91). The training is started as soon as possible after surgery. Crutches can be used for 1–2 weeks so that the operated leg is relieved of some weight. Loading the knee joint to the pain threshold is allowed.

Healing and complications

An athlete who has been operated on for a meniscus injury should not return to his ordinary training until he has regained almost full mobility and strength of the knee joint. This usually takes 4–8 weeks following surgery and 2–4 weeks after transarthroscopic surgery. *Even after he has returned to his sporting activity he should continue training the quadriceps and hamstrings muscles.*

Some months after surgical removal of the meniscus a new meniscus of somewhat weaker connective tissue is sometimes formed in the knee joint. This meniscus in its turn can tear, giving symptoms similar to those of the original meniscus injury.

People who have had a meniscus operation can, after many years' loading of the knee joint, be affected by degenerative changes in the articular cartilages caused by increased wear on the surfaces.

Articular cartilage surface injuries

Injuries to the articular cartilage surfaces of the knee joint can affect the joint surfaces of the femur, the tibia and the patella. Such injuries are often disregarded as they can be difficult to identify. They may occur in connection with direct impact against the knee joint but can also occur in association with meniscal and ligament injuries. Indeed, any condition that leads to excessive repetitive forces can cause symptoms. Cartilage damage can result in large cracks and defects on the joint surfaces and continued degeneration. The end result can be premature osteoarthritis.

Symptoms and diagnosis
— Swelling in the knee joint because of recurrent effusions.
— Pain which occurs during exertion and can mimic a meniscal injury.
— The injury can be confirmed by examination of the joint with an arthroscope.

Treatment
The *athlete* should:
— train the thigh musculature;
— use a heat retainer.

The *doctor* may:
— operate, for example, by removing the damaged cartilage which is gradually replaced by less elastic fibrocartilage;
— recommend that the injured person change to a sport which makes fewer demands on the knee joints.

Osteochondritis dissecans (release of bone fragments and cartilage into knee joint)

The release of fragments of bone and cartilage into the knee joint is a condition which often afflicts young people between the ages of twelve and sixteen years, permanently affecting the articular surface of the femur. The location of the injury is often obvious (see diagram on page 302). The condition causes the cartilage and bone to disintegrate in an area which may be as large as a hazelnut. Gradually the whole of the altered

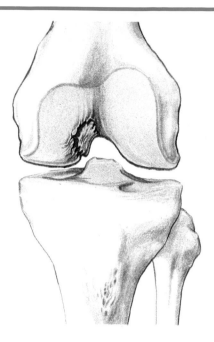

Release of a fragment of bone and cartilage in the knee joint.

area or parts of it can break away from the underlying bone and give rise to loose bodies in the joint. The result is locking and recurrent effusions.

Symptoms and diagnosis

— Pain during and recurrent aching after knee exercise which involves the knee joint. The pain is often widespread.
— Locking of the knee joint.
— Recurrent effusions in the joint.
— An X-ray examination confirms the diagnosis.
— Inspection of the joint with an arthroscope can be of help in deciding upon appropriate treatment. Any loose bodies can be removed via the arthroscope.

Treatment

The *doctor* may:
— prescribe rest when the injury is slight;
— immobilize in a plaster cast if the athlete is young and has a short history of symptoms;
— operate in symptomatic cases. The operation involves pinning the fragments of bone and cartilage in an attempt to prevent further disintegration of the articular surface. Fresh bodies may be pinned; old loose bodies are removed.

Healing

The affected athlete may return to sporting activity 3–6 months after the operation, but only after having consulted a doctor. Before returning, the athlete should have built up muscular strength and mobility by training.

Patello-femoral pain syndrome (chondromalacia patellae)

Damage to the articular surface of the patella usually occurs in individuals aged ten to twenty-five years and is associated with pain, especially on walking up and down hills and stairs and when squatting.

It is quite common for pain to occur in the knee joints when walking up and down hills and stairs. Compared with the normal flexion of the joint on flat ground, knee flexion increases considerably during these activities, thereby increasing compression between the patella and the femur. Walking *up* hills and stairs causes less pain than walking *down*, because during ascent the knee joint is flexed at an angle of about 50° under load, while on descent it is flexed at an angle of about 80° under load. In contrast to the situation when walking uphill, the body does not lean forward when walking downhill, so knee flexion is controlled by the quadriceps muscles alone, resulting in an increase in the compression forces between the patella and the femur.

The mechanism of this condition is unknown, but in some cases it is probably the result of repeated minor impacts or occasional major impacts on the knee joint, including direct falls and prolonged static or dynamic load on the knee joint during such pursuits as sailing, downhill skiing, weightlifting and strength training.

There may well be no evidence that the patella has been subjected to external impact, and other factors which may contribute to the condition include:

— a protruding patella;
— underdeveloped patella;
— constricting structures lateral to the patella;
— deep knee bends causing excessive cartilage loads;
— a patella which dislocates totally or partially;
— q-angle over 20° (this is the angle formed between a line through the line of action of the rectus femoris muscle and a similar line through the patellar tendon) which results in lateral movement of the patella;
— incorrect functioning of the extensor mechanism of the knee joint (malalignment);
— increased outward turning (pronation) of the foot and thereby increased inward rotation of the lower leg which alters both the q-angle and the direction of pull of the quadriceps;
— weak quadriceps muscles;
— fracture of the patella;
— increased angle between the tibia and femur (genu valgum).

The cartilage lining the articular surface of the patella can soften, fray and roughen with the formation of cracks and blisters (see diagram on page 304). Because of its lack of nerve supply, the cartilage itself is not painful, but pain can be caused when the patella slips and presses against the surface of the femur when the protective function of the cartilage has been eroded. Pain can also be caused by inflammation of the joint capsule.

Symptoms and diagnosis

— Widespread pain in the joint and behind the patella during exertion or load, for example when the affected person is sitting with the knee bent.

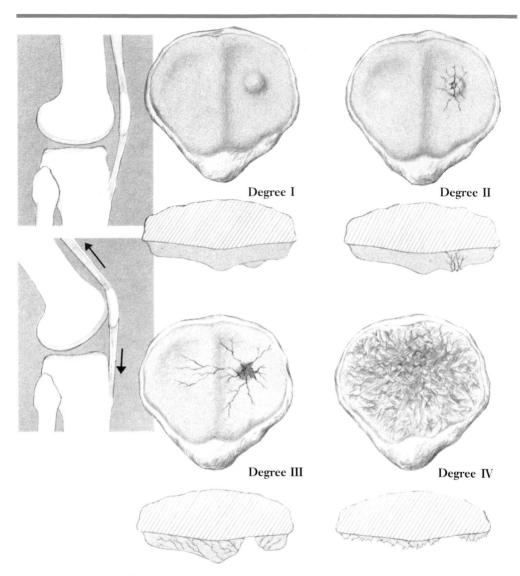

Degree I

Degree II

Degree III

Degree IV

The diagrams left show the location of the patella in relation to the thigh bone during extension (top left) and flexion (bottom left). During flexion the patella is pressed hard against the thigh bone. The diagrams above and right show the cartilage of the inner surface of the patella. **Degree I**: softening and blistering. **Degree II**: continued softening and crack formation. **Degree III**: crack formation down to the underlying bone and undermining of surrounding cartilage tissue. **Degree IV**: total destruction of the cartilage and the exposure of bone.

— The problems are accentuated when walking or running on hills and stairs, especially during descent.
— Pain and stiffness can be felt on rising from a sitting to a standing position. The problems are made worse by squatting.
— Pain when the patella is compressed against the femur.
— Tenderness around the patella.
— 'Creaking', during flexion and extension of the knee, from behind the patella.

— Sometimes a slight effusion in the knee joint is noticeable; also laxity and a tendency of the patella to subluxate.
— Increased (above 20°) q-angle;
— Malalignment of the lower limb including increased pronation of the foot, malrotation of the tibia, genu valgum (increased angle between tibia and femur), increased anteversion of the neck of the femur, increased rotation of the femur and so on, may be significant factors.
— Incorrect foot position and weakness of the thigh muscles, particularly the lower fibres attached to the inner side of the patella, may be significant.
— X-rays of the knee joint from a variety of angles can be carried out.
— Inspection of the joint with an arthroscope confirms the diagnosis.

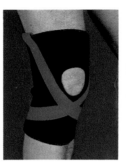 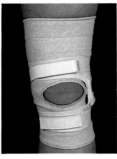

Two types of knee pad. Both prevent the dislocation of the patella and also injuries to the joint between the patella and the thigh bone.

Treatment

The *athlete* should:
— rest from painful activities;
— apply local heat;
— use a supportive brace or a heat retainer with a notch and a support for the patella (see photograph above);
— train the quadriceps and hamstring muscles by static exercise (see page 91) and also practise stretching.

The *doctor* may:
— prescribe rest and physiotherapy;
— prescribe anti-inflammatory medication when the condition is in its acute stage;
— carry out arthroscopy in order to make the diagnosis;
— operate in cases of prolonged symptoms which are difficult to treat. Sometimes degenerative articular cartilage can be removed from behind the patella during arthroscopy 'shaving'.

Healing

The problems caused by patello-femoral pain (chondromalacia patellae) can disappear spontaneously, though this can take up to 1 or 2 years. An affected athlete must often change training habits and sporting activity, above all avoiding movements that trigger pain.

Dislocation of the patella

Dislocation of the patella can occur as a result of violent impact on a normal patella, for example in soccer, and also after a minor or indirect impact on a small, underdeveloped patella, or patellar groove, for example

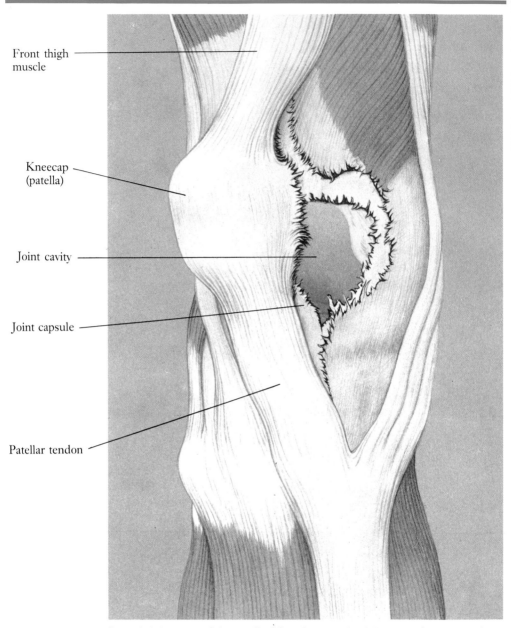

Front thigh muscle

Kneecap (patella)

Joint cavity

Joint capsule

Patellar tendon

Lateral dislocation of the patella. Note the extensive injury to soft tissues with ruptures in and around the knee capsule.

when an athlete changes direction of movement and then straightens his leg. The dislocation usually occurs outwardly (laterally). Fragments of bone and cartilage may be dislodged and become loose in the joint, and a tear of the joint capsule on the inner (medial) ridge of the patella can occur. The injury often affects young people aged fourteen to eighteen years and is not uncommon among athletes over the age of twenty-five. It is sometimes combined with a meniscus and medial collateral ligament injury and can also be confused with them. In cases of dislocation of the patella the injured person should be taken to hospital.

Symptoms
— Bleeding causing swelling in the knee joint.
— Tenderness over the medial ridge of the patella.
— Impaired mobility in the knee joint.
— Displacement of the patella.

Treatment
The *doctor* may:
— reduce the patella under anaesthetic if it has not already slipped back by itself, and request an X-ray examination;
— examine the joint by arthroscopy in order to evaluate the extent of the injury; loose fragments of bone and cartilage can then be removed;
— operate, when the patella is normally developed, if there are loose fragments of bone in the joint or fragments of bone torn away from the articular surface. At the same time the joint capsule is sutured. As an alternative, a knee immobilizer or a cast alone could be considered. When the patella is small and underdeveloped the dislocation has a tendency to be recurrent, so more extensive plastic (reconstructive) surgery must be considered in this case. A recurrent dislocation is, however, unusual in athletes over the age of twenty-five years.

Local inflammation of tendon and muscle attachments around the patella

Local inflammation of tendon and muscle attachments around the patella is caused by overuse, and most often affects the insertion of the quadriceps muscle into the patella. The hamstring insertions into the back and sides of the knee joint can also be affected.

Symptoms and diagnosis
— Pain in the knee during and after exertion. Pain is triggered on contraction of the muscles involved.
— Stiffness the day after a training period or a competition.
— Local tenderness in the tendon or muscle attachment.

Treatment
The *athlete* should:
— rest, which should clear the symptoms within a few weeks;
— apply local heat and use a heat retainer.

The *doctor* may:
— administer a local steroid injection and prescribe rest;
— prescribe anti-inflammatory medication;
— apply a plaster cast for some weeks.

Rupture of the lower part of the quadriceps femoris muscle

Muscle ruptures around the knee most commonly affect the quadriceps muscle in the front of the thigh. Part of the muscle, usually the rectus femoris, can rupture where it joins the tendon above the patella, or the tendon itself can become detached from its insertion in the patella.

Symptoms and diagnosis
— Tenderness and swelling where the muscle merges into the tendon above the patella or where the tendon inserts into the patella.
— A gap can be felt where the rupture has occurred.
— The injured person cannot actively extend the knee.

Treatment
The *doctor* :
— may treat with bandaging and gradually increasing strength and mobility training;
— should not operate in cases of a partial rupture as the injury usually does not lead to any noticeably impaired function in the long run;
— may operate in cases of major ruptures in young athletes when the tendon is avulsed from the patella;
— may operate on old injuries of this type.

Injury to the patellar tendon ('jumpers knee')

The patellar tendon runs between the patella and a protuberance on the upper anterior surface of the tibia (the tibial tuberosity). An injury to this tendon characteristically affects athletes involved in jumping and throwing sports, badminton, volleyball and basketball players and weightlifters, and it consists of a partial rupture of the tendon, often at the point of its attachment to the patella. In adolescents there may be a calcification of the attachment on the patella (apophysitis). In middle-aged and elderly athletes, microruptures may occur in a degenerative, damaged tendon. In its acute stage this injury is seldom noticed, but if the injured athlete resumes sporting activity before it has healed, inflammation occurs and can lead to prolonged and recurrent problems.

Symptoms and diagnosis
— Pain over the tendon (often at its point of attachment to the lower pole of the patella) during exertion, for example knee bending with load.
— Pain, aching and stiffness after exertion. The injured person can enter a typical cycle of pain (see page 41).
— Pain is triggered if the quadriceps is contracted, loading the kneecap and the tendon.
— Tenderness often distinctly located at tendon attachment to the patella.
— An X-ray examination of the soft tissues may show swelling and calcification (in adolescents) and support the diagnosis as can an ultrasonic examination of the tendon.

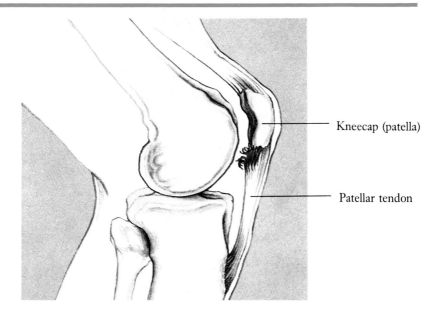

Kneecap (patella)

Patellar tendon

'Jumper's knee' – a partial rupture of the top posterior portion of the patellar tendon.

Treatment

The *athlete* should:
— cool with ice in the acute phase;
— apply ice massage;
— rest until there is no pain under load;
— apply local heat and use a heat retainer after the acute phase.

The *doctor* may:
— use plaster immobilization in the acute phase;
— prescribe anti-inflammatory medication;
— operate if the injury has not healed after a period of rest, or in chronic cases. The ruptured part of the tendon is removed so that healing is facilitated. After surgery the knee joint should be in a plaster cast for 4–6 weeks.

Healing

After the plaster cast treatment has finished the injured athlete should devote 2–4 months to rehabilitative training, at first in the form of flexibility training and carefully planned strength training initially using only the weight of the body as the load. Only after thorough rehabilitation should the athlete return to sport-specific training.

Osgood-Schlatter's disease (traction periostitis of the tibial tuberosity)

Osgood-Schlatter's disease describes the condition in which the tibial attachment of the patellar tendon becomes the seat of inflammation and

309

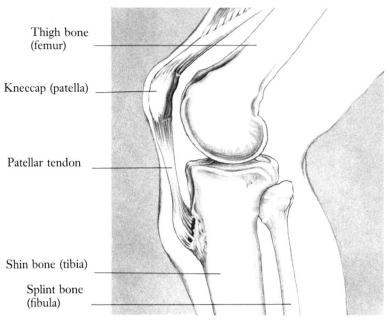

Thigh bone
(femur)

Kneecap (patella)

Patellar tendon

Shin bone (tibia)

Splint bone
(fibula)

Osgood-Schlatter's
disease. The bone is
inflamed and broken
up at the attachment of
the patellar tendon to
the shin bone.

disintegration of bone. The causes are unclear, but the condition is probably due to traction periostitis caused by overuse. It is primarily boys aged
between ten and sixteen who are affected.

**Symptoms and
diagnosis**

— Pain at the attachment of the tendon to the tibia during and after
exertion.
— Pain that can be triggered on contraction of the quadriceps against
resistance.
— Swelling and tenderness over the attachment of the patellar tendon to
the tibia.
— An X-ray examination may show fragmentation of the bone and inflammatory changes in the tibial tuberosity.

Treatment

The *athlete* should:
— rest;
— apply local heat and use a heat retainer;
— avoid movements that trigger pain.

The *doctor* may:
— apply a plaster cast for 3 weeks when pain is severe. This can result
in resolution of symptoms at least for a period of time;
— recommend change in type or level of activity.

**Healing and
complications**

Osgood-Schlatter's disease heals spontaneously. The problems can,
however, recur with further overloading of the patellar tendon in
adolescents, though this seldom occurs after the leg is fully developed at
seventeen to eighteen years of age. Problems that appear in older athletes
may be caused by loose bodies having formed in the bursa under the
patellar tendon. These can be removed by surgery with good results.

Bursitis around the knee joint

Around the knee joint there are a number of bursae (synovial sacs that can produce fluid) each of which can be damaged and/or become the site of inflammation. When the bursa anterior to the kneecap (patella) is involved the condition is often called 'housemaid's knee' and when the bursa below the knee is involved 'carpet-layer's knee'.

It is common for the pre-patellar bursa (anterior to the patella) to be

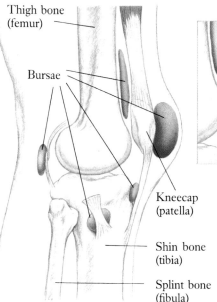

Thigh bone (femur)

Bursae

Kneecap (patella)

Shin bone (tibia)

Splint bone (fibula)

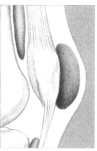 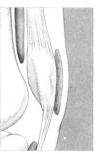 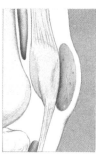

Left: schematic diagram of the location of the bursae around the knee joint. The diagram also shows acute bleeding in the anterior bursa of the kneecap. **Above left**: untreated bleeding, adhesions and loose bodies. **Above middle**: residual condition with scar tissue and adhesions after bleeding. **Above right**: chronic inflammation caused by adhesions and loose bodies.

affected by injuries, and bleeding can occur into it after impact and cause haemobursa or bursitis. Repeated movement and pressure can also cause acute or chronic bursitis. The other bursae around the knee joint may be similarly, but perhaps less often, affected.

The first symptoms of injuries to bursae and of bursitis are swelling, caused by bleeding, and tenderness. Pain is triggered when the knee joint is bent or straightened. If haemobursa has been present small loose bodies can later form in the bursa as a result of blood clots. These loose bodies can cause inflammation and effusion. Chronic irritant conditions in the bursae can also cause similar problems, and sometimes stop participation in sport, for example, in wrestlers who load the patella with the knee bent.

Symptoms and diagnosis
— Persistent pain from the area where the bursa is located, mainly on exertion of the knee joint.
— Tenderness and swelling over the bursa.
— Sometimes the skin over the bursa is hot and red.
— A spongy resistance on pressure against the bursa indicates an effusion.

Treatment
The *athlete* should:
— treat acute bursa problems according to the guidelines given on page 47;
— use a protective brace to unload the bursa.

The *doctor* may:
— aspirate and drain the bursa;
— administer a steroid injection into the bursa after it has been drained;
— operate in case of prolonged problems in order to remove loose bodies from the bursa or to remove the bursa itself;
— apply a compression bandage.

Distended bursa behind the knee, Baker's cyst, popliteal cyst

A distended bursa in the hollow behind the knee (the popliteal space) is a relatively uncommon condition which manifests itself as a swelling of the posterior joint capsule of the knee joint. The bursa is connected with the joint (see diagram below), and when an irritant condition is present with an effusion in the joint, synovial fluid can be pressed out into the bursa so that it becomes distended.

Symptoms and diagnosis

— A sensation of pressure which mainly affects the popliteal space but which may also be transmitted down into the calf muscles.
— Difficulties in bending and straightening the knee joint completely.
— Aching and tenderness after exertion of the knee joint.
— The distended bursa appears as a rounded, fluctuant swelling, usually the size of a golf ball but sometimes up to the size of a tennis ball when the knee joint is held in extension.

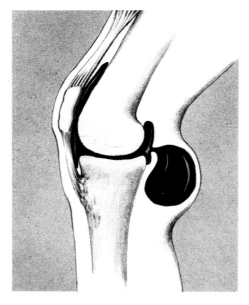

The bursa in the hollow of the knee (Baker's cyst).

— An X-ray examination of the knee joint with a contrast medium (arthrography) can show filling of the bursa.
— Arthroscopy can reveal the cause of the effusion in the knee joint.

Treatment

The *athlete* should:
— rest. The symptoms may then disappear by themselves.

The *doctor* may:
— treat any cause of the effusion in the knee joint;
— remove the bursa by surgery if it is causing problems.

Healing

The injured athlete can return to his sporting activity 8–12 weeks after surgery. Baker's cyst often disappears spontaneously in children.

'Runner's knee' (the ilio-tibial band syndrome)

'Runner's knee' is the everyday name of a painful condition which is located in the lateral side of the knee joint over the epicondyle of the femur and which affects athletes who undertake prolonged running practice. Runners with excessive pronation of their feet have an increased risk of being affected by this injury (see page 356); also runners who run on cambered roads.

Symptoms and diagnosis

— Pain which usually starts after the athlete has run a certain distance and which then increases so that it becomes impossible to continue. After resting for a while the pain disappears, but it recurs if running is resumed. The problems often increase when running downhill.
— Local tenderness in the lateral side of the knee joint over the femoral epicondyle and anterior to the origin of the lateral collateral ligament.
— On flexion and extension of the knee joint, the strong lateral band called the ilio-tibial band, slides across the lateral side of the epicondyle of the femur causing local inflammation (synovitis/bursitis).
— Signs of increased foot pronation.

Treatment

The *athlete* should:
— avoid running downhill or on the side of the road;
— apply ice in the acute phase;
— rest actively;
— apply local heat after the acute phase and use a heat retainer;
— practise static stretching (see page 96) of the tissues on the lateral aspect of the thigh.

The *doctor* may:
— prescribe anti-inflammatory medications;
— administer a local steroid injection and prescribe rest;
— prescribe shoe insertions (orthotics) in cases of increased pronation;
— resort to surgery.

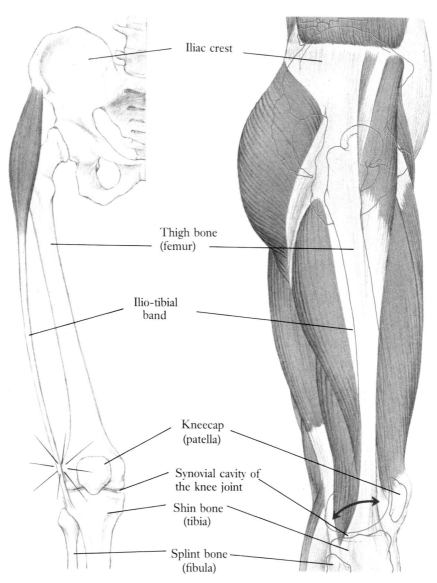

Iliac crest

Thigh bone
(femur)

Ilio-tibial
band

Kneecap
(patella)

Synovial cavity of
the knee joint

Shin bone
(tibia)

Splint bone
(fibula)

'Runner's knee'. **Right:** this shows how the ilio-tibial band lies close to the lateral side of the femur; **left:** this shows how the ilio-tibial band slips backwards and forwards over the lower, lateral part of the femur when bending and straightening the knee joint.

Inflammation of the popliteal tendon

Inflammation of the popliteal tendon is a relatively uncommon injury, but it is one cause of pain on the outer side of the knee joint. The popliteal tendon has its origin on the lateral (outer) aspect of the femur (the lateral condyle) and first runs beneath the lateral collateral ligament, then backwards to attach to the tibia. The popliteus muscle and its tendon are called into action when beginning to bend the knee and when the tibia is rotated inwards. This injury is experienced by runners.

Symptoms and diagnosis
— The characteristic symptom of inflammation of the popliteal tendon is pain on the lateral side of the knee joint when it is bent at an angle of about 15–30° and under load. The pain occurs above all when walking or running downhill and downstairs.
— Local tenderness on palpation over the tendon attachment on the lateral aspect of the femur just anterior to the lateral collateral ligament. This tenderness is most apparent if the injured person sits down after the examination and holds the knee joint of the injured leg at an angle of 90° with the foot placed on the knee joint of the healthy leg.
— Pain can occur when rotating the lower leg inwards.
— Before the diagnosis is made the doctor should check that there is no injury to the lateral meniscus.

Treatment
The *athlete* should:
— rest actively;
— apply local heat and use a heat retainer;
— run on an even and level surface and also avoid hills and cambered roads.

The *doctor* may:
— prescribe anti-inflammatory medication;
— administer a local injection of steroid and prescribe rest;
— operate in cases of prolonged and severe problems.

Injury to the biceps femoris muscle

The biceps muscle in the thigh is one of the hamstring muscles and is a knee flexor which can be affected by partial or total rupture and also by injuries due to overuse. The most frequent injury in the knee joint region occurs where the muscle inserts as a tendon into the head of the fibula (see diagram on page 316), and fragments of bone can sometimes be torn away. The injury may occur in combination with a tear of the lateral collateral ligament and is seen in contact sports and also sometimes among wrestlers, track and field athletes and others.

Symptoms and diagnosis
— Local tenderness and swelling over the insertion of the biceps into the posterior aspect of the head of the fibula.
— Pain starts when the knee joint is bent against resistance.
— Absence of muscle function in cases of total rupture.
— In cases of injury due to overuse a typical pain cycle is present (see page 41).
— An X-ray examination can sometimes show that fragments of bone have been torn loose.

315

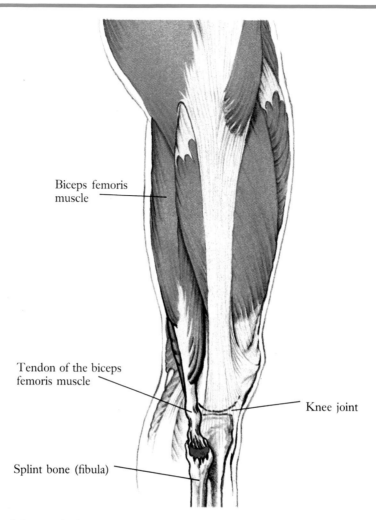

Biceps femoris muscle

Tendon of the biceps femoris muscle

Knee joint

Splint bone (fibula)

Injury to the biceps femoris muscle at its insertion in the fibula.

Treatment

The *athlete* should:
— apply ice and bandage in the acute phase;
— rest, apply local heat and use a heat retainer until there is no pain under load;
— carry out strength and stretching exercises after the acute phase.

The *doctor* may:
— prescribe anti-inflammatory medication;
— apply a plaster cast in cases of rupture;
— operate when there is a total rupture.

Fractures of the patella

The patella can be cracked by transverse or longitudinal fractures or shattered by stellate fractures. The injury often occurs as a result of falls on to the knee. When the fragments are displaced, surgery is required followed by about 4 weeks' plaster cast treatment. When there is no displacement a plaster cast will usually suffice. A transverse patellar fracture often requires no more than bandaging. The patient should subsequently be instructed in isometric thigh muscle training.

INJURIES OF THE LOWER LEG

The lower part of the leg comprises the shin bone (tibia) and the splint bone (fibula) and is connected at the top to the knee joint and at the bottom to the ankle joint.

Fractures

Fractures of the lower leg occur most frequently in Alpine skiers but also cross country skiers, riders and players in contact sports such as American football, soccer, rugby and ice hockey.

In Alpine skiing, the injury occurs most frequently in skiers aged approximately nineteen years and there is no difference in incidence by sex. Snow conditions are an important consideration in tibial fractures. In a study in Vermont, it was found that on icy or hard packed surfaces, the incidence of tibial fractures was low while it was high on powder snow. These data demonstrate the need for efficient release bindings. Modern

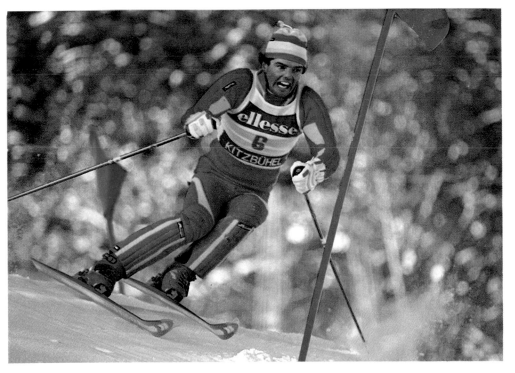

Fractures are not uncommon among downhill skiers. *Photo: Dan Ljungsvik.*

ski boots end above the middle lower leg and so called 'boot top' fractures can occur at this level. A contributory factor may be that the binding of the ski has not released. Improved equipment in recent years has resulted in a decrease in the number of lower leg fractures. Tibial fractures are relatively unusual in cross country skiing but they do occur. Inability of the skier to free the heel from the binding in a weighted twisted fall may result in transmission of damaging torque from the ski to the lower leg.

Soccer fractures can occur when the lower leg is kicked by an opponent while the foot is loaded. Rugby tackles or an opponent tripping over an outstretched leg may also cause fractures.

The tibia and fibula may fracture simultaneously or separately. As a rule the injury is more serious if both bones are affected, particularly if the broken ends penetrate the skin causing a compound fracture. The different types of fracture can be seen on page 18.

Fractures of the tibia and fibula

Symptoms and diagnosis
— Intense, instantaneous pain in the injured area.
— Tenderness and swelling over the fracture.
— Inability to use the injured leg.
— The normal contour and alignment of the lower leg can be deranged as a result of displacement of the fractured bones.

Treatment
When treating fractures it is important to remember that the soft tissues around the injury are also damaged. Guidelines for emergency treatment can be found on page 64.

The *trainer* should:
— cover an open wound as soon as possible with a sterile compress or something similar. If qualified medical staff are expected to arrive shortly, further measures should wait;
— transport the injured athlete to hospital as soon as possible. If no suitable means of transport is immediately available, an attempt can be made, with the utmost care, to put the leg into its correct position and, if possible, to splint it;
— do not give the injured athlete anything to eat or drink as this can delay his treatment on arrival at hospital. If an anaesthetic is required, it may be delayed for several hours if the patient has eaten or taken fluids.

The *doctor* may:
— examine the injured area and nerve function and circulation distal to the injury;
— X-ray the injury;
— realign the bones if necessary and put the leg in a plaster cast which, for the first 4–8 weeks, should include the foot, the lower leg and the thigh right up to the groin. Thereafter a Patellar Tendon Bearing plaster is applied up to the knee joint. The plaster treatment usually lasts for 8–12 weeks or sometimes longer;
— operate if necessary. The bone ends can be fixed with steel wire or a plate and screws. After surgery, plaster may be applied for 4–12 weeks, if necessary.

Healing and complications	After the period of plaster treatment there follows a period of roughly the same length during which mobility and strength are improved by training. A return to competitive sports is usually not possible for at least 6 months after the injury. In cases of a fracture of the tibia there can be complications such as non-healing with false joint formation (pseudoarthrosis). This condition is difficult to treat and often requires surgery followed by several more months' plaster treatment.

Fractures of the fibula alone

When the fibula is fractured, a simultaneous injury occurs at the moment of injury to the syndesmosis, that is, the strong ligaments that unite the fibula and the tibia at the ankle joint (see diagram on page 346). It is therefore important that the ankle joint is examined for stability by a doctor and X-rayed.

Symptoms and diagnosis	— Pain and tenderness over the fracture. — Pain when the leg is under load. — When the syndesmosis is damaged the ankle joint shows swelling, tenderness and instability.
Treatment	A *doctor* may X-ray the lower leg and also the ankle joint and examine the stability of the latter. An isolated fracture of the fibula without displacement often requires only rest and no plaster treatment, but when the syndesmosis is injured surgical repair of the ligaments is necessary.
Healing	The healing time varies between 4 and 6 weeks, depending on the extent of the fracture. If an injury of the syndesmosis is present the deltoid ligament can be ruptured (see page 346).

Pain in the lower leg

The musculature of the lower leg is enclosed in four tight, inflexible compartments of connective tissue which are anchored to the tibia and fibula. A cross-section through the lower leg about 4 in (10 cm) below the knee joint shows that the four compartments are clearly defined (see diagram on page 320). In front, between the tibia and the fibula, there is an anterior compartment which contains the tibialis anterior muscle, the toe extensors and the blood vessels and nerves which supply the anterior aspect of the lower leg and foot. At the back the lower leg is divided into two compartments, one deep and one superficial. The deep one, which is located between the tibia and the fibula and behind the tight connective tissue band (interosseus membrane) that connects the two, contains the long toe flexors (flexor digitorum longus and flexor hallucis longus) and the tibialis posterior muscle. Nerves and blood vessels pass to the back of the lower leg and the sole of the foot through this deep compartment. The posterior superficial muscle compartment at the back contains the broad, deep calf muscle (the soleus) and the superficial calf muscle (the gastrocnemius). On the lateral aspect of the leg, around the fibula, is a lateral compartment which encloses the long and short muscles that arise from that bone (the peroneus longus and the peroneus brevis).

Compartment syndromes in general

Compartment syndromes are painful conditions caused by increased pressure inside the different muscle compartments. They may be acute or chronic.

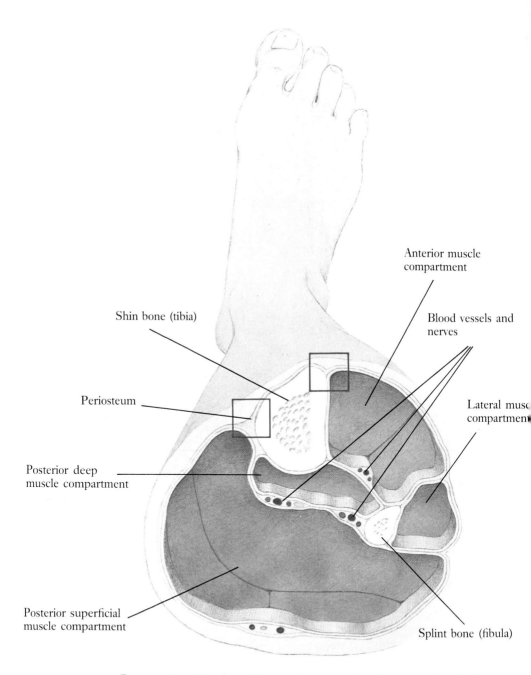

Anterior muscle compartment

Shin bone (tibia)

Blood vessels and nerves

Periosteum

Lateral muscle compartment

Posterior deep muscle compartment

Posterior superficial muscle compartment

Splint bone (fibula)

Cross-section of lower leg. The muscles are enclosed in four well-defined muscle compartments. The squares indicate common sites of tenderness at the anchor points of muscle compartments to the periosteum of the shin bone.

Acute compartment syndromes

Acute compartment syndromes can arise as a result of:

— external impact which causes a soft tissue injury with bleeding inside a compartment;
— a muscle rupture with bleeding inside a compartment;
— overuse, for example, from running on a hard surface without having prepared for or adjusted to it.

Chronic compartment syndromes

Chronic compartment syndromes can occur as a result of the increase in muscle bulk following prolonged training. The increase in bulk causes the musculature to grow larger than is allowed for by the surrounding fasciae since these tight membranes are not particularly elastic. When the muscles are at rest there is no problem, but during muscular work thousands of small blood vessels dilate in order to increase the blood flow and thus increase the bulk of the muscles too. Pressure is increased if a muscle in the lower leg is then required to work for any length of time and the blood flow is obstructed, causing a relative lack of oxygen. This changes the cell environment by the formation of lactic acid, and fluid begins to leak from the capillaries. Swelling (oedema) occurs within the muscle and this further increases the pressure on the muscle compartment, impairing blood flow even more. This vicious circle continues unless exercise ceases. Muscular contraction within the compartments can also exert traction on the periosteum, causing it to become inflamed (periostitis).

Compartment syndromes can give symptoms at the front, at the back and on each side of the lower leg.

Pain in the front of the lower leg

Anterior compartment syndrome

Acute anterior compartment syndrome can occur as a result of direct impact, for example a kick or a blow, to the tibialis anterior muscle. This is, however, uncommon as the muscle lies well protected at the side of the tibia. Acute bleeding in the anterior compartment of the lower leg can lead to greatly increased pressure which in turn impairs the blood flow in blood vessels that pass through the muscle compartment. Of most importance is the artery which supplies the anterior part of the dorsum of the foot, and this artery can become completely blocked, an acute condition requiring surgery. The operation involves opening the muscle compartment and removing blood and debris. See also the section on muscle haematoma on page 31.

Acute anterior compartment syndrome due to overuse can be triggered by the athlete training or competing too intensively, perhaps on a hard surface and without being properly prepared.

Symptoms and diagnosis

— A characteristic symptom is acute pain which gradually increases until it becomes impossible to continue running.
— Weakness can occur when the foot is bent upwards.
— A sensation of numbness extending down into the foot may be felt.

— Local swelling and tenderness can be present over the tibialis anterior muscle.
— Pain can be triggered when the foot or toes are passively bent downwards (plantar flexion).

Treatment

The *athlete* should:
— rest actively;
— cool the injured area.

The *doctor* may:
— prescribe diuretics;
— prescribe anti-inflammatory medication;
— check the effectiveness of the treatment by measuring the pressure in the muscle compartment;
— operate to divide the fascia if the pressure in the muscle compartment does not diminish. Treatment should be started early as the increased pressure can cause permanent damage to muscle and other soft tissues in the muscle compartment.

Chronic anterior compartment syndrome mainly affects athletes who do a lot of running, or specialized sports such as walking. These athletes have increased the bulk of their lower leg muscles by hard training, and the muscles have thus become larger than the surrounding fasciae will allow. At rest, the muscles fill the whole compartment. During exertion, the extensive capillary network opens up, and the resulting increase in blood flow in turn increases the pressure in the muscle compartments. This causes obstruction first to the venous blood supply and then the arterial flow. The resultant pain is due to lack of oxygen and tension which gradually gets worse until the athlete can no longer go on with his track training, either because of the pain itself or because of deterioration of muscular function which makes him simply too weak to run.

Symptoms and diagnosis

— Pain which increases under load and which finally makes continued muscle work impossible.
— The pain disappears after a short period of rest but recurs when physical activity is resumed.
— A sensation of numbness in the cleft between the big toe and the second toe, weakness in the foot and marked difficulty in raising the front of the foot (dorsiflexion).
— Local swelling and tenderness over the muscle belly on the lateral side of the tibia is often present.
— Pain and muscle weakness when bending the foot upwards can be provoked by muscle work.
— Passive plantar toe flexion will provoke pain.
— The pressure in the muscle compartment can be measured at rest and during muscle work until pain is triggered. Increased pressure is present in cases of chronic anterior compartment syndrome.

Treatment

The *athlete* should:
— rest until pain has resolved;
— apply local heat and use a heat retainer;

— analyse running surfaces, running technique, training, type of shoes, and so on.

The *doctor* may:
— treat the injured athlete with diuretics and anti-inflammatory medication;
— operate in order to divide the fascia and give the enlarged muscle more space.

Inflammation of the tendon sheath of the tibialis anterior muscle (tibialis anterior syndrome)

An acute inflammation in the tendon sheath of the tibialis anterior muscle often arises from acute overuse of the ankle joint, for example from jumping and running (especially on a hard surface), in racket sports and so on. It is dorsiflexion of the ankle joint which precipitates the problem.

Symptoms and diagnosis
— Local pain when flexing (dorsiflexing) the ankle joint upwards.
— Creaking (crepitus) over the tendon on moving the ankle joint.
— Temperature increase, skin redness and swelling may be present over the lower anterior part of the tibia.
— Tenderness over the tendon and its sheath on direct pressure over the lateral side of the tibia and also when the foot is bent up and down. If the hand is placed over the tendon, crepitus sometimes can be felt.

Treatment
The *athlete* should:
— rest actively;
— apply cooling both in the acute stage and later, when it may be alternated with heat treatment.

The *doctor* may:
— prescribe anti-inflammatory medication;
— prescribe crutches for 2–3 days to take the weight off the leg. As a rule, plaster treatment is not needed when the injury is acute, but in case of prolonged symptoms such treatment can sometimes be of value.

Pain on the medial (inner) side of the lower leg

Pain on the medial side of the lower leg can arise from the tibia (stress fracture), from the posterior deep muscle compartment or from the periosteum (periostitis).

Stress fractures

Both tibia and fibula can be the site of stress fractures. They occur after prolonged and repeated loading, for example long-distance and cross-country running and repeated jumping. In the tibia, stress fractures are often located in the upper two thirds of the bone while in the fibula they usually occur 2–3 in (5–7 cm) above the tip of the lateral malleolus.

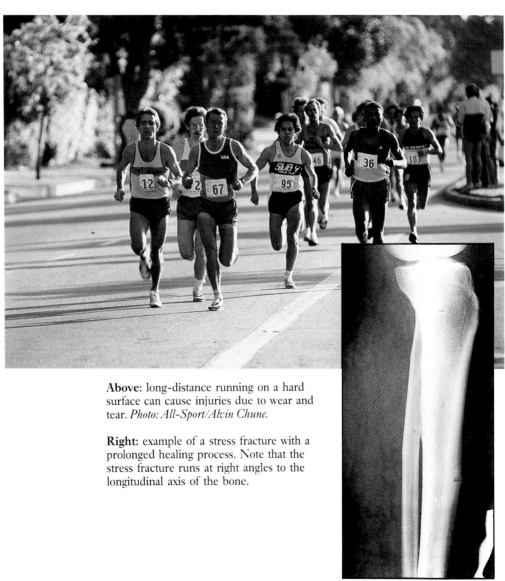

Above: long-distance running on a hard surface can cause injuries due to wear and tear. *Photo: All-Sport/Alvin Chune.*

Right: example of a stress fracture with a prolonged healing process. Note that the stress fracture runs at right angles to the longitudinal axis of the bone.

Symptoms and diagnosis

— Pain usually occurs after running long distances, without a history of impact.
— Local tenderness and swelling over the fracture.
— When the injury is recent, the line of the fracture can be so fine that it does not show on an X-ray. When there are persistent problems with pain on exertion and tenderness a repeat X-ray examination

should be taken 2–4 weeks after the first. Often the fracture can then be seen to be healing.

— If new periostal bone formation along the tibia or the fibula is seen on an X-ray it should be interpreted as a sign of a stress fracture.

— Examination with radioactive isotopes at an early stage gives a definite confirmation of the diagnosis. A localized accumulation of isotopic material is apparent in the area in question.

Treatment

Generally the treatment consists only of rest. When the pain is troublesome and also when the fracture is located in the middle part of the tibia, plaster treatment for a month may be employed. Otherwise there is a risk of delayed healing, which may give rise to treatment problems.

Since stress fractures can be recurrent, the afflicted athlete should avoid the load elements which have caused the injury. He should discuss his training programme with his coach and perhaps also with a doctor. The healing of the fracture should be checked by X-ray before sporting activities are resumed.

Posterior deep compartment syndrome

The *acute posterior deep compartment syndrome* can occur as a result of external impact or acute overuse of the muscles; for example during running and jumping, when the front of the foot and the toe flexors are strained, especially when taking off from a surface. An injury such as this may affect all the muscles simultaneously or one, for example tibialis posterior, flexor hallucis longus or flexor digitorum longus in isolation. It can be difficult – sometimes impossible – to decide which muscles have been affected, but certain clues can be found if each muscle group is tested individually. If bending the big toe downwards against resistance triggers pain, the flexor hallucis longus tendon is involved. If bending the whole of the foot downwards and inwards against resistance triggers pain, the tibialis posterior muscle is primarily involved and if bending all the toes downwards against resistance triggers pain, the long toe flexors are involved.

In the case of a *chronic posterior deep compartment syndrome*, increased pressure will be present in the muscle compartment after provocation of pain. When the muscles are working, this pressure, in addition to the increased muscle contraction, can cause traction on the attachment of the muscle compartment to the periosteum on the inside edge of the tibia. The result may be an inflammation of the periosteum (periostitis).

The cause of chronic posterior deep compartment syndrome is an increase in muscle bulk due to prolonged, intensive training.

Symptoms and diagnosis

The examination should always be performed after provocation.

— Pain on kicking or taking off from the surface and also on heel-raising. The pain starts insidiously and gradually intensifies until physical activity is rendered impossible.

— A sensation of numbness in the foot and weakness on taking off from the surface.

325

— The symptoms abate after resting for a while but recur when there is renewed exertion.

Treatment   The treatment is the same as in cases of chronic anterior compartment syndrome (see page 320).

Medial tibial stress syndrome
(Periostitis of the medial margin of the tibia 'shin splints')

Periostitis is a common complaint in athletes who often change surfaces and types of shoes, alter their techniques, or subject themselves to intensive hard training on hard tracks, streets or floors. Periostitis of the medial margin of the tibia can be triggered by running and other sports with elements of jumping, the main cause of the pain being repeated take-offs from a hard surface. Runners who run on tip-toe, run with their feet turned outwards, or use spiked shoes can suffer from these complaints. Increased pronation (see page 356) or a high instep (see page 366) can be contributory causes.

Symptoms and diagnosis
— Tenderness over the distal medial margin of the tibia. The tenderness is especially pronounced over the lower half of the bone.
— A certain degree of swelling can be felt and seen.
— The pain ceases at rest but returns on renewed loading. The injured athlete can enter the pain cycle (see page 41).
— Pain is triggered when toes or ankle joint are bent downwards.
— Local tenderness in the lower half of the tibia. A certain degree of irregularity can sometimes be felt along its edge.
— An X-ray examination should be carried out in cases where symptoms are prolonged, to exclude fatigue fracture. The examination shows changes neither in the skeleton nor in the soft tissues.
— There is normal pressure in the compartment.

Preventive measures
Every change of surface should be made gradually while the intensity of training is adjusted accordingly.
— The correct clothing and equipment should be used. Shoes should be chosen to suit the surface; those with studs, for example, should not be used when training on asphalt. Orthotics may be required.
— The technique should be adjusted to the surface.
— Careful warm-up.

Treatment   The *athlete* :
— should interrupt training and competition and rest as early as possible. The sooner training is given up, the more rapidly the injury will heal. A chronic condition can then be avoided. Pain is a warning which should signal rest;
— should not start training again until there is no pain under load and the tenderness over the tibia is gone;
— can often maintain a certain degree of physical fitness by cycling or swimming. If cycling, the pedal should be held under the heel rather than the front of the foot;
— can apply local heat and use a heat retainer. Sometimes alternating heat and cooling can be of value;

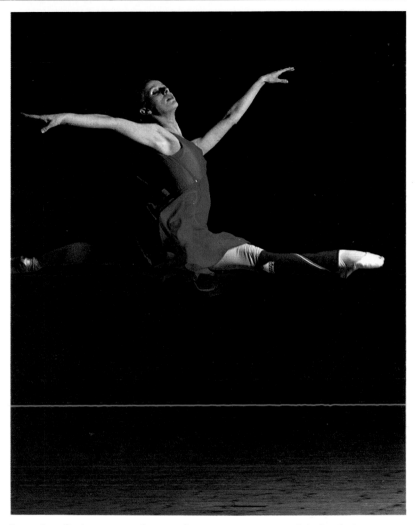

It can be of value to use a heat retainer to prevent or treat injuries during activities involving hard and repeated loading.

— should see a doctor if the complaints are persistent.

The *doctor* may:
— prescribe anti-inflammatory medication or diuretics;
— administer steroid injections under the periosteum;
— prescribe ointments;
— measure the pressure in the posterior deep muscle compartment during provocation in cases of persistent complaints to exclude deep posterior compartment syndrome;
— analyse malalignment as a cause. Examine the anatomy of the lower leg and the foot, particularly with regard to pronation and a high longitudinal arch (instep);
— operate in order to divide the periosteum from the medial margin of the tibia.

Miscellaneous Periostitis can occur as an isolated condition but can also be one of the symptoms of a chronic posterior deep compartment syndrome.

If the above (conservative) treatment fails to relieve pain due to loading within a couple of weeks then a stress fracture should be suspected and excluded by X-ray or bone scan.

Pain in the back of the lower leg

Posterior superficial compartment syndrome

In cases of posterior superficial compartment syndrome, the muscle compartment contains the broad deep calf muscle (the soleus) and the superficial calf muscle (the gastrocnemius) which is affected. Symptoms, diagnosis and treatment are in principle the same as for anterior compart-ment syndrome (see page 320).

Rupture of the gastrocnemius muscle ('tennis leg')

Ruptures of the calf musculature usually occur at the point where the Achilles tendon merges with the inner belly of the calf muscle. The injury occurs most frequently in tennis, badminton, squash, volleyball, basketball and handball players and also in the jumping sports.

Symptoms and diagnosis
— A sudden pain in the calf. The athlete sometimes thinks he has been struck on the leg from behind.
— In middle-aged and elderly individuals a muscle rupture in the calf can be misinterpreted as thrombosis.
— Difficulty in contracting the calf muscle and walking on tiptoe.
— Local tenderness over the injured area.
— Effusion of blood in the region of the rupture.
— A gap can be felt in the muscle tissue over the injured area.

Treatment
The *athlete* should:
— immediately treat the injury by cooling, apply a compression bandage and elevate the leg according to the guidelines given on page 68;
— rest.

The *doctor* may:
— in cases of minor ruptures and when the injury has affected elderly people prescribe a support bandage and the early introduction of mobility and progressive strength training;
— operate when the injury is extensive and has affected a young, active athlete. Blood is removed and the muscle end is stitched to the tendon (see page 329).

Healing and complications
As a rule, the injured athlete can return to training 4–8 weeks after a minor rupture. After surgery, rehabilitation will demand another 6–8 weeks.

An untreated muscle rupture leads to scarring which carries with it the risk of a repeated rupture if the muscle is overexerted.

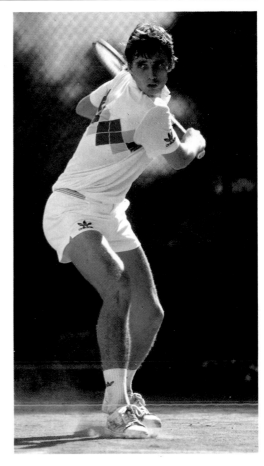

Right: Ruptures of muscles and tendons are common in dynamic sports with rapid movements. *Photo: Adidas.*

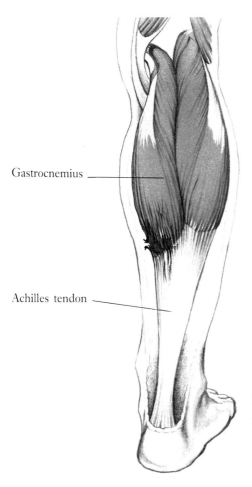

Gastrocnemius

Achilles tendon

Left: rupture of the inner belly of the gastrocnemius muscle at the merger of muscle and tendon – 'tennis leg'.

Rupture of the soleus muscle

On vigorous take-offs or jump-ups the soleus muscle deep in the calf can be overloaded and rupture. As a rule, such ruptures are only partial.

Symptoms and diagnosis

— Pain which is located deep down in the calf and which recurs on repeated loading.
— Pain is triggered when the foot is bent down against resistance and also when attempting to walk on tiptoe.
— Bleeding which most often makes itself felt only some 24 hours after the injury has occurred. Bruising then becomes visible on the inner side of the upper and middle part of the shin.
— Deep local tenderness over the rupture.

329

Treatment

The *athlete* should:
— immediately treat the injury by cooling, apply a compression bandage and elevate the leg according to the guidelines given on page 68;
— keep the bandage on for a week and train with active unloaded movements;
— thereafter train the muscle to the pain threshold with increasing load.

The *doctor* may:
— prescribe further strength and mobility training;
— prescribe anti-inflammatory medication.

If the bleeding accompanying the muscle rupture is extensive, acutely increased pressure can occur in the posterior superficial muscle compartment (see the section on page 328).

Healing

The injured athlete should not return to his regular training until there is no further pain during movements under load.

Pain in the lateral side of the lower leg

In the lateral side of the lower leg pain can occur in the fibula as a result of stress fractures (see page 324) and also in the lateral muscle compartment as a result of acute or chronic lateral compartment syndrome.

Lateral compartment syndrome

Acute lateral compartment syndrome can occur as a result of external impact or from sudden overuse of the muscles. Symptoms, diagnosis and treatment are in principle the same as for cases of acute anterior compartment syndrome (see page 321).

Chronic pressure increase in the lateral muscle compartment occurs mainly in runners and is often associated with deficient ligaments on the lateral aspect of the ankle joint. The muscle group of the lateral compartment acts to stabilize the lateral side of the ankle joint and can be overloaded in cases of stretching and instability of the joint. Symptoms, diagnosis and treatment are the same as for chronic anterior compartment syndrome (see page 321).

Injury to the common peroneal nerve

Injuries to the peroneal nerve in its course down the lateral aspect of the upper part of the fibula can occur as a result of impact — a blow, a kick or a fall — in the region or as a result of external pressure in the form of a tape or plaster cast.

Symptoms and diagnosis

— The pressure on the nerve causes paralysis creating a weakness in dorsiflexion of the ankle joint and eversion (pronation) of the foot.
— The skin in the area may lose some sensitivity.

Treatment

— Strength and mobility training.

330

— Taking the weight off the injured area.
— A bandage can keep the foot in its normal position, if necessary.
— Electrical stimulation by a physiotherapist in order to reduce muscle wasting in cases of paralysis.
— Anti-inflammatory medication is sometimes used.

Healing

The function of the ankle joint usually returns after a period that varies in length from a few days to several months. The function usually returns if the nerve is damaged only by pressure.

Rupture of the Achilles tendon

A rupture of the Achilles tendon is one of the commonest of the tendon injuries that occurs in sport. The tendon rupture can be total or partial, and the injury mainly afflicts football, handball, volleyball, basketball, tennis, squash and especially badminton players and also athletes such as runners and jumpers.

Total rupture of the Achilles tendon

The tendons begin to show degenerative changes at the early age of twenty-five to thirty years. The changes bring about weakness in the tendons but to some extent they can be prevented or at least delayed by regular physical activity. Total ruptures of the Achilles tendon usually occur in degenerated tendons which are subjected to increased load. Those affected are often athletes who, after a brief or lengthy interruption in training, have resumed their training or started sporting activities in order to keep fit.

Symptoms and diagnosis

— Intense pain over the ruptured area of the Achilles tendon in the acute phase. The injured person will state that 'it cracked like a gun shot' or that he had a blow or a kick from behind at the moment the pain began. The pain diminishes, however, after the acute phase and the athlete experiences an improvement of the condition. Attention must be focused on the functional impairment.
— The injured athlete cannot walk normally on the foot or on tiptoe.
— Increasing swelling because of bleeding which can gradually cause bruising over the lower part of the leg and the foot.
— Distinct tenderness over the ruptured area which is often located about 1–2 in (2–5 cm) above the heel bone (calcaneus).
— A gap in the tendon can be felt.
— Impaired ability to bend the foot downwards (plantar flexion).
— Thompsen's test gives a positive result. In this test the injured athlete lies on his stomach with the knee joint of the leg in question slightly bent. When the examining doctor compresses the calf muscle of the injured leg with one hand, the foot is bent downwards (plantar flexed) if the Achilles tendon is intact but remains in its initial position if the tendon is torn (see photograph on page 332).

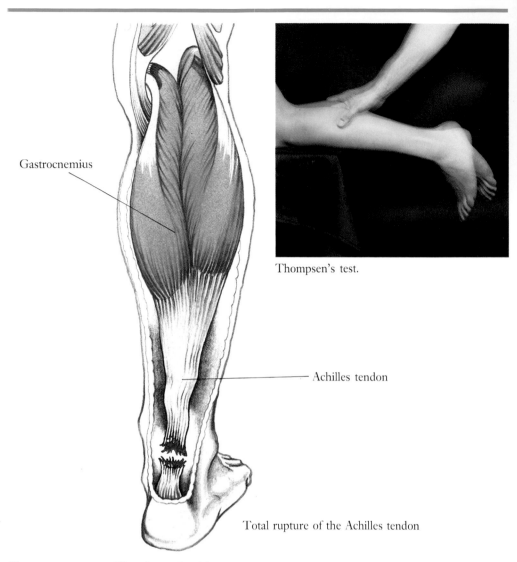

Gastrocnemius

Thompsen's test.

Achilles tendon

Total rupture of the Achilles tendon

Treatment

The *doctor* should:
— operate by suturing the ends of the tendon together. After the operation there follows about 6 weeks' plaster cast treatment. Sometimes plaster treatment alone may be sufficient in the elderly and less active, but a careful rehabilitation is required under those circumstances.

Healing and complications

Convalescence is usually at least as long as the plaster treatment, that is, 6–8 weeks. After the plaster has been removed the doctor can give directions to the patient on mobility training for the ankle joint. When the athlete has regained full mobility of the leg, strength training (see page 454) can be commenced. After initial surgery, some stiffness may be experienced for a time. After immobilization in a plaster cast only, there is an increased risk of rerupture.

In cases of a total rupture of the Achilles tendon, it is usually necessary to allow 6–8 months' break in competition after surgery and at least 9–12 months' break after plaster cast treatment only.

Partial rupture of the Achilles tendon

A partial rupture of the Achilles tendon occurs in runners, jumpers, throwers and others and also in racket sports, and can lead to scar formation which is liable to cause inflammation. This often becomes chronic and can cause prolonged problems.

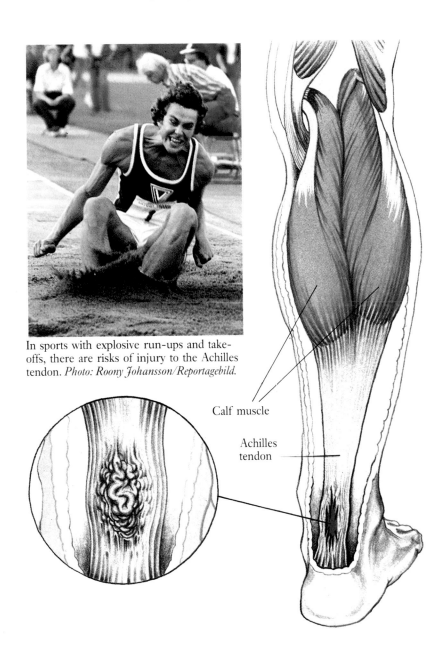

In sports with explosive run-ups and take-offs, there are risks of injury to the Achilles tendon. *Photo: Roony Johansson/Reportagebild.*

Calf muscle

Achilles tendon

Partial rupture of the Achilles tendon. The enlarged picture shows how inflammatory tissue can form in the injured area after a rupture.

Symptoms and diagnosis

— Most patients experience a sudden onset of pain at the time of injury. Some may, however, not always notice pain at the actual moment of rupture. The pain then becomes more evident after the completion of the activity.

— When physical activity is resumed, the injured athlete feels an intense shooting, cutting or stabbing pain.

— During the following training period the symptoms may disappear for a while after warm-up, but they return with even greater intensity when the training is over. The result can be that the injured person enters a vicious cycle of pain (see page 41) in which the condition becomes progressively more painful and progressively more difficult to treat.

— Stiffness in the morning and also before and after exertion.

— When the injury is in its acute stage, a defect can be felt in the tendon (sometimes no larger than the tip of the little finger) over which there is extreme tenderness.

— When the healing process has started a small, local swelling is often found over which a distinct tenderness is present when the area is pressed from the sides. The swelling is usually very slight but can sometimes cause a change in the contour of the tendon.

— If the injured athlete is in severe pain there is often tenderness when the swollen area is touched directly from behind.

— In cases of prolonged symptoms there is often a decrease in the strength and size (atrophy) of the calf muscle.

— An electromyograph (electrical recording of muscle activity) can support the diagnosis.

— An X-ray of the soft tissues is of value in showing local swelling of the ruptured area and swelling (oedema) of the adjacent soft tissues.

— If the rupture is located in the attachment of the tendon to the heel bone (calcaneus), an X-ray of the deep bursa with a contrast medium (bursography) can be of value.

Treatment

The *athlete* should:
— rest and treat with ice in the acute phase;
— use crutches if pain is severe;
— use shoes with ½ in (1 cm) heel-wedges;
— consult a doctor.

The *doctor* may:
— when the rupture is small and acute, apply a plaster cast for 4–6 weeks, in the slight plantar flexion;
— in cases of prolonged symptoms operate in order to remove scar tissue. The treatment after surgery is a plaster cast which is worn for 5–6 weeks. A careful progressive rehabilitation programme is necessary (see page 452).

Treatment should start early as the injury will otherwise be difficult to manage.

Healing and complications

Convalescence is usually 10–12 weeks, that is, twice as long as the time for which the plaster cast is worn. The injured athlete should not resume competition for at least 4–6 months.

Achilles tendinitis

Inflammation can occur in the Achilles tendon and its surrounding tissues as a result of prolonged repeated loading. This injury causes great problems for long-distance runners among others, often during winter training and when training on a hard surface. The inflammation can be acute and, if left untreated, can gradually deteriorate and become chronic.

Acute inflammation of Achilles tendon

Acute Achilles tendinitis often occurs in untrained individuals who start training too intensively but also in well-trained athletes who change surface, type of shoe or technique or who train in cold weather. Running on a very soft surface (sand) and running uphill can trigger pain.

Symptoms and diagnosis
— Pain on using the Achilles tendon.
— Diffuse swelling over the Achilles tendon.
— Intense, diffuse tenderness and impaired function.
— In cases of severe inflammation skin redness appears over the tendon.
— When the fingers are pressed on the tendon during ankle joint movement, a creaking sensation (crepitus) can be felt.

Preventive measures
Warm-up and stretching exercises are important. Well-designed training and competition shoes of good quality should be used. A heel wedge of $\frac{1}{2}$ in (1 cm) will relieve tension in the Achilles tendon.

Treatment
The *athlete* should:
— rest; in the acute phase, crutches may be helpful;
— cool with ice to reduce pain and swelling;
— use $\frac{1}{2}$ in (10 mm) heel wedge;
— apply local heat after the acute phase and use a heat retainer;
— consult a doctor if the complaints do not abate after a few days.

The *doctor* may:
— prescribe anti-inflammatory medication;
— apply a plaster cast in severe cases;
— prescribe a training programme after the acute phase which should include strength training and static stretching (see page 96). Eccentric exercises which put high load on the tendon should be part of the programme when healing so allows.

Healing
When treatment of acute inflammation of the Achilles tendon has been started early the prognosis is good, and the injury heals in 1–2 weeks. The risk of recurrence is small if the injured athlete does not return to his sporting activity too early.

> An acute inflammation of the Achilles tendon can change into a chronic condition which is very difficult to treat. It is therefore of the utmost importance that athletes should rest where there are signs of Achilles tendinitis.

Chronic inflammation of Achilles tendon

Chronic inflammation of the Achilles tendon occurs in athletes (often elderly) who have been training intensively on a hard surface for a long time and who have ignored warning pains. These pains at first tend to disappear after the warm-up exercises before a training period so that the affected athlete can continue his training. The symptoms return after training is over and gradually become more and more severe. Sooner or later continued running is impossible, and the athlete is trapped in the pain cycle (see page 41).

Symptoms and diagnosis

— Pain, aching and stiffness in the Achilles tendon before, during and after exertion.
— There is diffuse swelling in the tendon.
— The tendon is tender to touch (palpation) in places.
— The athlete may suffer pain in the Achilles tendon when walking, especially uphill and upstairs.
— In cases of persistent Achilles tendon problems a partial rupture should be suspected, and investigations should then be carried out by a doctor.
— An X-ray examination of the soft tissues allows a comparison with the undamaged side to be made.

Treatment

The *athlete* should:
— rest;
— apply local heat and use a heat retainer;
— use shoes with ½ in (1 cm) heel wedge.

The *doctor* may:
— analyse the injured athlete's training and then consider especially the design of the shoes and the type of surface he uses for training;
— prescribe an exercise programme with strength training and stretching (page 91). The strength training should include eccentric exercises (see page 91).
— prescribe anti-inflammatory medication for a short time;
— prescribe medicated bandages (containing ointment which stimulates the blood flow and controls the inflammation);
— apply a plaster cast for 3–6 weeks if there is severe pain or malfunction;
— operate in prolonged cases, releasing the tendon from the surrounding scar tissue which is then removed.

Healing

Chronic Achilles tendinitis is a very persistent condition which is very difficult to treat. It is therefore essential that pain in the Achilles tendon is considered a warning signal. Inflammation of the Achilles tendon should be treated at an early stage.

Achilles bursitis

Bursitis over the calcaneus (heel bone) can occur in a superficial bursa located under the skin and in a deep bursa located between the tendon and the calcaneus — the retrocalcaneal bursa.

Between the skin and the posterior surface of the Achilles tendon lies a superficial bursa which is vulnerable to pressure from shoes and which often becomes inflamed. Between the Achilles tendon and the calcaneus there is a deeply located bursa which can become inflamed if it is irritated either by external pressure or by a partial tendon rupture. If prolonged pressure against the tendon attachment, for example repeated dorsiflexion, is the cause of the inflammation of the bursa, a bony prominence often appears on the posterior aspect of the calcaneus, which further increases the risk of the area being subjected to pressure.

Symptoms and diagnosis

— Redness and thickening of the skin occurs over the calcaneus on the lateral side of the Achilles tendon attachment if the superficial bursa is involved.
— Pain can be experienced when running uphill or on soft surfaces.
— There are often symptoms such as tenderness and swelling which make it difficult for the athlete to wear ordinary shoes.
— When the deep bursa is pressed from both sides of the Achilles tendon, a spongy resistance can be felt.
— An X-ray with a contrast medium (bursography) and an X-ray of the soft tissues confirm the diagnosis.

Right: contrast X-ray (bursography) of the bursa at the calcaneus. The X-ray shows a normal bursa seen from the front and side.
Below: inflammation of the bursa at the attachment of the Achilles tendon to the calcaneus.

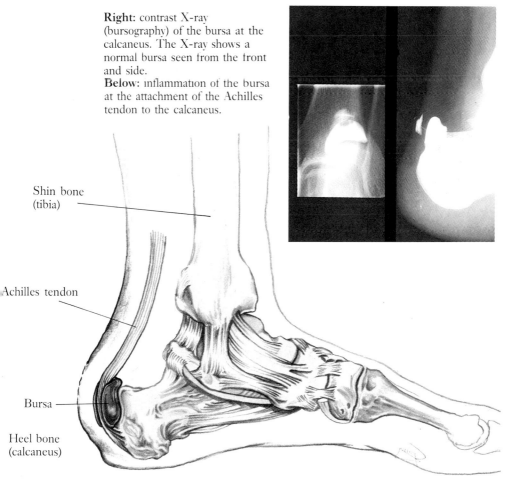

Shin bone (tibia)

Achilles tendon

Bursa

Heel bone (calcaneus)

Treatment

The *athlete* should:

— relieve the calcaneus of pressure, immediately symptoms begin, for example by wearing shoes without backs such as sandals or wooden clogs;

— relieve the area when the superficial bursa is inflamed with a foam rubber ring which is placed around the bony prominence if one has formed;

— adjust the shoes, for example by raising the heel and softening the counter in order to avoid pressure against the area;

— apply local heat.

The *doctor* may:

— prescribe anti-inflammatory medication;

— give ultrasound treatment;

— give a local steroid injection and prescribe rest;

— operate when the inflammation in the bursa has become chronic and a bony prominence has appeared. During the operation the bursa and the prominence are removed.

Apophysitis calcanei

In active individuals aged eight to fifteen years the Achilles tendon attachment (apophysis) to the calcaneus can become the site of fragmentation, a condition which is probably caused by overloading and can be seen on X-ray examination (compare Osgood Schlatter's disease, page 309).

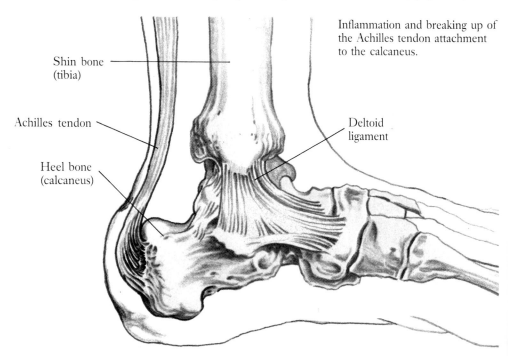

Shin bone (tibia)

Achilles tendon

Heel bone (calcaneus)

Inflammation and breaking up of the Achilles tendon attachment to the calcaneus.

Deltoid ligament

Symptoms and diagnosis	— Pain in the calcaneus when running and walking. The complaints often remain after exertion when stiffness sets in and causes a limp. — Some swelling and tenderness over the Achilles tendon attachment to the calcaneus. — An X-ray confirms the diagnosis.
Treatment	The *athlete* should: — rest until the pain has gone (the symptoms, however, often return); — use shoes with ½ in (1 cm) heel wedge which can alleviate the symptoms as the Achilles tendon is relieved from tension. The *doctor* may: — apply a plaster cast for about 3 weeks, which can give permanent pain relief.
Healing	The condition resolves spontaneously when the afflicted athlete reaches the age of sixteen to eighteen years and ossification of the skeleton is complete.

Tibialis anterior tendinitis

The tendon of the tibialis anterior muscle runs down the front of the lower leg and across the ankle joint and bends the ankle joint upwards. This tendon can become inflamed in any part of its course. The inflammation can occur as a result of overloading or external pressure, often because of shoes or skating boots which are laced too tightly. The injury occurs in ice hockey, team handball and basketball players and also in runners.

Symptoms and diagnosis	— Pain which is triggered when the foot is bent up (dorsiflexed) at the ankle joint. — Tenderness, swelling and sometimes redness over the tendon in the acute phase and impaired function. — Tendon creaking (crepitus) can be felt when the foot is bent up and down when the injury is in its acute phase.
Treatment	The *athlete* should: — rest; — apply ice massage in the acute phase (alternately with heat treatment); — apply local heat and use a heat retainer after the acute phase; — relieve the tendon by distributing the pressure of the shoe or skating boot over the surrounding parts of the foot, for example by putting foam rubber between the lacing and the tendon. The *doctor* may: — apply a plaster cast when the injury is in its acute phase; — prescribe anti-inflammatory medication and ointments; — prescribe an exercise programme after the acute phase.

ANKLE JOINT INJURIES

The ankle joint comprises the tibia, fibula and talus. The tibia and the fibula are held together by strong ligaments, a syndesmosis or fibrous joint, and together form the so-called ankle joint mortise against which the talus rests. The ankle joint is stabilized by the joint capsule and by strong ligaments.

Fractures of the ankle joint

The ankle joint is one of the areas which most frequently suffers fractures in sports. Well-functioning ankle joints are a basic requirement for almost all sports, so much care should be devoted to their injuries.

As the bones and surrounding ligaments cooperate to maintain stability in the ankle joint, combination injuries are common.

The mechanism of injury The commonest mechanism of injury is an inward turning of the sole of the foot and the front of the foot (supination – inward rotation). Depending on the force of supination, different injuries can occur:
— tearing of the ligament between the talus and the fibula;
— fracture of the fibula on a level with the joint line;
— fracture of the medial malleolus;
— dislocation of the talus.

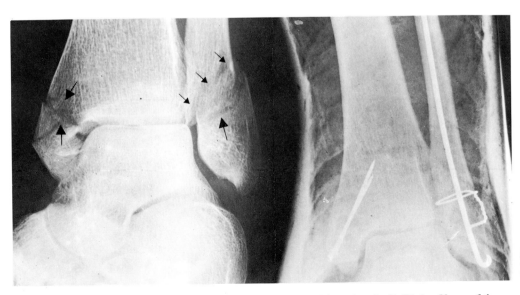

Left: X-ray of fractures of the medial and lateral malleoli. **Right:** X-ray of the same injury after surgery. The lower fragment on the lateral malleolus is held in place by a steel wire (cerclage) and a long pin. The torn off fragment on the medial malleolus is held in place by two shorter pins. The bone is surrounded by plaster.

Another common injury is an outward turning of the sole of the foot and the front of the foot (pronation – outward rotation). Again, different injuries occur depending on the force of pronation:

— tearing of the deltoid ligament or a fracture of the medial malleolus;
— tearing of the syndesmosis;
— fracture of the fibula above the ankle joint;
— dislocation of the talus.

Other mechanisms of injury are also possible.

Symptoms and diagnosis

— Intense aching and pain when the foot is under load.
— Tenderness and considerable swelling.
— Sometimes visible displacement.
— An X-ray shows a skeletal injury.

Treatment

The *athlete* should:

— immediately cool the injury, apply a compression bandage and elevate the foot according to the guidelines given on page 68;
— consult a doctor.

The *doctor* may:

— apply a plaster cast for 4–8 weeks if there is no displacement and the ankle joint is judged to be stable;
— operate in cases of a fracture with displacement or where there is instability of the ankle joint.

Healing and complications

The convalescent time is about as long as the plaster treatment period, that is, 4–8 weeks. After the plaster has been removed the injured athlete can start a range of motion and strength training exercises for the ankle joint (see page 454 for training exercises), and proprioceptive training.

An ankle joint fracture needs at least 2–3 months to heal to full stability, and the injured athlete should allow a break from competition of at least 4 months. When training is resumed a support bandage should be used.

After surgery during which the injured bone has been realigned to its exact position, the healing prognosis is good. If there is a slight displacement in the fracture during healing it can, however, result in wearing of the cartilage and impaired future functioning due to osteoarthrosis.

Ligament injuries of the ankle joint

Ligament injuries of the ankle are among the commonest of all sports injuries and occur in most ball sports, jumping sports, and so on. The injuries can in principle be total or partial. For a background to this type of injury see the section 'Joint ligament injuries' on page 22.

Every sprain in which the range of movement of the ankle joint has been exceeded causes damage to the stabilizing tissues with bleeding, swelling and tenderness and should be considered as a ligament injury. In cases of sprains and dislocations it is mainly the lateral and medial ligaments of the ankle joint that tear. Sometimes a small portion of bone is torn away at the point of ligament attachment, whilst the ligament itself remains intact. This type of avulsion injury is found in young growing athletes with very strong ligaments and also in elderly individuals with brittle bones.

Ligament injuries in the ankle joint should never be neglected, as correct treatment often ensures complete recovery. A return to sporting activity should not be made until there is no pain and normal mobility and strength is restored to the ankle joint. The injured athlete therefore must allow 4–12 weeks' break from training, depending on the degree of severity of the injury. When starting to strengthen the ankle joint by training, the joint should be protected by a support tape or bandage (see page 162).

When instability is present in the ankle joint after the treatment of the injury has ceased or after repeated trauma to the joint, surgery may have to be performed.

Tear of the anterior talofibular ligament

The ligament in the ankle joint that is most often injured runs between the fibula and the talus. Its main function is to prevent the foot from slipping forwards in relation to the tibia. In about 70 per cent of all cases of ligament injuries in the ankle joint this ligament alone is injured. In about 20 per cent of the cases, there is a combination injury with a tear of the talofibular ligament as well as calcaneofibular ligament, which runs between the fibula and the calcaneus. The mechanism of injury is usually a supination – inward rotation of the foot.

Symptoms and diagnosis

— Pain when the ankle joint is loaded and moved.
— Swelling and tenderness in front of the lateral malleolus.
— Effusion of blood which later results in bruising around the injury.
— Instability in cases of a total ligament tear can be tested by pulling the foot forwards in relation to the tibia, the so-called anterior drawer test (see photograph on page 344).
— An X-ray examination with an anterior drawer test confirms the diagnosis.

Treatment

The treatment depends on whether the injury is a total tear with instability or a partial tear with preserved stability which the doctor decides on the basis of the joint's stability tests.

The *athlete* should:
— when he suspects a ligament injury, stop all sporting activities;
— apply immediate cooling, a compression bandage and elevation according to the guidelines given on page 68.

The *doctor* may:
— X-ray the ankle joint in order to determine whether there is a fracture or an avulsion injury. In cases of an avulsion injury a fragment of bone has been torn away from its origin at the point to which the ligament is attached;
— prescribe early mobility training, including extension and flexion of the

ankle joint in cases of a partial injury with relatively limited bleeding or swelling; start proproceptive training;

— fix the ankle joint with adhesive strapping or a plaster cast for about 1–3 weeks if the injury is a partial tear with extensive bleeding and swelling, or for about 6 weeks if the tear is total;

— prescribe anti-inflamatory medication and physiotherapy;

— operate in cases of a total ligament tear in a young active athlete, or if both the lateral ligaments are torn. The operation is followed by plaster treatment for 5–6 weeks;

— in cases of an avulsion injury operate in order to replace the detached piece of bone in its original position. In this way, the function of the ligament is restored.

Healing and complications

The healing of a ligament injury in the ankle joint can take 2–8 weeks depending on the severity of the impact and the extent of the injury. Problems, however, can remain for 8–10 months after the incident. When the injured athlete has no pain on moving the ankle joint and has good mobility, rehabilitation training can start (see page 454). Proprioceptive training is extremely important, otherwise the ligament is liable to be injured again. Strengthening of the peroneus longus and brevis should also be carried out. During the training period which can extend over 6–8 weeks the ankle joint should be protected from further overstretching with the help of an adhesive strapping, an elastic bandage or tape.

An untreated ligament injury can result in stretching of the ligament which can lead to permanent instability with recurrent sprains.

If a ligament injury still causes problems with instability 4–6 months after it occurred, the ligament can be sultured together or reconstructed by surgery.

Tear of the calcaneofibular ligament

On supination of the foot an isolated injury can occur to the ligament which runs between the fibula and the calcaneus, although it is more usual for the anterior talofibular ligament to be injured at the same time (see diagram on page 345).

Symptoms and diagnosis

— Swelling and tenderness over the injured ligament, distal to the lateral malleolus.

— Pain when moving and loading the ankle joint.

— Effusion of blood which later causes bruising behind and below the lateral malleolus.

— Exaggerated ability to turn the foot inwards (increased supination) compared with the undamaged ankle joint.

— An X-ray with supination provocation can confirm the diagnosis.

Treatment

The *athlete* should:

— give the injury emergency cooling, apply a compression bandage and elevate the foot according to the guidelines given on page 68;

— consult a doctor.

The cause of injury, the injury itself and a stability examination: the ligament between splint bone and ankle bone. **Right:** the cause of injury. A vigorous inward rotation and supination of the foot can cause a rupture of the ligament between the fibula and talus. **Below:** examination of the stability of the foot in cases of suspected injury to the anterior talofibular ligament. The hand should grasp the heel bone and ankle bone as it is essential to test the stability of the joint between the tibia and fibula and the talus. The examiner should try to pull the foot forwards in relation to the lower leg.

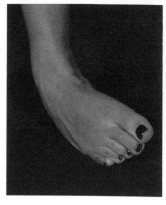

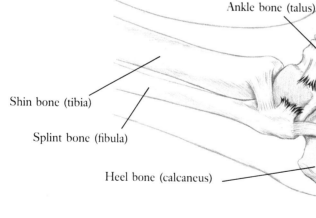

Below: a tear of the ligament between fibula and talus.

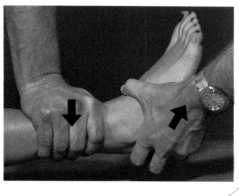

Ankle bone (talus)

Anterior talofibular ligament

Shin bone (tibia)

Splint bone (fibula)

Calcaneofibular ligament

Heel bone (calcaneus)

The *doctor* may:
— support the ankle joint with an adhesive strapping, an elastic bandage or plaster cast for about 3 weeks if stability is maintained;
— operate in cases of instability in the ankle joint, especially in combination injuries.

For a rehabilitation programme, see page 454.

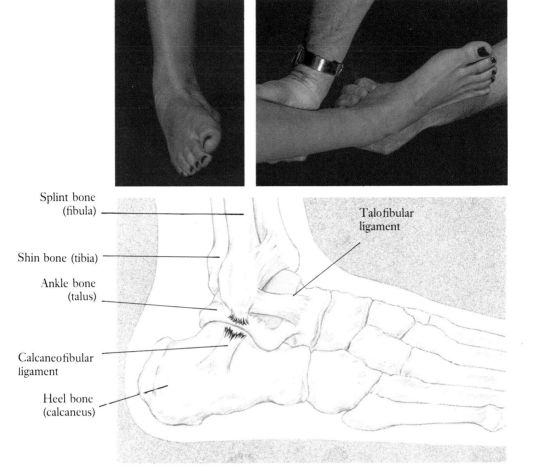

Splint bone
(fibula)

Talofibular
ligament

Shin bone (tibia)

Ankle bone
(talus)

Calcaneofibular
ligament

Heel bone
(calcaneus)

The cause of injury, the injury itself and stability examination: the ligament between fibula and calcaneus. **Top left:** the cause of injury. A vigorous supination of the foot can result in a rupture of the ligament between fibula and calcaneus. **Top right:** examination of the stability of the ankle joint in cases of suspected injury. **Above:** a rupture of the ligament between fibula and calcaneus.

Tear of the the deltoid ligament

In less than 10 per cent of all cases of ligament injuries in the ankle joint the deltoid ligament is damaged. Usually the tear is partial and injury occurs during pronation when the sole of the foot is turned outwards.

Symptoms and diagnosis

— Pain on moving and loading the ankle joint.
— Swelling and tenderness over the course of the ligament below the medial malleolus.
— When the tear is total there is increased pronation in comparison with the range of movement of the undamaged joint.

Treatment The *athlete* should:
— give the injury emergency cooling, apply a compression bandage and elevate the foot according to the guidelines given on page 68;
— consult a doctor.

The *doctor* may:
— in cases of partial tear and maintained stability, support the ankle joint with an adhesive strapping, an elastic bandage or a plaster cast for 3–4 weeks;
— when it is difficult to decide if instability is present, examine the joint by TV fluoroscopy. When the joint is unstable the injury should be operated on, after which it is immobilized in plaster for 6 weeks.

Injury to the ligaments between the tibia and the fibula (the syndesmosis)

The syndesmosis comprises the anterior and posterior tibiofibular ligaments and the interossoeus membrane.

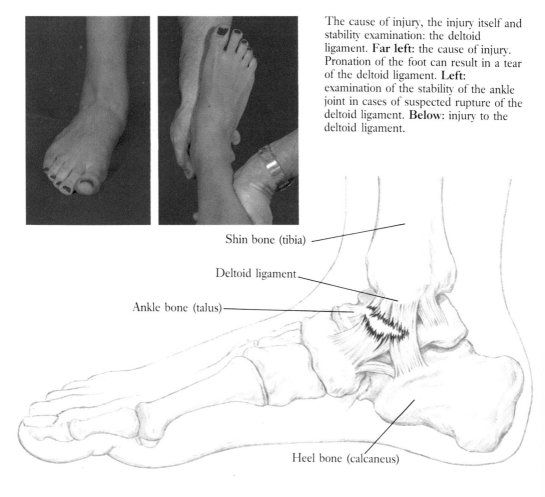

The cause of injury, the injury itself and stability examination: the deltoid ligament. **Far left:** the cause of injury. Pronation of the foot can result in a tear of the deltoid ligament. **Left:** examination of the stability of the ankle joint in cases of suspected rupture of the deltoid ligament. **Below:** injury to the deltoid ligament.

Shin bone (tibia)

Deltoid ligament

Ankle bone (talus)

Heel bone (calcaneus)

A tear of the syndesmosis can occur in combination with deltoid ligament injury when the foot sustains pronation – outward rotation. The syndesmosis can be injured in combination with a fracture of the fibula above the ankle joint or a fracture of the medial malleolus. An injury to the syndesmosis can later cause lateral subluxation of the talus if it is not treated.

Symptoms and diagnosis
— Tenderness and swelling at the junction of the tibia and the fibula.
— Pain on moving and loading the ankle joint.
— Instability in the ankle mortise (see diagram on page 348) which can cause the talus to slip laterally in relation to the tibia.
— A widening of the ankle mortise can be observed on an X-ray with simultaneous stability testing.

Treatment
The *athlete* should:
— apply cooling and a compression bandage and elevate the foot according to the guidelines given on page 68.
— consult a doctor.

The *doctor* may:
— in cases of minor injuries with maintained stability support the ankle joint with an adhesive strapping or a plaster cast for 3 weeks.
— operate in cases of instability.

Osteochondritis dissecans of the talus

Osteochondritis dissecans of the talus may result from a pronation or supination injury of the ankle joint. In a pronation injury, osteochondritis is located on the medial aspect. It may appear as an osteochondral fracture with a minimal dislocation, or as a detached fragment. The articular surface may even turn 180° so it faces the bone surface of the talus.

Symptoms and diagnosis
— Pain during and after excercise.
— Swelling and tenderness of the ankle.
— Locking sensation in the joint.
— Limited ankle movement.
— X-ray will confirm the diagnosis.

Treatment
The *athlete* should:
— rest.

The *doctor* may:
— immobilize in an acute, non-displaced fracture;
— use arthroscopy, which may be of value in chronic cases;
— operate in dislocated acute cases and disabling chronic cases.

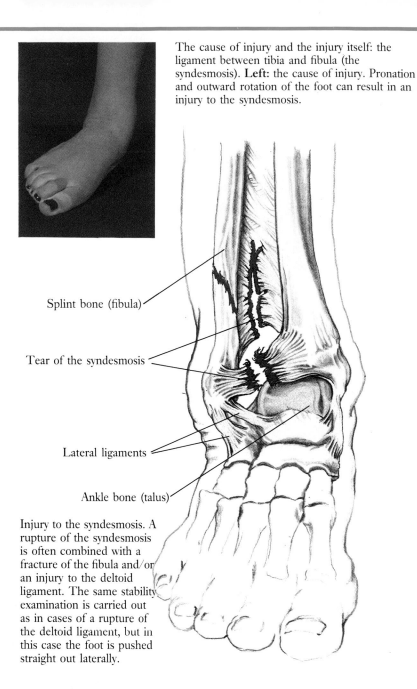

The cause of injury and the injury itself: the ligament between tibia and fibula (the syndesmosis). **Left:** the cause of injury. Pronation and outward rotation of the foot can result in an injury to the syndesmosis.

Splint bone (fibula)

Tear of the syndesmosis

Lateral ligaments

Ankle bone (talus)

Injury to the syndesmosis. A rupture of the syndesmosis is often combined with a fracture of the fibula and/or an injury to the deltoid ligament. The same stability examination is carried out as in cases of a rupture of the deltoid ligament, but in this case the foot is pushed straight out laterally.

'Footballer's ankle'

In cases of untreated acute overstretching, and also after repeated over-stretching of the ankle joint, changes can occur in the form of bony deposits (osteophytes) anteriorly where the joint capsule is attached. The condition is not uncommon and mainly affects athletes who for many years have been participating in football, cross-country running, orienteering and so on. The cause may be hyperextension or hyperflexion of the ankle joint which causes traction in the attachment of the joint capsule or minor fractures due to impacts between the bone surfaces (see diagram on page 350). The bony deposits can cause inflammation in the joint capsule and tendon sheaths.

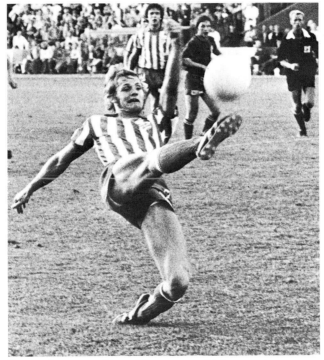

Repeated overstretching of ligaments and joint capsule can cause 'footballer's ankle'.

Symptoms and diagnosis
— Tenderness when pressing with the fingers over the front of the ankle joint. Sometimes the bony deposits (osteophytes) can be felt.
— Pain as a band across the ankle joint, for example when making ankle kicks in soccer.
— Pain when the foot is bent up or down.
— Often slightly impaired mobility in the ankle joint.
— Bony deposits (osteophytes) show up on an X-ray.

Treatment

The *athlete* should:
— carry out strength and mobility training and also do static stretching exercises;
— use a heat retainer;
— apply tape.

The *doctor* may:
— administer a steroid injection into the tender spot and prescribe rest;
— operate in cases of pronounced problems, paring away the bony deposits (osteophytes).

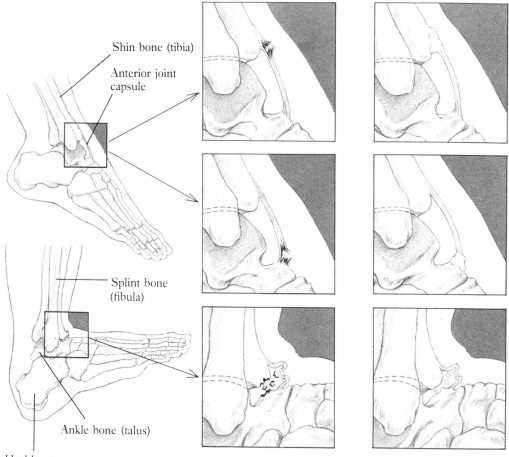

Shin bone (tibia)

Anterior joint capsule

Splint bone (fibula)

Ankle bone (talus)

Heel bone (calcaneus)

'Footballer's ankle': possible mechanisms of bone changes at the front of the ankle joint. **Top left:** overstretching in passive plantar flexion. **Top right:** overstretching in passive dorsiflexion. The middle diagrams show alternative injuries in their acute stages, and the diagrams to the right show residual conditions.

Dislocation of the peroneal tendons

The peroneal tendons run behind the lateral malleolus. These tendons contribute to dorsiflexion and outward rotation (pronation) of the ankle joint. If the ankle turns, the connective tissue band (retinaculum) which holds the tendons in their compartments behind the lateral malleolus can be torn, allowing the tendons to slip forwards across the lateral malleolus. Recurrent dislocation of the tendons results in inflammation which may cause chronic problems. The injury occurs in athletes with unstable ankle joints, in downhill skiers, and in athletes who take part in jumping sports.

Symptoms and diagnosis
— Pain on pronation (turning the sole of the foot upwards and outwards).
— Pain when the tendons slip forwards out of their usual position. This can occur if the foot is pronated at the same time as being bent upwards (dorsiflexed), and also when the tendons are pressed from behind with the thumb against the lateral malleolus.
— Tenderness behind the lateral malleolus.
— Swelling and bruising in cases of acute injury.

Treatment
The *doctor* may:
— apply a plaster cast for 3–4 weeks in cases of acute injury;
— operate in order to suture the retinaculum and then apply a plaster cast for 4 weeks;
— in cases of chronic problems reconstruct the retinaculum or, in some other way, prevent the tendons from slipping forwards.

Tibialis posterior syndrome

The tibialis posterior muscle arises from the back of the tibia and fibula, and merges into a tendon enclosed in a sheath which runs behind the tibia and the medial malleolus and is attached to the boat-shaped navicular bone on the inside of the foot. Increased pronation of the foot results in increased load and tension on the tendon of the tibialis posterior muscle, leading to inflammation of the tendon or its attachment or the tendon sheath. These are subjected to mechanical pressure behind the medial malleolus where they run in a narrow groove. The injury is common, causing problems primarily in running but also in skating and skiing.

Symptoms and diagnosis
— Pain when the tendon slides in the sheath during movements.
— Pain when the tendon is subjected to passive loading and active exercises.
— Tenderness can occur, as a rule, over the attachment of the tendon to the navicular bone but also over the course of the tendon behind the medial malleolus.
— Swelling sometimes occurs.
— Tendon creaking (crepitus) can be felt when the injury is in its acute stage.
— Increased pronation of the foot may be present.

Treatment   The *athlete* should:
— give up loading the foot for a couple of weeks;
— apply cooling when the injury is in its acute stage and after that apply local heat, for example by using a heat retainer;
— apply tape to the injured area;
— use a semi-firm shoe support which supports the longitudinal arch and reduces the pronation of the foot.

The *doctor* may:
— prescribe anti-inflammatory medication;
— give a steroid injection into the tendon sheath — never, however, into the tendon — and, in addition, prescribe rest;
— apply a plaster cast for 3 weeks;
— operate if the tendon sheath has become constricted so that the tendon can no longer glide normally in it.
The physical proximity of the inside edge of the tibia and the tendon of the tibialis posterior muscle can make it difficult to distinguish between the tibialis posterior syndrome and medial tibial periostitis.

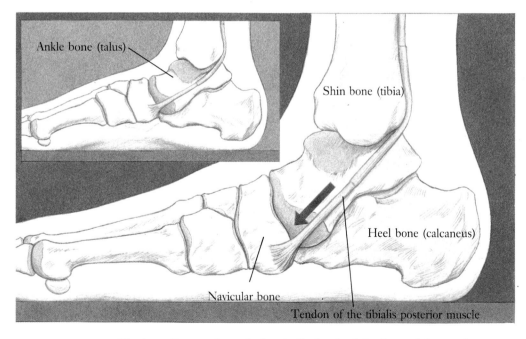

The inset diagram shows the longitudinal arch of the foot and the attachment of the tendon of the tibialis posterior muscle in an unloaded state. The main diagram shows the foot in a loaded state with increased pronation. The tendon of the tibialis posterior muscle is now extended.

FOOT INJURIES

The foot is the part of the musculo-skeletal system that receives and distributes the body load when walking, jumping and running. Most sports contain elements of running or jumping during which the strains on the lower extremities of the body increase sharply. The forces that are created when the foot is put down in running, for example, are two or three times the body weight and have to be distributed over the tissues, the shoes and the running surface. A runner can take more than 5,000 steps an hour with each leg which means that overloading problems can arise from even a slight deviation from normal body build or correct running technique.

Anatomy and function

The lower extremities should be seen as functional units in which different parts cooperate. Deviations from the normal anatomy of the foot, for example, can cause problems in the knee and/or hip joints or vice versa.

The foot is composed of twenty-six different bones which are interconnected at about thirty joints and held together by ligaments and joint capsules. Some thirty tendons, including those of the muscles of the lower leg and those of the muscles of the foot itself, are involved when the foot moves.

The foot can be divided into three parts. The back, or heel, consists of the talus (ankle bone) and the calcaneus (heel bone). The middle consists of the navicular bone, four other bones (the cuboid and three cuneiform bones) and the metatarsal bones. The front part consists of the five toes. The big toe, like the thumb, consists of only two phalanges while the other toes consist of three. The length and shape of the toes can vary considerably which can cause problems for athletes. When the toes are loaded the big toe is pressed against the surface while the other toes make a grasping movement.

There are two arch systems in the foot: a transverse, anterior arch and a longitudinal arch which follows the inside of the foot from the calcaneus to the basic joint of the big toe. The front arch is held together by ligaments which in an unloaded state maintain the shape of the arch, and in a loaded state are stretched as the arch is pressed against the surface. When the foot is loaded the plantar aponeurosis (the arch ligament, see diagram on page 362) which runs along the arch from the calcaneus and out into the toes is also stretched. The more the arch is loaded, the tighter the ligament becomes.

Many movements of the foot and toes are controlled by muscles which have their origins in the lower leg and whose tendons are attached to the foot. Movements of more precision are controlled by muscles which have both their origins and insertions in the foot itself.

Foot movements

The foot has two axes round which movements can be made. One runs horizontally through the talus and is the axis for vertical movements at the ankle joint. The other axis runs diagonally from behind, through the lower part of the calcaneus and forwards and upwards through the talus.

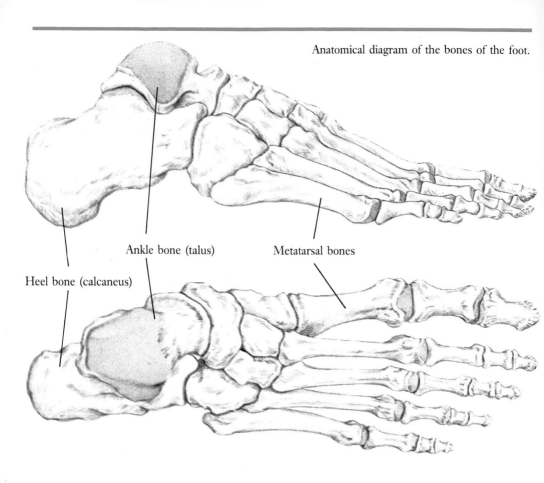

Anatomical diagram of the bones of the foot.

Ankle bone (talus)   Metatarsal bones

Heel bone (calcaneus)

The movements the foot makes round this axis are known as pronation and supination (see diagram on page 357). Pronation means that the sole of the foot is turned outwards and that the main part of the inside of the foot has contact with the surface, that is, the position of a flat foot. Supination means that the sole of the foot is turned inwards so that the medial border of the foot is higher than the outer one.

Running and walking

During running, the foot is slightly supinated just before it is placed down. The foot is usually placed on the surface with the outside of the heel touching first. Then the arch is loaded and flattened and pronation begins which, together with contraction of the calf muscles, causes the forces generated to spread through the whole foot and leg. The flattening of the longitudinal arch continues until the arch ligament (plantar aponeurosis) is tightened. By this time the forces generated by the body weight have passed through the foot, and preparations for take-off have started. The foot is in pronation for about 40–70 per cent of the supporting phase and then gradually changes into supination. The latter stabilizes the front of the foot so that a better lever is available for the take-off.

The angle of the foot

The angle of the foot in relation to the lower leg is important. The angle can be checked against skin markings which are made along the tibia and should be parallel to a vertical axis through the talus and the calcaneus. This vertical axis should, in its turn, be at right angles to a line through the anterior arch.

Causes of injuries

The causes of foot injuries in running, for example, are factors which influence the distribution of load, including anatomical features, body weight, shoes, surface, training programme and technique (see diagram below).

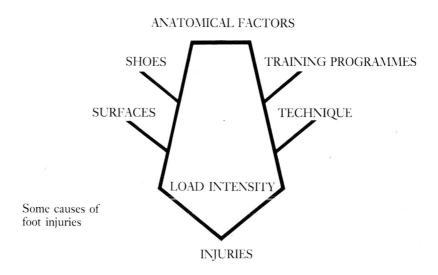

Some causes of
foot injuries

Anatomical factors

Significant deviations from the normal anatomical structure of the foot (for example, excessive pronation or flat-foot, and pes cavus or claw-foot) can cause injuries, but even minor variations can be sufficient to do so if subjected to prolonged or repeated loading.

Pronated foot ('flat-foot') A certain degree of pronation is normal in a foot that is loaded, but excessive pronation is a compensatory movement caused by an incorrect relationship between heel and foot or between leg and foot. It is common for the relationship between leg and foot to be slightly imperfect, and the result can easily be inadequate balance. During loading, the soles of the feet can be forced against the surface by excessive pronation.

During running, excessive pronation — or pronation maintained for too long in the supporting phase — is associated with increased stress on the supporting structures of the foot, and also causes increased work for the muscles, so injuries due to overuse can occur. Excessive pronation may also be a mechanism by which the body compensates for other slight anatomical defects and deviations.

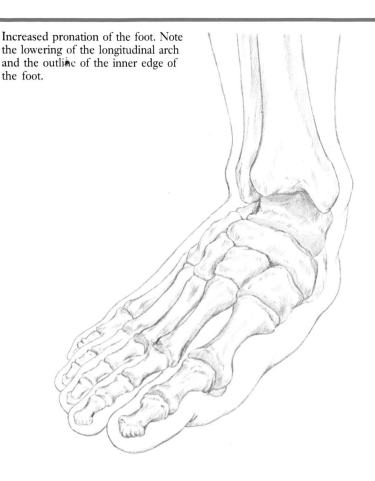

Increased pronation of the foot. Note the lowering of the longitudinal arch and the outline of the inner edge of the foot.

Flat-footedness or excessive pronation can be confirmed by the 'wet foot test'. The foot is dipped in water and a walking footprint is made on a smooth, dry surface. The footprints then show the load distribution across the foot (see diagram opposite). When the foot is normal the longitudinal arch does not leave a print, but if excessive pronation is present a print of the whole foot appears.

Excessive pronation may cause increased load on the whole of the lower extremity since it results in an increased inward rotation of the lower leg. This can lead to a change of the biomechanical work pattern of the thigh musculature (see diagram opposite) so that the lower leg, the knee joint and the hip joint are subjected to increased load. This can be the cause of overuse injuries and other painful conditions in these areas.

Injuries which are associated with excessive pronation include chondromalacia patellae, tibialis posterior syndrome, plantar fasciitis and trochanteric bursitis. It is, however, important to stress that the anatomical changes bear no direct relationship to a specific diagnosis.

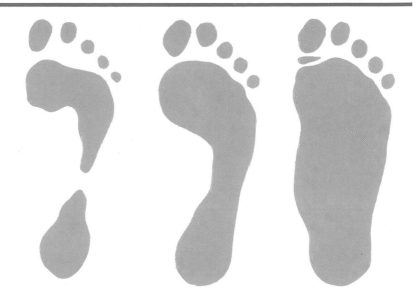

Footprints of loaded feet. **Left:** a foot with a high instep (pes cavus or claw-foot). **Middle:** a normal foot. **Right:** a foot with increased pronation (flat foot).

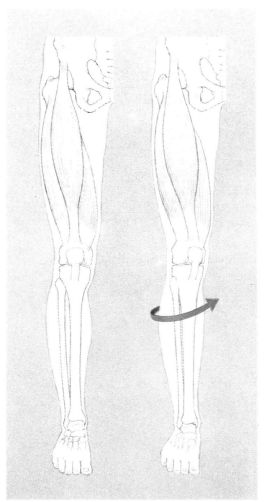

Left: a normal leg. **Right:** a leg where the foot is in a position of exaggerated pronation resulting in an increased inward turn of the lower leg.

357

**Pes cavus
(claw-foot)**

A claw-foot has a high longitudinal arch and is relatively inflexible, being combined with tight calf musculature and tight ligaments of the sole of the foot. Because of the reduced weight-bearing foot surface there is an increased risk of, for instance, pressure concentration, incorrect load distribution, heel pains and tendinitis. Claw-feet are dealt with more thoroughly on page 366.

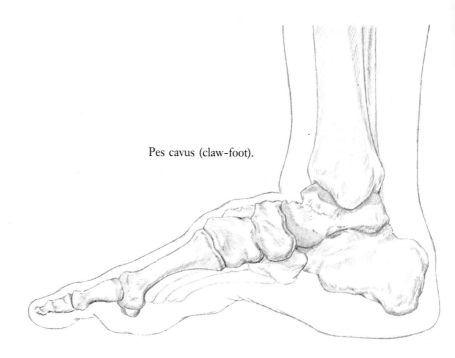

Pes cavus (claw-foot).

Training programmes

Mistakes in training are a prime cause of injuries. The commonest errors among runners are running too far, training too intensively with inadequate time for recovery, running on hilly ground and changing from one surface to another.

Surfaces

The period during which athletes support the foot against the surface is very short — in sprinters it is, for example, 0.11 seconds, in middle-distance runners 0.14 seconds and in high-jumpers on take-off 0.21 seconds. During this time a shock wave is generated and followed by compression waves. The force of the shock wave has to be distributed between the surface, shoe and body tissues. If the surface is too hard there are increased demands on the shoes as the body tissues should be spared as far as possible. Too soft a surface checks the force of the shock wave and can in its turn cause problems. Soft sand, for example, can trigger problems from the Achilles tendon since the heel sinks down into the surface and the foot slips on take-off. Wet, icy and slippery surfaces can be a contributory cause of muscle-tendon injuries, above all in the groin and the thigh and also of injuries to ligaments in the knee and ankle joints.

The average main road has a drainage slope of 7–9°, and anyone who trains on a main road and always runs on the same side can be affected by an artificial 'long leg–short leg' condition which can cause overuse problems.

Running uphill is especially trying for athletes with short calf muscles and tense Achilles tendons which can as a result be affected by overuse. Running downhill is trying for the knee joints and sometimes causes overloading problems around the patella and the lateral side of the knee.

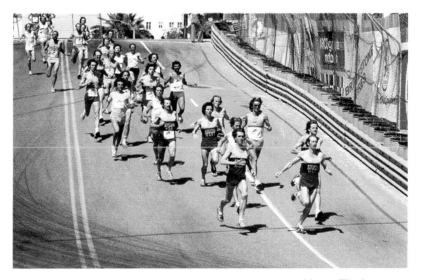

Running uphill as well as downhill can sometimes cause problems. The knee joints are particularly susceptible when running downhill. *Photo: All-Sport/Tony Duffy.*

Footwear

The relationship between shoe, foot and surface is of the utmost significance to the frequency of injury in runners. In most sports the shoes are the most important items of equipment. They have to distribute the load so that as little as possible of the shock wave is transmitted to the body tissues, and if the working surface is hard, the shoes should have soles with good shock-absorbing properties. In sports in which the risk of injury due to training or accidents is high, the stabilizing qualities of shoes are of value. Good shoe design is described on page 111.

Technique

Running technique varies from one sport to another. Long-distance runners generally strike first with the heel, followed by the toe, while short-distance runners tend to be mid-foot strikers or to run on their toes only. The commonest technique faults are to strike too hard with the heel or to run flat-footed, and they can result in overuse injuries. Repeated incorrect running or jumping technique always results in such injuries.

Body weight

Overweight causes increased load on the tissues which then tire more easily. The result can be the development of overuse injuries.

Foot injuries due to overuse

Injuries due to overuse can occur when a tissue is subjected to repeated normal or high load which leads to microscopic ruptures and tissue injury. The response of the body to tissue injury is an inflammatory reaction. The pain which is the most outstanding feature of the tissue injury is often of a temporary nature. It can disappear completely during the warm-up phase before a training period or a competition which the injured athlete can then carry out with relatively little trouble. Later, however, the pain returns with increased intensity. It usually disappears after rest but recurs at the next training session or competition, only to disappear yet again, in most cases, in the course of the warm-up exercises. There is a high risk that the injured athlete will enter a pain cycle (see page 41) which is difficult to break. The pain will ultimately become continuous during rest as well as physical activity.

'Painful heel cushion' (bruised heel)

The heel cushion is divided into small compartments containing fat and surrounded by fascia of connective tissue which are attached to the skin. Unlike the skin on the dorsum (top) of the foot, the skin on the sole of the foot cannot slide backwards and forwards over the tissues beneath. Repeated jumps landing on the heels, as performed by hurdlers, long-jumpers and triple-jumpers, can cause a rupture in these connective tissue bands. The fat compartments are pressed outwards from the area of the heel which contacts the running surface, and this causes the protective effect of the fat cushion to be reduced. Thus the skin lies in close opposition to the bone which becomes more sensitive to pain during loading.

As long as the ruptures in the connective tissue bands are not too extensive and have occurred only recently there is only local tenderness in the heel cushion, but in prolonged cases the underlying bone can be felt beneath the skin. Once it has arisen, the condition is very difficult to

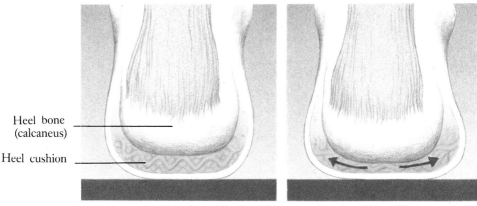

Heel bone
(calcaneus)

Heel cushion

Left: normal heel cushion. The bone is protected by fatty tissue. **Right:** a painful heel cushion. The fatty tissue is pressed out towards the sides of the heel impairing the protection for the heel bone.

treat. It must therefore be prevented, partly by using the correct technique, but more especially by using shoes that are suitable for the surface and have a heel which absorbs as much of the force of the shock wave as possible and distributes the remainder well. When signs of painful heel appear, the athlete can use shoes with an insert in which there is a notch for the painful area.

Inflammation of the bursa under the calcaneus

Between the calcaneus and the heel cushion there is a small bursa which can become painful after impact — in basketball, for example. Running and sometimes even walking then becomes an impossibility for the affected athlete and rest is recommended. A shoe insert with a notch for the painful area under the heel may be effective. In cases of prolonged problems, a doctor can give a steroid injection which should be followed by rest.

Plantar fasciitis ('heel spur')

The arch ligament or plantar aponeurosis (fascia) is a fibrous band that runs forwards from the plantar medial part of the calcaneus, blending with ligaments which are attached to the toes (see diagram on page 362). When an athlete lifts his heel during take-off, the angle between the different parts of the foot increases and the aponeurosis is drawn distally. As the toes are bent, the aponeurosis is stretched and the longitudinal arch is stabilized.

During a vigorous take-off, a rupture can occur in the origin that is common to the plantar aponeurosis and the short flexors of the toes. Injuries can also occur during a fast turn which causes marked pressure on the tissues of the sole of the foot.

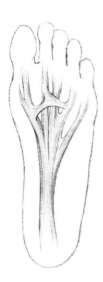

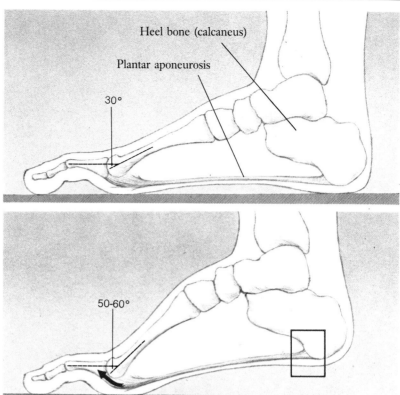

Top: the foot and plantar aponeurosis (fascia) when the whole foot is loaded against the surface. The diagram above shows how the plantar aponeurosis is stretched during take-off. The ringed area indicates the seat of inflammation at the origin of the plantar aponeurosis from the heel bone. **Far left:** the plantar aponeurosis seen from underneath.

Athletes who have an excessive pronation in the ankle joint develop inflammation in the origin of the plantar aponeurosis more often than others. When, as a result of the pronation, the arch is stretched and the toes spread out, the aponeurosis is subjected to increased strain. Prolonged sporting activity in shoes which do not provide sufficient support for the arch can also cause heel pain.

Symptoms and diagnosis
— Pain at the origin of the aponeurosis from the calcaneus under load. At rest the problems abate.
— Morning stiffness and limp.
— Marked tenderness on pressure and sometimes swelling over the calcaneus.
— Pain when the injured athlete is standing on tiptoe and walking on his heels.
— Numbness along the outside of the sole of the foot.
— An X-ray sometimes shows an oedema and a bony outgrowth which arises as an irritant reaction to the stretching of the ligament attachment. The find is fortuitous, since heel spurs are often present without symptoms, yet are often lacking in problem feet.

Treatment	The *athlete* should: — rest; — treat the injury by cooling when it is in its acute phase; — take the weight off the injured foot with crutches; — tape to unload the area or apply a heat retainer sock or insole; — check whether it is the sports shoes that increase the load on the aponeurosis; the shoes can be too stiff, for example, or too soft; — carry out static stretching exercises as a preventive and rehabilitative measure. The *doctor* may: — prescribe arch supports (orthotics) with a notch corresponding to the painful area; — prescribe anti-inflammatory medication; — operate if rupture and/or prolonged problems are present.
Healing and complications	The injury should be treated at an early phase as the problems can otherwise be very prolonged. Some cases involving extensive disruption of the aponeurosis have been described. Most of these ruptures have occurred after patients have been treated with local steroid injections. An extensive rupture of the aponeurosis is exceedingly difficult to treat.

Entrapment of nerves

Tarsal tunnel syndrome	Just below the medial malleolus lies a passage through which pass the medial and the lateral plantar nerves. In cases of excessive pronation of the foot the load increases on the tissues that surround the flexor tendons, and inflammation can occur and cause swelling which results in trapping of these nerves (the tarsal tunnel syndrome). The affected athlete feels pain arising from the area of entrapment. It radiates distally along the inside of the foot and along the sole towards the toes, that is, the area that the nerves supply. The treatment of this injury with arch supports (orthotics) and heat gives good results, but sometimes surgery has to be undertaken.
Entrapment of the medial calcaneal nerve	The medial calcaneal nerve passes from a deep connective tissue layer to a more superficial level at the inner edge of the heel where the thick heel skin meets the thinner skin on the medial side of the foot. When there is excessive pronation or increased pressure from the shoes over this area the nerve on the medial side of the calcaneus can be trapped. Pain radiates from the medial side of the heel out towards its centre. The treatment is rest, local symptomatic measures and heat. If this treatment has no effect, surgery can be performed.

Stress fractures of calcaneus, navicular and metatarsal bones

Stress fractures are found in otherwise healthy individuals from the age of seven years onwards in normal bone and under normal physical conditions without the bone having been subjected to trauma.

Stress fractures can occur as a result of prolonged and repeated load on the legs. Long-distance runners and athletes who train intensively or are badly prepared are particularly susceptible to this type of injury. In athletes, stress fractures occur mainly in the lower leg, for example in the calcaneus, the navicular and the metatarsal bones. A stress fracture of the second or third metatarsal bone is sometimes called a 'march fracture' as it often occurs in infantrymen.

Symptoms and diagnosis
— Pain in the affected bone during activity.
— Very distinct tenderness and local swelling.
— An X-ray of the injury shows no fracture in about half the cases. If there is still a suspicion that the injury is a stress fracture, another X-ray should be taken 2–3 weeks later. Healing tissue (callus) can then be seen around the fracture.
— If the X-ray does not prove the existence of a fracture, an examination with radioactive isotopes (bone scan) can confirm the diagnosis.

Treatment
The weight is taken off the injured foot, usually with crutches. The treatment otherwise is as described on page 55.

Healing
The injured athlete can resume his sporting activity to its full extent when he is free of symptoms, as a rule 6–8 weeks after their onset.

Fractures

Fractures of the talus

The talus (ankle bone) can be fractured in football, downhill skiing, ski-jumping, high-jumping and indoor sports. The injury is rare and difficult to treat, and is likely to be complicated by injuries to blood vessels which can prejudice healing.

Fractures of the calcaneus

In cases of trauma and accidents in sports which involve falls from a high altitude, for example parachuting, fractures of the calcaneus can occur. The injured person then finds it difficult to stand on his foot because of pain and severe swelling. The treatment consists of rest with a varying degree of relief from weightbearing; sometimes surgery is considered. A fracture of the calcaneus can cause prolonged, sometimes permanent problems with pain when the heel is under load.

Metatarsal problems

Insufficiency of the longitudinal arch

Excessive pronation and low arches

Feet show many individual differences. The longitudinal arch may be flat, but the foot is still functional. If the foot is under load, for example during sporting activity on a hard surface, and is pressed down because of incorrect loading, excess body weight or prolonged standing, the arch can collapse, resulting in a flat foot. In cases of excessive pronation or very low arches, the medial edge of the foot is lower than the lateral edge, and at the same time the metatarsal bones and the toes are rotated outwards.

Symptoms and diagnosis

— Often there are no problems at all.
— Pain can occur due to overuse and aching in the feet and lower leg.
— When there is repeated load, for example during running, pain can occur in the feet, lower leg, knee joint and groin.
— A feeling of fatigue in the feet.
— Calluses can form on the sole of the foot in areas of increased load.

Preventive measures

— Flexibility training of the ankle joints and static stretching exercises of the calf muscles.
— Foot exercises with toe movements.
— The athlete should use shoes with a good construction of the outer sole, inner sole and heel counter.

Treatment

— Arch supports (orthotics, see below).
— Taping.
— Active rest. In certain cases the affected athlete must take a break from running but can still maintain physical fitness by, for example, swimming or cycling.

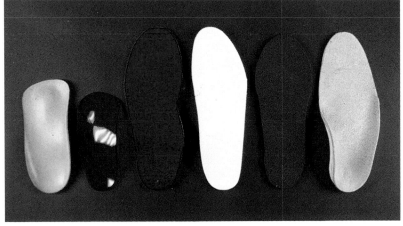

Different types of arch supports (orthotics). The supports to the left have a pad at the front as a support for the front arch.

Insufficiency of the anterior transverse arch

The normal function of the anterior transverse arch is considered to be the provision of elasticity. The middle metatarsal bones and the toes flex down towards the surface when the anterior transverse arch is stressed in the supporting phase and in take-off. A slackening of the ligaments between the metatarsal bones could then occur, and if this happens the arch loses its arched shape and load-absorbing ability. The foot becomes broader and the metatarsal bones as well as the toes acquire a fan-like spread.

Symptoms and diagnosis
— Pain when the anterior transverse arch is loaded.
— Calluses from under the ball of the foot as a result of the skin being exposed to increased pressure.
— Eventually the big toe can deviate and come to lie across the other toes (hallux valgus – see page 368).
— Pressure can cause a bursa and a bony outgrowth to form on the medial side of the big toe. Continued pressure, for example from shoes, can lead to inflammation occurring in the bursa (bunion).
— The condition can cause 'hammer toe', that is, all the toes except for the big toe lie in a permanently bent position. This causes increased pressure on the nerve supplying the cleft between the third and fourth, and the second and third toes (Morton's metatarsalgia), and painful calluses (corns) can appear on top.

Treatment
— Shoe orthotics with a pad for the anterior transverse arch (see photograph on page 365).
— In cases of hallux valgus with bursitis and hammer toe surgery may be necessary.
— Gripping exercises with the toes.
— General exercise programme.

Pes cavus (claw-foot)

A foot with a high longitudinal arch is called pes cavus (claw-foot), and is a congenital abnormality. A claw-foot is relatively inflexible and has a limited articular range. It is often combined with a tight calf musculature and usually with a tight plantar aponeurosis. The weightbearing surface is relatively small, so there is a risk of concentration of pressure and abnormal load conditions.

Symptoms and diagnosis
— The foot is inflexible, and its arch is hardly flattened at all under load.
— Hammer toe develops, that is, the toes are bent and cannot be straightened.
— The big toe is displaced downwards which often leads to the formation of painful calluses.
— Pain on prolonged exertion. Obvious claw-feet do not usually tolerate long-distance running very well.

Treatment
— Specially made arch supports with good shock-absorbing properties should be used. Shoes with ½ in (1 cm) heel wedges of a semi-hard material can be of value in order to relieve calloused areas.

— Static stretching is an important type of training for all types of claw-foot. The exercises can be carried out on a board which is inclined at an angle of about 35°. The toes and the heel should then be slanted downwards alternately.

— Any calluses that form should be pared down and relieved from pressure.

Bunions on the foot

Sometimes bunions (bony prominences or exostoses) occur on the top or sides of the foot. A bunion can increase in size or become inflamed. As a rule, they are caused by pressure from shoes which are laced too tightly. The bunions most often appear on the top (dorsum) of the foot anterior to the ankle, and are sometimes composed of separate bones. Foot mobility is often normal, but the affected person cannot walk in shoes. Tenderness can be caused by inflammation in a bursa which has formed over the bunions. X-ray shows either a small bony bunion, or sometimes an extra bone.

The treatment for an bunion which causes problems is often an alteration of the shoe. Sometimes it can be removed surgically.

Inflammation of the flexor tendons of the toes (flexor tendinitis)

The tendons which bend the toes run along the top (dorsum) of the foot and merge with muscles which are attached to the anterior aspect of the tibia. When these tendons are subjected to increased pressure from sports shoes which are ill-fitting or laced too tightly, they can become inflamed. The symptom is pain on the top of the foot, which is worse during running. Tenderness can be felt along the course of the tendons. In cases of acute tendinitis, crepitus can sometimes occur.

Treatment
— Active rest.
— Anti-inflammatory medication.
— Altering the shoes. Sometimes a piece of felt or foam rubber with a notch for the painful area can prevent pressure from the tongue of the shoe.
— When the problems are prolonged a steroid injection may be necessary, and should be followed by rest.
— In exceptional cases surgery is performed.

Fractures of the metatarsal bones

A fracture of one or more of the metatarsal bones is the commonest of the fractures that can affect the foot. The injury can occur when, for example, the foot is trodden on in some ball sport. Because of the pain, the injury is treated with plaster for a few weeks. In cases of fracture with displacement of two or more metatarsal bones, surgery may be considered. As a rule, the injury heals without causing any future disability.

Fractures of the base of the fifth metatarsal bone can occur as a result of twisting or avulsion injuries. The peroneus brevis is attached to the base and may cause non-union of the fracture by pulling the bones apart. Treatment in a plaster cast is recommended. In cases of displacement, surgery is needed.

Inflammation or rupture of the tendon of the peroneus brevis muscle

Inflammation and partial ruptures of the fifth metatarsal bone attachment of the tendon of the peroneus brevis muscle are not uncommon in football players. Sometimes the tendon sheath can be inflamed, resulting in crepitus. Pain is felt over the upper part of the fifth metatarsal bone. When the injury is in its acute stage, anti-inflammatory medication are used. If necessary a plaster cast is applied. In other respects the injury is treated according to the advice given on page 43.

Toe problems

Hallux valgus

The big toe can normally be angled outwards by up to 10°. If the angle is greater the condition is called hallux valgus. In such cases of displacement an exostosis forms on the medial side of the foot where the angle is greatest. The outgrowth is covered by a bursa which can sometimes be inflamed and extremely sore as a result of being exposed to pressure (a bunion).

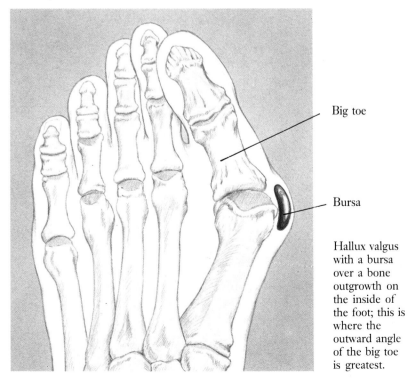

Big toe

Bursa

Hallux valgus with a bursa over a bone outgrowth on the inside of the foot; this is where the outward angle of the big toe is greatest.

One cause of hallux valgus is a depressed anterior arch. Excessive pronation, and imbalance and contractions of the muscles of the big toe, can be of importance in the appearance of hallux valgus. Other contributory factors are thought to be ill-fitting shoes and a displacement of the first metatarsal bone.

Symptoms and diagnosis
— The big toe is angled more than 10° outwards and may be pressed against the second toe, which in its turn may be pressed against the third so that an increasingly faulty foot posture is present.
— A callus often occurs on the sole of the foot under the second metatarsal bone.
— Problems when wearing shoes.
— Skin redness and tenderness can occur on the medial edge of the foot where the angle is greatest.

Treatment
The *athlete* should:
— wear wide-fitting shoes with moderate heels;
— put a piece of soft felt or a rubber pad between the big toe and the second toe.

The *doctor* may:
— prescribe arch supports with pads under the anterior transverse arch;
— prescribe shoes shaped to match the exostosis;
— operate. Surgery should, however, only be carried out when the problems are severe.

Hammer toe

The proximal interphalangeal joint in the toes may become contracted into a flexed position, caused by an insufficiency of the anterior transverse arch (see page 366) or too small shoes. Painful corns will appear over the prominent joint. The pressure can be relieved by wearing shoes with a deep and spacious toe box and a support for the anterior transverse arch. Occasionally, surgery is necessary.

Hallux rigidus

Hallux rigidus (stiff big toe) can occur after repeated minor injuries to the articular surfaces of the metatarsophalangeal joint of the big toe. The mobility of this joint is then impaired, and the affected athlete finds it difficult to run and walk normally. Long-distance runners may complain that pain from the big toe makes them unable to run the required distances. An X-ray of the metatarsophalangeal joint of the big toe can sometimes show changes due to wear.

The symptoms of hallux rigidus are tenderness over the metatarsophalangeal joint of the big toe and also impaired mobility of the toe, above all in upward bending (dorsiflexion). The affected athlete's foot should be examined for any features which could be corrected with the help of shoe arch supports (orthotics). Sometimes the athlete has to change to another sport like cycling or swimming so that the toe joint is relieved. Occasionally operative treatment of hallux rigidus can be necessary.

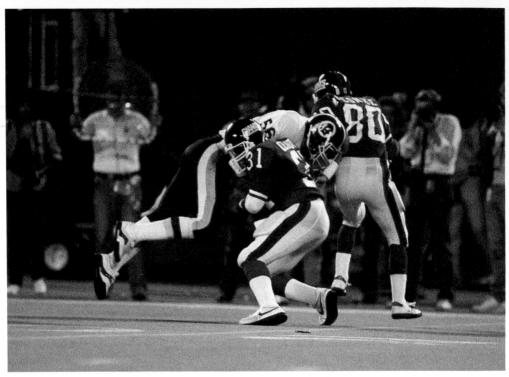

'Turf toe syndrome' can occur as a result of sporting activity on an artificial surface. *Photo: All-Sport/David Cannon.*

'Turf toe syndrome'

In playing soccer or American football on an artificial all-weather surface, or squash, the player's shoe grips the surface during a sudden stop, while the foot slides forwards in the shoe, resulting in vigorous upward bending (dorsiflexion) of the big toe. The ligaments are stretched, the articular surface is injured and the joint capsule is stretched or torn. The injury is becoming increasingly common as artificial surfaces are more widely used. The symptoms are swelling and pain in the base joint of the big toe (metatarsophalangeal joint) and also tenderness on stretching or bending the toe.

An athlete affected by 'turf toe syndrome' should be X-rayed to check whether there is a fracture. Emergency treatment includes cooling, compression bandaging, elevation of the foot, relief from weightbearing and rest. After 2–4 days the injured athlete can again bear weight. During the rehabilitation period the big toe can be protected with a stiff, firm sole which is long and broad enough to prevent the toe from making exaggerated movements. The injured joint can also be stabilized by taping. In cases of 'turf toe syndrome' the injured athlete should allow at least 2–4 weeks' rest from his sporting activity.

Fractures of the sesamoid bones

Fractures can affect the sesamoid bones of the foot, and the two sesamoid bones under the metatarsophalangeal joint of the big toe are generally the most vulnerable. These sesamoid bones are attached to the tendon of the flexor of the big toe. A fracture usually affects the medial sesamoid bone, when the big toe is forced to bend vigorously upwards, for example on take-off accompanied by impact on the foot. Sometimes inflammation can occur in the tendon surrounding the sesamoid bones due to uneven pressure distribution in the area.

Symptoms and diagnosis
— The athlete cannot run on tiptoe and has pain on take-off.
— Local tenderness and swelling.
— Pain occurs when the toes are bent upwards.
— If there is a fracture, an X-ray confirms the diagnosis.

Treatment
— Plaster cast should be worn for several weeks.
— If the injury does not receive medical attention until a late stage and the fracture has by then healed badly, surgery may be considered. The sesamoid bone is removed.
— The injury often affects athletes with high arches and a tight arch

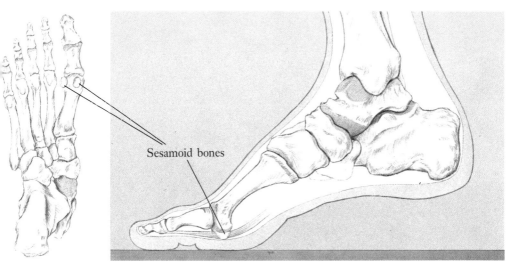

Sesamoid bones

In the ball of the foot under the big toe there are sesamoid bones which can be injured, particularly on take-off.

ligament. Surgical measures can sometimes be taken to reduce the tension in the arch ligament.

Morton's syndrome

The sensitivity in the toes is transmitted to the brain by nerves. Each nerve transmits the sensitivity from the lateral side of one toe and the medial side of the adjacent toe. The metatarsal bones can sometimes be compressed, as a result of wearing ill-fitting shoes, for example, or having a depressed anterior arch. The plantar digital nerves often join between the metatarsal head and may become compressed, which results in a local nerve swelling (neuroma), usually between the third and fourth metatarsal. This causes a painful condition known as Morton's syndrome.

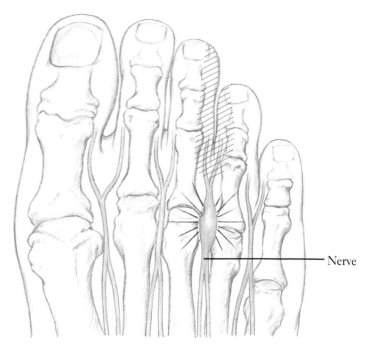

Nerve

The nerves of the toes. When the front arch is weak, a nerve can get trapped between the bones. The nerve then swells, increasing pressure which in turn may cause radiating pain and numbness in the toes (shaded areas).

Symptoms and diagnosis

— The injured athlete usually complains about recurrent pain from the lateral side of one toe and the medial side of the next. It is generally the third and the fourth toes which are affected.
— The symptoms are often compared to an electric shock.
— Sensitivity can be impaired on the other sides of the two affected toes.
— The problems can occur spontaneously when they are least expected.
— The injured athlete can be completely without pain when walking barefoot so pain can be relieved by taking off the shoes.
— By compressing the metatarsal bones, pain can be triggered in the affected toes.
— Local tenderness may be felt between the toes when a thin object, for example the back of a pen, is pressed against the skin.

Treatment

The *athlete* should:
— rest and relieve pressure on the toes;
— wear wide-fitting shoes.

The *doctor* may:
— prescribe anti-inflammatory medication for a couple of weeks;
— prescribe an arch support (orthotic) with a pad which can spread the metatarsal bones and thereby ease the pressure on the nerve;
— prescribe physiotherapy, using a faradic current to stimulate the transverse portion of the adductor hallucis and increase arch support.
— operate, which is a very effective treatment.

Fractures of toes

Fractures of toes can occur in most sports, for example when players kick the ball. Fractures of the big toe are the most serious, especially if a joint is involved. If there is displacement, the bone ends must be realigned after which the injury is treated with a plaster cast for about 4 weeks. Fractures of other toe bones heal without any treatment other than rest, provided there is no displacement. A 3–5 weeks' break in training is necessary.

Toe-nail problems

Ingrowing toe nails

An ingrowing toe nail is a common complaint among athletes, usually caused by ill-fitting shoes pressing the skin against the edge of the nail. The big toe which has a broad nail is most often affected.

Preventive measures are essential. Shoes should be big enough, well-fitting and comfortable, and tight socks should not be worn. Careful foot hygiene is necessary. The toe nails should be cut regularly, at least once a week, and cut off straight, as they can grow down into the nail fold if the sides of the nail bed are trimmed to a curved outline. Nails that are too thick should be thinned.

In cases of ingrowing toe nails, bacterial infections can invade the cuticles and cause extreme discomfort. Such infections should be drained and the area kept dry and treated with a local antiseptic and possibly an antibiotic powder. Antibiotics taken by mouth may also be of value. If ingrowing toe nails cause persistent problems, surgery can be resorted to. A number of different approaches may be used, but it is usual for either a 'wedge' of nail or the whole nail to be removed depending upon the length and severity of problems and on previous treatment. Excision of the nail bed (from which new nail growth arises) ensures that the nail does not regrow.

Black nails ('tennis toe', 'soccer toe')

Black nails (black because of bruising) can occur as a result of a blow to the nail, being trodden on, wearing shoes that are too narrow or the toe nails being left too long. Bleeding occurs in the nail bed and appears as a black spot or patch under the nail. Bruised nails occur in most sports; in running they can be caused by the toe nails being pressed against the front part of the shoe especially when the shoes are too small and when running downhill.

Bleeding in the nail bed tends to be painful because the blood which gathers under the nail exerts pressure on the tissues. It can be released, after first cleaning the nail, by making a hole with a clean, sharp knife or with a red-hot needle or straightened paper clip. This is by no means as alarming as it sounds. The blood drains out spontaneously through the hole which is then protected with a dressing to prevent the nail bed becoming infected. This procedure preserves the nail, which would otherwise fall off after 2–3 weeks because of disruption of its blood supply. Once an injured nail becomes loose and begins to separate from its attachment to the cuticle, there is a risk of infection occurring and it is wise to seek medical advice.

Anyone who has had a bruised nail should consider how the injury occurred, and if the shoes are at fault, should change them.

Bony outgrowth under the nail (subungual exostosis)

In cases of repeated impact to a toe, for example when a basketball player has his toe trodden on repeatedly, a bony outgrowth (exostosis) sometimes develops at the outer extremity of the affected toe and impinges on the nail bed. This usually affects the big toe and is very painful and highly sensitive to pressure and further impact. In many cases the nail has to be removed in order to relieve the pressure, an alternative being to remove the exostosis surgically.

Skin conditions which affect the feet

Calluses

The skin thickens in response to pressure and calluses form. Pressure on the feet can be caused by shoes that are laced too tightly or are too narrow or by some anatomical variation. Calluses can occur at many different sites, the commonest being:
— the heel;
— the ball of the foot, especially in those who push off with the second toe;
— the top surface of 'hammer' or otherwise bent toes; and
— the medial side of the big toe where there is an exostosis at that point.

Calluses on the foot are treated by relieving pressure. If necessary they can be trimmed with a sharp knife or filed with a foot file and this can be done by a chiropodist. Sometimes calluses are recurrent, and then treatment is a question of removing the triggering cause, for example an exostosis, or altering or replacing faulty shoes. This usually prevents further problems.

Skin outgrowths

Skin outgrowths are a kind of callus which form between the toes, usually the fourth and fifth toes, as a result of pressure from shoes that are too narrow. Treatment consists of wearing shoes with a wider fitting at the same time as protecting the affected area from further pressure by the use, for example, of rings of felt or foam rubber placed around the outgrowths.

'Athlete's foot'

When foot hygiene is inadequate, and when the feet are not dried thoroughly after showers or baths, fungal infections may develop. The fungus causes the skin between the toes to become soggy, cracked and whitish in appearance and often to smell offensive. The condition is infectious and can spread from one individual to another via floors on which people walk barefoot such as those of locker rooms, showers and swimming baths.

Preventive measures

— Regular washing of the feet with soap and water followed by thorough drying.
— Regular, frequent changes of socks.
— Porous shoes that allow circulation of air and evaporation of moisture.
— Avoidance of walking barefoot in locker-rooms, etc.

Treatment

The *doctor* may:
— prescribe a fungicidal preparation. The application should be used regularly as directed and treatment continued for a couple of weeks after the skin appears to have returned to normal.

Verrucas or warts

Verrucas (or warts) are caused by a virus and can be transferred from one individual to another via the floors of showers and locker rooms where people walk barefoot. The incubation period is 1–6 months. Verrucas are most often located on the sole of the foot, are round or oval in shape and have a crack or dark spot in the middle. They can generally be distinguished from calluses though this may be difficult when a verruca appears in a weightbearing area and both conditions are present.

Verrucas cause pain when pressed against underlying tissue, and can also be painful when pressed from the sides. They may become infected by bacteria and rarely this infection may spread to the bloodstream.

Verrucas will disappear spontaneously after 2–4 years, but treatment should be commenced as soon as they are discovered in order to prevent spread.

Any unusual lump or bump which appears on the skin, especially if the diagnosis is not obvious and the skin is discoloured or bleeds, should prompt a consultation with a doctor.

Treatment

The *athlete* should:
— file or rub down the verruca with an emery board as far as possible, perhaps after 10–15 minutes' hot foot-bath, and then treat the verruca with a proprietary wart preparation which contains salicylic acid. The instructions for use should be followed with care and the normal surrounding skin protected. Treatment may have to be continued for several months.

The *doctor* may:
— cut or burn away verrucas if necessary.

HEAD INJURIES AND UNCONSCIOUSNESS

Head injuries occur in most sports, but mainly in contact sports and among riders, downhill skiers and boxers. There is also a risk of their occurring when heading a football, especially if faulty technique is used. A kicked football in flight can reach a speed of 60 mph (100 km/h) and weigh about 1 lb (400 g) (even more if it is wet), so considerable forces can be transmitted from the ball to the head.

Unconscious-ness

A distinction should be made between unconsciousness caused by head injuries on impact (for example, a fall or collision) and those triggered by some other cause, such as inadequate circulation during long-distance running. It is up to the person providing assistance to determine the cause and act accordingly.

Unconsciousness caused by a blow to the head

Whether or not the injured person is unconscious at the time of examination, head injuries should always be considered potentially serious as grave complications can ensue.

Although a serious injury can occur without any loss of consciousness, in general terms the period of unconsciousness is directly related to the severity of the injury. An attempt should therefore be made as soon as possible after an incident involving a blow to the head to decide whether unconsciousness has indeed occurred. Unconsciousness is usually associated with some loss of memory and the easiest way of assessing the situation is to ask the injured person what happened before, during and after the accident.

After a head injury, the following situations may develop:

1. *Head injury without unconsciousness.* The injured person has no loss of memory but may complain of a headache, nausea and/or dizziness and may also be pale and generally upset. The nausea can lead to vomiting.

   Athletes who are in this state should stop their sporting activity immediately. They should be kept under observation, must not be left alone and should consult a doctor for advice.

2. *Head injury with unconsciousness of short duration (less than 5 minutes).* If there has been a short period of unconsciousness and the injured person is complaining of symptoms such as headache, nausea, vomiting and/or dizziness and is generally upset, a serious injury may well have occurred. The injured person should be transported to a doctor or hospital for further management. As a rule, the symptoms settle without any further problems, and observation in hospital, if it is felt necessary, will be unlikely to last for much longer than 24 hours.

3. *Head injury with unconsciousness of long duration (more than 5 minutes)* should be considered very serious. The injured person should be taken to hospital as soon as possible for diagnosis, observation and treatment.

Measures at the scene of injury in cases of unconsciousness

It is of vital importance to ensure immediately that the unconscious person has *free air passages* and is breathing normally. Obstruction of the airways in an unconscious individual due to any condition can cause death, and, if breathing or heart activity stops for longer than 3–5 minutes, permanent brain damage occurs.

If the injured person is breathing of his own accord he should be placed on his side. In order to ensure that the air passages are kept open, the unconscious person should be placed in what is often known as the 'recovery' position. He is turned on to his left side with his left arm behind his back and his left leg bent to a right angle at both the hip and knee. His right arm is placed across his body with the hand on the ground, and his right leg kept straight. In this position he is prevented from falling on to his face.

If the injured person is not breathing of his own accord, artificial respiration must be commenced, using mouth-to-mouth resuscitation. The injured

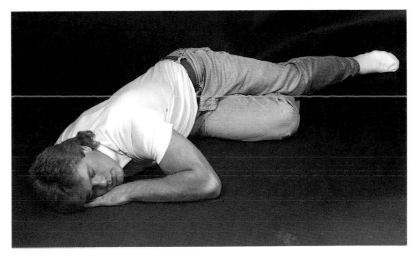

The recovery position.

person is placed on his back with his head tilted backwards, and the following measures are taken before artificial respiration is started:
— *the mouth cavity is cleared* of objects such as dentures, loose teeth, soil, and vomit.
— *the head is tilted backwards and the lower jaw is pulled up.* The tongue of an unconscious person can fall against the back wall of the throat and obstruct breathing. Backward tilting of the injured person's head and support of the chin is usually sufficient to free the air passages. One hand is then put on the injured person's forehead while the other supports the neck so that the head is supported in the extended position and the mouth opens.

Mouth-to-mouth resuscitation (the kiss of life)

To administer mouth-to-mouth resuscitation, take a deep breath, open your mouth wide and press it as closely as possible to that of the injured person. If it is an adult, pinch his nostrils closed and breathe out strongly into his mouth at the same time. (The patient's chest should heave if this is done correctly.) Then lift your head, turn it sideways and breathe in while the patient breathes out. Blow in at a rate of about 12 times a minute for adults, that is, once every 5 seconds. If the patient is a child, blow in more frequently, more gently and preferably through the patient's nose and mouth simultaneously. Don't stop until the patient begins to breathe on his own.

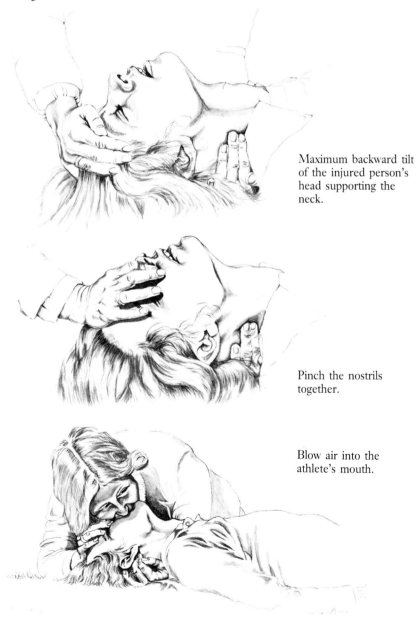

Maximum backward tilt of the injured person's head supporting the neck.

Pinch the nostrils together.

Blow air into the athlete's mouth.

— *The unconscious person should be taken to hospital as soon as possible.*
— While waiting for transport *he should be kept covered* and something warm, for example a blanket, placed beneath him.
— *Give nothing to drink* to a person who is or has been unconscious.
— *Never leave anybody who is, or has been, unconscious alone.*

Note that if there is suspicion of an injury to the neck the injured person's head should *not* be bent back to free the air passages. Instead this should be achieved by raising his lower jaw. Even in a situation in which an injured person should not be moved until expert medical staff arrive, his air passages must be kept open effectively.

Head injuries with unconsciousness should be considered serious, and may be followed by complications.

Mouth-to-mouth resuscitation is the only effective method of artificial respiration when no aids are at hand. The method should be mastered by everybody.

Complications In cases of head injury, *internal bleeding* may occur. This is the result of rupture of blood vessels, which can happen with or without bony injury to the skull, and if it continues it gradually compresses the brain. The increased pressure on the brain tissues can affect the centre which controls breathing with the result that breathing stops. Only an immediate operation to stop the bleeding and relieve the pressure will give the injured athlete a chance to recover.

Bleeding from the ears or bleeding with a simultaneous flow of fluid

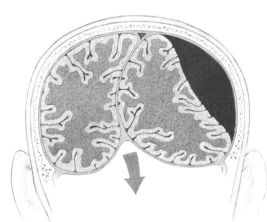

Bleeding between the bones of the skull and brain. The increased pressure is transmitted down towards the base of the skull.

from the injured person's nose suggests that a fracture of the base of the skull may have occurred, and this may involve injury to a number of important nerves.

In cases of head injury, it may take hours or days for evidence of complications to appear. A variety of different techniques may be used for investigation including X-rays, specialized scans and ultrasound.

Unconsciousness without head injury

Unconsciousness may occur during long-distance races, especially in hot weather, even when the athlete is relatively well-trained. Fluid loss leading to a reduction in blood volume and thus a poor blood supply to the brain is the usual cause, but unconsciousness may also follow an abnormal heart rhythm or a marked fall in blood sugar levels.

Treatment
— *Make sure that the air passages are clear* in the unconscious person.
— *Keep the injured person covered* (but not overheated) and place something warm beneath him.
— *Lift the injured person's legs* so that the blood flow to the brain increases.
— *Do not give* an unconscious person *anything to drink.*
— *Call a doctor* or arrange *immediate transport to hospital.*

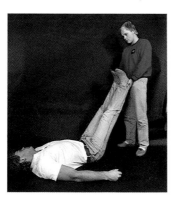

Unconsciousness without head injury; the patient's legs should be lifted to increase the blood flow to the brain.

FACIAL INJURIES

Open wounds

Wounds on the forehead and scalp may occur in association with injuries to underlying tissues. Such injuries often occur in contact sports, such as ice hockey, rugby, and soccer, but also among riders, downhill skiers and others.

When there is a risk of skeletal injuries and/or there is copious bleeding, the injured person should see a doctor.

Wounds must be thoroughly cleaned. For general treatment see page 56.

Fractures of the maxillary bone (upper jaw)

Fractures of the upper jaw bone (maxillary bone) occur in contact sports such as football, ice hockey, rugby, handball and also boxing. This injury should be suspected if:

— the upper jaw has been subjected to a blow;
— the teeth are out of alignment and there is pain when the injured person clenches his teeth;
— one half of the cheek feels numb;
— a tender irregularity can be felt in the bone edge along the lower border of the eye-socket;
— there is double vision.

Fractures of the upper jaw are most often treated by surgery and heal in 6–8 weeks.

Fractures of the zygomatic bone

The zygomatic bone runs between the cheek and the ear, and a fracture should be suspected if:

— the zygomatic bone or the upper jaw have been subjected to a blow;
— there is tenderness with swelling over the zygomatic bone;
— chewing is painful.

If an X-ray shows that the fractured zygomatic bone is pressed inwards, the injury is operated on and heals in about 4 weeks.

Fractures of the mandibular bone (lower jaw)

A fracture of the lower jaw should be suspected if:

— the chin has been subjected to a blow, for example a punch in boxing;
— pain occurs when the injured person opens his mouth or clenches his teeth;
— the teeth are out of alignment;
— there is local tenderness in front of the ear.

Surgery is necessary if displacement has occurred. The lower jaw will be fixed to the upper jaw by wiring the teeth for 6–8 weeks.

NOSE INJURIES

Nosebleeds

A nosebleed is caused by rupture of one or more blood vessels in the nose, and is common in contact sports such as handball, ice hockey, football and also boxing and riding. Note that a broken nose should be suspected when bleeding occurs after a blow.

Treatment

The *athlete* should:
— sit upright if possible;
— place thumb and index finger over the nose and pinch the nostrils together for about 10 minutes after which bleeding will have stopped in nine out of ten cases. Keep the head bent forward rather than backwards;
— put a ball of cotton wool or a compress in the nostril for about 1 hour. Make sure that it cannot be inhaled and do not forget to remove it;
— see a doctor if the bleeding continues in spite of the above measures.

The *doctor* may:
— insert a compress with vessel-contricting agents;
— insert a pressure balloon in cases of severe bleeding;
— cauterize the ruptured blood vessel.

Fractures of the nasal bones

Fractures of the nasal bones occur in contact sports and also among riders and boxers. The injury is not particularly serious but as a rule requires treatment so that the fracture can be re-aligned surgically, bearing in mind the future appearance and function of the nose.

EAR INJURIES

Injuries to the outer ear

Injuries to the outer ear are not common in sport. Repeated blows or repeated pressure against the ear, for example in boxing and wrestling can, however, cause bleeding which, if it is not treated, can result in a 'cauliflower ear'. A similar acute injury is seen in rugby players.

Emergency treatment with cooling and compression should be applied in order to reduce the swelling to a minimum. Bleeding in the outer ear should be treated to prevent later deformity.

Injuries to the middle ear and the inner ear

If a blow to the side of the head is followed by pain from the ear, slight bleeding or impaired hearing, a rupture of the eardrum should be suspected. These symptoms should always lead to a medical examination since injuries to the eardrum can result in permanently impaired hearing.

Those involved in shooting should always use effective ear muffs in order to avoid damage of this sort.

EYE INJURIES

The area around the eye is constructed in such a way as to give the eye the greatest possible protection against external impact. Direct impact against the eye from a large object, for example a football, can result in bleeding and swelling in the eyelid and surrounding soft tissues but seldom injures the eye itself. Blows from small or pointed objects, such as elbows, fingers, sticks, rackets, squash balls and pucks can, on the other hand, cause direct injuries to the eyeball.

Corneal abrasions

One of the commonest eye injuries in sport is a small wound on the cornea (that is, the clear central part of the eye which covers the iris). The wound can be caused by a finger nail, a foreign body in the eye or a contact lens. The affected person complains of pain and a gritty sensation in the eye, especially in bright light and when blinking. Increased tear flow is a common symptom.

If a wound on the cornea is suspected, a doctor should be seen for advice since the injury can affect the sight. The treatment is usually ointment or eyedrops and rest, and an eye pad may be applied for a day or so.

Bleeding into the anterior chamber of the eye

A blow to the eye with a blunt object can cause bleeding in front of the iris. The blood forms a fluid level between the iris and the cornea at the bottom of the anterior chamber of the eye.

The treatment is immediate rest, since the bleeding may otherwise increase. The injured person should see a doctor for examination and observation. The condition often heals spontaneously without any permanent disability, but in exceptional cases the sight may be permanently damaged.

Inflammation and bleeding in the conjunctiva

The eye is relatively resistant to irritation, but swimmers can be affected by inflammation of the conjunctiva (which covers the whole of the eyeball) because of the chlorine in swimming pool water. The complaint can also be triggered by oversensitivity or overexposure to sunlight. It is harmless, and the problems can be relieved by eyedrops. Swimmers can prevent the complaint by using protective goggles.

Bleeding in the conjunctiva is not uncommon after blows to the eye but is seldom serious and disappears spontaneously within a few days or weeks. If the sight is affected, a doctor should be consulted.

Detached retina

The retina (that is, the lining at the back of the eye upon which sight depends) can be detached by a hard blow to the eye, and this should be suspected if the injured person has impaired sight within a limited field of vision. The injury should be examined by a doctor.

A doctor should be consulted in all cases of eye injuries, especially if signs of bleeding or impaired sight are present after a blow.

INJURIES TO THE MOUTH

Tongue injuries

The tongue can sometimes be bitten accidentally during sporting activity, and a wound with bleeding then occurs. The injury is painful but not serious, and a gash that is less than ½ in (1 cm) long does not need any treatment. More extensive wounds may need careful stitching by a doctor.

Dental injuries

Dental injuries are especially common among children. A quarter of all dental injuries in children occur during physical training or sporting activities. Collisions with opponents during contact sports are the commonest cause, but direct blows from equipment, for example hockey sticks or cricket balls may be to blame.

In the majority of cases it is the front teeth of the upper jaw that are affected, and in half of these cases more than one tooth has been damaged.

Dentists usually classify dental injuries in the following way:
— fracture of the crown of the tooth affecting the enamel only;
— fracture of the crown of the tooth affecting both enamel and dentine;
— fracture of the crown of the tooth with exposed pulp;
— injury of the attachment of the tooth in the jaw;
— injury of the root of the tooth;
— combination of fracture of crown and root;
— a lost tooth.

It is rare that a dental injury heals spontaneously without treatment. Dental injuries in children are considered as serious, since injuries to teeth and jaws that are not fully developed can lead to their being adversely affected for life.

Treatment

The injured person should *immediately* (the prognosis worsens with every hour's delay) see a dentist in cases of the following types of dental injuries:
— a broken tooth;
— a tooth that is knocked out;
— a tooth that is loose and bleeding.

A tooth that has been knocked out should be kept, since it can sometimes be re-implanted successfully into its correct position. The likelihood of this occurring depends on the length of time for which the tooth has been out of its socket and the degree to which the periodontal membrane has dried out. During the journey to the dentist the tooth should be kept moist, for example under the tongue or in a saliva-soaked handkerchief, so that drying of the periodontal membrane is minimized.

Preventive measures

Different types of gum shields for athletes have been constructed, including those suitable for use in ice hockey and boxing (see page 117). Unfortunately in some sports there is resistance among top-level players to using these shields which sets a bad example to young people. It should be a matter of course that all ice hockey and rugby players, for example, use this form of protection.

NECK INJURIES

Injuries to the larynx

The larynx (voice box) is hollow and is composed of elastic cartilage lined with mucous membrane. Air which is breathed in passes between its vocal cords to reach the lungs.

When a neck chop is dealt in wrestling or a blow is delivered by an arm, a stick or a ball to the front of the neck, the cartilage of the larynx can be bent inwards quite sharply. When the impact ceases, the cartilage springs back as a result of its own elasticity, and when that happens the mucous membrane may be torn loose. Bleeding can then occur between the cartilage and the mucous membrane and can spread to affect the vocal cords which become swollen and cause hoarseness of the voice. The swelling can gradually increase until it obstructs the opening between the vocal cords which impedes breathing. Children are particularly prone to this injury.

Blows against the front of the neck followed by hoarseness should prompt a visit to a doctor. Injuries to the larynx usually, however, heal with no treatment other than rest and observation.

Wounds to the neck region

Wounds to the neck can involve the large blood vessels running to and from the heart. Injuries of this type are uncommon but serious. They can occur, for example, in ice hockey when a skate hits the neck, and during accidents in motor sports. Profuse bleeding occurs and must be stopped immediately by pressing a towel against the wound and applying constant hard pressure. The injured person should be transported to hospital as soon as possible.

Injuries to the neck (see page 239)

CHEST INJURIES

Fractured rib

Fractured ribs are common in sport and especially in contact sports. They can occur after a direct blow with a blunt object, such as the handle of a stick, or as a result of forceful compression of the chest during a hard body tackle, for example, in rugby.

Symptoms and diagnosis
— Pain over the fracture area, especially when breathing deeply, coughing or sneezing.
— Tenderness and swelling over the fracture area.
— Compression of the whole chest causes pain over the fracture area.
— An X-ray of the chest confirms the injury and excludes underlying lung damage.

Treatment
Fractured ribs generally do not require any treatment other than pain relief, and heal spontaneously. Binding or strapping is discouraged as it prevents complete expansion of the lungs.

Very occasionally, if several ribs are fractured, and there is a possibility of interference with normal respiration, the injured person may be admitted to hospital for observation.

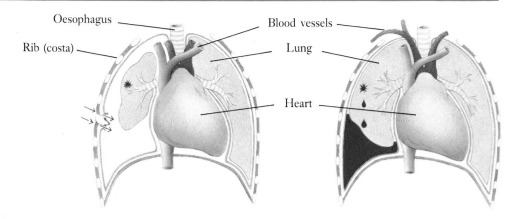

Oesophagus

Blood vessels

Rib (costa)

Lung

Heart

Left: an open injury where the sharp end of a broken rib has punctured the lung and caused leakage of air and at the same time collapse of the lung (pneumothorax). **Right:** an injury which has caused bleeding from the lung to pass into the pleural sac (haemothorax). Pneumothorax and haemothorax can occur together.

Healing and complications

In cases of a fracture without complications the injured athlete can return to his sport after 3–6 weeks depending on the symptoms.

Occasionally the sharp end of a fractured rib can puncture the lung and cause leakage of air (pneumothorax) or bleeding (haemothorax) from the lung into the pleural sac which surrounds it. Increasing breathing difficulties should arouse suspicion that one of these complications may have occurred. If it has, treatment will include draining the pleural cavity by means of a tube inserted through the chest wall.

ABDOMINAL INJURIES

Injuries to the abdomen are rare in sport, but their outcome can be catastrophic. They can be the result of falling off or being kicked by a horse, and also occur in contact sports and among cyclists, downhill skiers and others.

Rupture of the spleen

The spleen is located in the upper left part of the abdomen, and the commonest cause of death among athletes with abdominal injuries is rupture of this organ. The injury may result from a direct blow to the abdomen, for example when a cyclist falls in such a way that the handlebars impact into the upper left part of the abdomen. Rupture occurs rarely in cases of fractured ribs. It is important to remember that a ruptured spleen can result from any violent blow to the left side. Athletes who have had infectious mononucleosis (glandular fever) recently are more at risk.

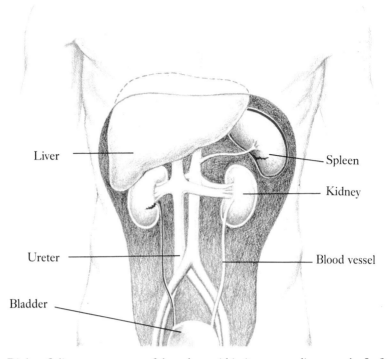

Liver

Spleen

Kidney

Ureter

Blood vessel

Bladder

Right of diagram: rupture of the spleen within its surrounding capsule. **Left:** rupture of a kidney. The bleeding caused by the rupture can pass blood into the urine.

Symptoms and diagnosis

A rupture of the spleen and its surrounding capsule causes bleeding into the abdominal cavity with ensuing pain and nausea and also tenderness and tenseness of the abdominal muscles. The injured person is at first affected only by pain, but after perhaps an hour begins to show signs of shock with a fast and weak pulse, pallor, sweating and sometimes drowsiness or loss of consciousness.

If the capsule remains intact, bleeding from the damaged organ occurs more slowly, and gradually distends and weakens the capsule. There is then a risk that rupture will be triggered by physical activity about 1–2 weeks after injury, and this occurs in 10–20 per cent of cases.

Treatment

The course of events and the results of the doctor's examination and investigations will determine the length of stay in hospital. If a rupture of the spleen is confirmed, it is removed immediately by operation. This has no significant consequences and does not lead to any later disability.

If symptoms such as nausea, fatigue, or pain in the left upper abdomen or left shoulder tip persist after a blow, a doctor should be consulted.

Rupture of the liver

The liver is located in the upper right-hand part of the abdomen below the rib cage. Its tissue is frail and it can rupture as a result of blows to this area. The injury occurs only rarely in sport.

A major rupture of the liver results in bile and blood flowing out into the abdominal cavity and causing peritonitis which may prove fatal. Pain and symptoms of shock occur soon after injury and the injured athlctc should be taken immediately to hospital. As a rule, surgery is necessary.

Kidney injuries

The kidneys are located above the pelvic girdle, one on each side of the spine. As a result of a violent impact, a kidney can rupture causing blood to appear in the urine. The injury is uncommon in sport. The bleeding often stops spontaneously and causes no further problems, but if disruption of a kidney is severe, and bleeding continues, it must be removed by surgery.

Blood in the urine after a blow in the kidney area should lead the athlete to seek medical advice.

After sustained vigorous physical exertion without impact, blood can appear in the urine. This does not necessarily indicate a kidney injury, but should be investigated by a doctor.

Injuries to the lower abdomen

A blow to the testes can cause bleeding and swelling which can disrupt the blood supply to the testes and cause sterility. The injury can be prevented by using a box, especially in contact sports.

Blows to the penis can cause painful cramp in the sphincter of the bladder which can make it difficult to pass water. The pain usually ceases once urination takes place.

Gynaecological injuries, for example a haematoma of the vulva can occur in water skiers. Wearing a wet-suit prevents such problems.

Acute winding

After blows to the abdomen it is not unusual for the athlete to be winded and remain lying doubled up on the sports ground. Helpful organizers and team mates will then run up and try to lift him. He will, however, recover more quickly if he is allowed to crouch so that his abdominal and respiratory muscles can relax.

Injuries during Specialized Activities

INJURIES ASSOCIATED WITH OUTDOOR LIFE

Prolonged activity in the open air, especially in winter, makes heavy demands on the individual who may be exposed to exertions he is not used to or has not allowed for.

Preventive measures

Basic physical fitness

Anyone going into remote places should first achieve a certain basic physical fitness. During preparation for a long hike, for example, unfamiliar aspects of the undertaking, such as carrying a packed rucksack, should be practised beforehand.

Equipment

The equipment carried during a long hike should meet the demands that the term implies. Shoes should always be well worn-in and the rucksack should fit well. Comfortable and appropriate equipment is a prerequisite for an enjoyable stay out in the open, and a change of clothes should always be carried in reserve.

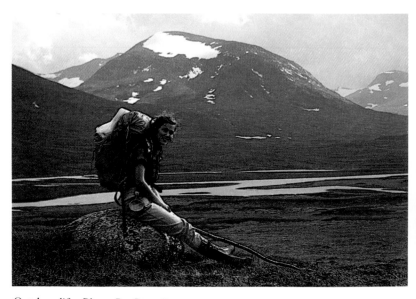

Outdoor life. *Photo: Per Renström.*

Health

A strenuous hike may not restore health and strength, but an excursion in the mountains often demands more than it gives in return. Anyone who has recently had a bad cold, bronchial catarrh or a similar infection should not indulge in a long demanding hike. In such circumstances, staying at a country hotel and taking short day trips with rests in between is more likely to be beneficial.

Body heat

It is vital to learn to conserve body heat, particularly in winter. Basic body heat is maintained by burning food and supplemented by muscular work. During stays out in the open, demands are increased, and a hungry person feels the cold more easily, so a high calorie intake should be aimed at. Alcohol and tobacco should be avoided, and damp clothes should not be allowed to dry on the body as this causes heat to be lost by evaporation.

Blisters and wounds

Blisters are a perennial problem on long treks. For comments on blisters see page 59, and for wounds see page 56.

Insect bites or stings

Insect bites often cause itching, but the urge to scratch them should be resisted. A locally applied anti-pruritic agent usually works well to prevent irritation, and if reaction is severe a doctor may prescribe an anti-histamine.

'Sprains' (ligament injuries to knee and ankle joints)

Ligament injuries to knee and ankle joints often occur during outdoor activities. For details on these injuries see page 286 and page 340.

Anyone who sprains his ankle while out in the countryside *should not take off his shoe* to examine the injury, particularly in winter. As a rule, nothing can be seen but swelling, and it is usually then impossible to replace the shoe because of the swelling and discomfort. High boots are in any case an excellent support for the ankle joint.

Healing of a ligament injury in the knee or ankle may be delayed considerably if the injured person walks on the leg in question.

In practice, this means that he or she should discontinue walking if at all possible. In cases of mild sprain, an elastic bandage (see page 162) gives good support.

Injuries due to overuse

During prolonged exertion, such as hill walking, overuse problems can occur, especially when the subject is unfamiliar with the type of activity involved.

Walking downhill, for example, may cause pain around the kneecap (Patello-femoral pain syndrome; see page 303), while long walks uphill and running on sandy beaches can result in an Achilles tendinitis (see page 335). If a heavy rucksack is carried during a long walking tour, the straps can press against the shoulders and exert increased pressure on the suprascapular nerve (see page 198).

Before any activity of this sort, careful preparations are essential. The equipment that is going to be used should be chosen carefully and well 'worn-in', and unfamiliar activities, such as carrying a packed rucksack for any length of time, should be practised in advance.

Fractures

For general symptoms and treatment, see page 18. Fractures should always be treated by a doctor, so during remote outdoor activities for example, it usually falls to the injured person's companions to arrange transport.

Fractures should be immobilized by splinting, and skis, sticks, straight branches, and so on, can be used in the absence of anything better. The splinting should include the joints on either side of the fracture. When the femur is fractured, for example, the hip joint and the knee joint should be stabilized, and the splint should extend from the armpit down to the foot. If a suitable splint is not available, a broken leg can be supported by strapping it to the other leg, and a broken arm can be strapped to the body. If it is badly displaced it may be necessary to realign a broken leg by straightening it longitudinally before transport takes place.

Apart from the splinting, as little as possible should be done to fractures out in the open, and transfer to hospital should not be delayed any longer than is necessary.

General rules for care and transport of injured people

If a severe injury occurs out in a remote area, the injured person should be placed in a sheltered position and kept warm. Something warm, for example an anorak or survival bag, should also be placed *under* him. If it is likely to be more than 4 hours before he reaches a hospital, the patient should be given something hot to drink and if necessary something to relieve the pain. While waiting for transport he should be reassured and calmed.

It is difficult to move a seriously injured person, and the transport should be carefully prepared. If a stretcher, sledge or boat is available it should be brought to the scene of the injury, and during the move the injured person should be made as comfortable as possible. Do not hesitate to call for helicopter help in cases of severe injury, such as fractures.

Frost-bite

Frost-bite is a collective name for injuries which are caused by exposure to low temperatures, which may mean temperatures above as well as below freezing point. The extent of the frost-bite depends on the temperature, the length of exposure and the wind chill factor. In temperatures above freezing, dampness is also important. 'Lifeboat foot', 'air-raid shelter foot', 'trench foot' and so on are all conditions caused by sitting still in cold and damp conditions.

Increased wind speed causes an increased likelihood of frost-bite, and the true temperature at different windspeeds is shown in the table below.

Temperature in °F (°C):

according to the thermo- meter	in still air	at 5 m/s	at 10 m/s	at 15 m/s	at 20 m/s
32° (0°)	32° (0°)	24° (−5°)	6° (−15°)	1° (−18°)	−5° (−20°)
14° (−10°)	14° (−10°)	−7° (−21°)	−20° (−30°)	−28° (−34°)	−33° (−36°)
−5° (−20°)	−5° (−20°)	−28° (−34°)	−51° (−44°)	−58° (−49°)	−64° (−52°)

When the outside temperature is 14°F (−10°C) and the weather is calm it is very tempting to go out skiing, but if the wind force is 10 m/s the effective temperature is −20°F (−30°C). Note that the same effect is exerted by wind rush in, for example, motor-cycle racing and Alpine skiing. Simply turning one's face into the wind gives a good idea of wind speed.

Local frost-bite

The following symptoms suggest frost-bite:

Symptoms of local frost-bite
— the skin becomes white and numb, though the victim does not always notice what is happening.
— usually there is a gradual onset of local stinging pain, but this may be absent if the cold is extreme.

Treatment of local frost-bite
The *injured person* should:
— shelter behind a companion, in a survival bag or something similar;
— use his body heat to warm the affected area. A warm hand can be placed against a frost-bitten cheek or nose. A chilled hand can be put in the armpit or on the warm skin of the abdomen. A chilled foot can be placed against a companion's abdomen;
— never use snow to rub or massage frost-bitten skin;
— never warm up in front of an open fire as the sensitivity in the frost-bitten part may have been impaired and severe burns can result.

Companions/leaders should:

— provide the injured person with dry, warm clothing and a hot drink;
— force the injured person to keep moving in order to increase his body temperature;
— take the injured person indoors, or, in cases of extensive frost-bite, take him to hospital.

In cases of local frost-bite the injured person can warm up by having a hot bath (40°C). This treatment should not be used, however, if he is suffering from general hypothermia.

Complications If blisters appear a few hours or days after the skin has suffered a local cold injury they should be left untouched. The surface of the blister is the best protection against infection.

The long-term effects of frost-bite can be extreme sensitivity to cold in the skin that has been damaged together with stinging pains and sweating.

General hypothermia

In cases of general hypothermia the patient becomes progressively weaker and more indifferent. He is overcome by tiredness, and can in fact fall asleep and ultimately die because of his reduced body temperature. For him, it may seem much more pleasant to submit and fall asleep than to fight and overcome the cold.

Treatment If the patient is conscious the following rules apply:

— he should be provided with dry, warm clothes next to his body;
— he should be *forced* to move his body and activate his muscles;
— a warm, sweetened drink may be given. Too hot a drink causes the blood vessels of the skin to dilate so that even more heat is lost, the core temperature is lowered further and the heart may be damaged;
— the patient should, if possible, be taken indoors as soon as possible;
— warming should be carried out slowly at normal room temperature. Local heat should not be applied; do not cover the patient with extra blankets when indoors;
— the patient should be taken to hospital as soon as possible.

If the patient is unconscious the following rules apply:

— under no circumstances attempt to give anything to drink;
— remove wet clothes;
— warm the patient slowly at room temperature with his head lower than his feet. Breathing and pulse should be checked;
— the patient should be taken to hospital as soon as possible where warming can be carried out under controlled conditions.

Sport in hot climates

Training and competition in hot climates can be great problem to athletes, and anyone training or competing in such environments should be well aware of the risks and preventive measures.

The temperature of the body, generated by muscle work and metabolic heat, is regulated by evaporation, radiation, and convection. Evaporation is the most important method of heat loss. For effective control of body heat by evaporation, the athlete must drink sufficient amounts of liquid. Heat loss is dependent on environmental conditions, such as the temperature of the air, humidity, wind speed, solar radiation and solar reflection from objects in the environment. Heat convection will cease in air temperatures above 38°C (100°F); evaporation will cease when water vapour pressure is over 40mm Hg; the slower the wind speed, the slower the rate of sweat evaporation.

An increase in body temperature has both physiological and psychological consequences for the athlete and may affect his or her ability to perform. Heat injury may occur in three forms: heat cramps, heat exhaustion and heat stroke.

Heat cramp

Heat cramps affect the muscles which work most intensively; for example, in runners and soccer players, the calf muscles are most commonly affected, and in racket players, the arm muscles are affected. The exact mechanism of heat cramps is unknown, but they may be due to intracellular water and electrolyte disturbances. Cramps are extremely painful and make further activity impossible.

Heat exhausation

There are two forms of heat exhaustion: water depletion and salt depletion, the former being the major threat to athletes. During strenuous muscle work in warm environments, the athlete may lose between 1–2 l body water per hour in sweat. If this water loss is not replaced by water intake, dehydration will occur. Intracellular fluid volume decreases and the osmolarity of the extracellular fluid increases drawing water from the cells into the extracellular space. Severe dehydration may cause circulatory collapse and kidney failure.

Symptoms | The athlete experiences fatigue, dizziness and muscle inco-ordination. He may become delirious and, in severe cases, become comatose.

Treatment | In the early stages, the athlete should drink water; in advanced cases of dehydration, fluid should be given intravenously. As a rule, there is no need to give the athlete electrolyte solutions during the early stages of dehydration.

Heat stroke

Heat stroke may occur if the rising body temperature is unchecked. It will cause tissue damage, including inactivation of enzymes, and damage to cell organelles and cell membranes. Heat stroke may occur to long-distance runners, cyclists, soccer players and especially American footballers, who wear protective paddings that interfere with evaporation.

Symptoms

The athlete may become confused and delirious. He may have convulsions, and become comatose. The body temperature will increase to 41–42°C (104–109°F) and the skin may look and feel dry and hot, due to the cessation of sweating.

Treatment

Cool down the athlete as soon as possible with tepid water and air movement. Send the athlete to a doctor or a hospital to continue the cooling-down process and to restore the water and electrolyte balance.

Complications

— Damage to the liver, with jaundice;
— Damage to the kidney, with renal failure and acidosis;
— Minor myocardial injury. Arrhythmia may be present;
— Hypotension and collapse of the circulatory system;
— Watery diarrhoea resulting from electrolyte imbalance.
— Damage to the brain.

Prevention

It is very important to prevent heat injuries. Strenuous sporting activity in high temperatures should not be allowed, especially when the vapour pressure exceeds 40mm Hg. The real danger is dehydration but it can be prevented by a sufficient intake of water.

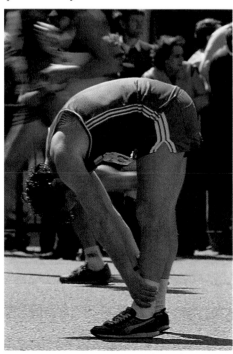

Heat exhaustion *Photo: All-Sport: Simon Miles*

Risks at high altitudes

Air density and barometric pressure decrease at high altitudes. The partial pressure of oxygen in the air decreases in proportion to the barometric pressure. This is of great importance to endurance sports. At an altitude of 3,000 m and above the partial pressure of oxygen falls to a level at which intellectual function may be affected, and at much lower altitudes the ability to do aerobic work is reduced. Anaerobic work and pulmonary ventilation increase, and lactic acid production will begin sooner.

These negative effects of high altitude can be decreased by acclimatizations, which increases the haemoglobin concentration in the blood. The optimal time for acclimatization varies depending on the altitude but usually athletes should arrive about 2–4 weeks before competition at a high altitude. In some sports the high altitude may improve the performance of the athlete, especially in sports where air resistance is normally a hindrance in achieving better results, for example in long jump and sprinting. However, this is not the case with technical sports and other sports where performance is limited by the need for oxygen.

Skin injuries from solar radiation

The solar radiation to which the skin is exposed during stays at high altitude and in summer is far more intense than the average athlete is used to. To avoid sunburn it is necessary to become accustomed to the sun gradually. Sunscreens or sun filter lotions with a high protection factor should be used for the skin and salve for the lips. Exposed parts such as the forehead and nose can be protected with a peaked cap or a piece of paper respectively.

Degrees of burns

First degree: the skin is red. Damage is confined to the superficial layers of skin and heals in a couple of days without treatment.
Second degree: blisters form in the skin. If they burst, a sterile bandage and possibly a medicated compress should be applied. If the burn covers a skin area greater than 2 in² (10 cm²) a doctor should be consulted.
Third degree: all the layers of the skin are destroyed, and the victim should definitely consult a doctor. During the early stages of a burn it can be difficult to judge whether it is second or third degree.

Sun- or snow-blindness

Sun- or snow-blindness is caused by ultraviolet rays and is manifest as an inflammatory reaction in the conjunctiva and the cornea of the eye. Visible sun light and ultraviolet radiation are not the same, and the ultraviolet rays penetrate even when the weather is hazy and cloudy. As a preventive measure, tight-fitting, preferably dark-coloured sunglasses with side shields should be used. The sunglasses should be used at all times as the eyes never grow accustomed to the strong ultraviolet radiation encountered during visits to snow-covered regions or when sailing.

Symptoms

— In cases of sun- or snow-blindness the affected person feels 'gritty' discomfort, swelling and pain in his eyes towards evening.
— The whites of the eyes become red, and the victim is disturbed by strong light, having to screw up his eyes which water constantly.
— When the injury is severe the affected person has to be led as if he were blind.

Treatment

The injured person's eyes must be protected from light. This is achieved by fitting his sunglasses with small pieces of cardboard in which holes have been made for the pupils so that he can only just see his way about.
— Eye drops or eye ointment which have a relaxing effect on the ring muscle of the iris may be prescribed.

Generally sun- or snow-blindness lasts for 2–4 days and does not normally result in any lasting disability.

INJURIES IN SPORTS FOR THE HANDICAPPED

Handicaps may be classified as follows:
— disability resulting from amputation, paralysis following birth injuries or injuries to the back or the nervous system;
— defects in, for example, sight and hearing, mental handicaps;
— medical handicaps, for example heart disease, respiratory disease, diabetes, haemophilia.

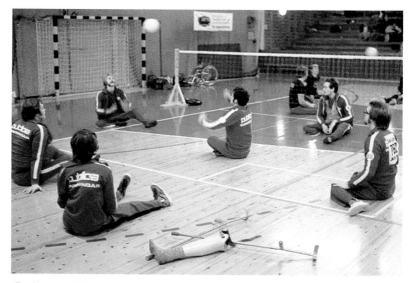

Prolonged sitting often results in pressure sores.

Despite the fact that a disabled person may have received excellent training in a hospital or special centre, he is still likely to have significant limitations, and when back in the community he may lose some of his acquired skills. Sport for the handicapped, graded according to level of skill and type of disability, offers a chance to continue training and acquiring new skills outside hospital quite apart from its enormous benefits in social and psychological terms. Sports activities for the disabled are arranged in most countries, and participation is generally free of charge. Most of the sports involved have been adapted to suit the handicapped and competition takes place up to international level.

Injuries in sports for the handicapped do not differ substantially from the injuries suffered in other sports. The commonest are pressure sores and blisters, crushing injuries and also ligament, muscle and skeletal injuries.

The disabled person's chances of avoiding injury depend on the nature of his disability, and certain handicaps, such as wasted muscles with impaired muscular strength or paralysis with loss of sensation, make recognition and diagnosis of injuries more difficult. Every disabled person should have the opportunity to take part in sporting activities, according to his own capabilities and qualifications, under appropriate medical supervision and in cooperation with physiotherapists or trained sports coaches.

Pressure sores

Disabled people with paralysed legs are often dependent on crutches or a wheel-chair and often have impaired sensitivity over the buttock area. Sitting for a long time causes pressure which can result in the development of pressure sores. These start as small red spots which do not look particularly ominous, but which, because of impaired sensitivity, may not at first be noticed and progress rapidly. The result can be an ugly deep sore which takes a long time to heal.

Obviously it is most important to prevent pressure sores. The athlete should not remain sitting for too long but should regularly lift himself out of his chair. *Before each competition or training session the coach should examine the athlete and look for signs of pressure sores.* If there is any skin redness, the area in question should be relieved from pressure, for example by using a 'rubber ring' or by using alternative sitting positions. The dubious skin area should be washed with soap and water, dried thoroughly, rubbed with surgical spirit and exposed to the air. If a sore has already appeared a doctor should be consulted. For blisters see page 59.

Blisters and sores

Many handicapped people have to use aids such as corsets, artificial limbs and various types of bandages. The pressure from these aids can cause redness and blisters, and the athlete should be examined for these conditions before and after training and competition. General principles concerning the treatment of blisters are to be found on page 59.

Contusion injuries

Many handicapped people have to use a wheel-chair, which may also be a part of their sporting activities, for example in athletics. When athletes

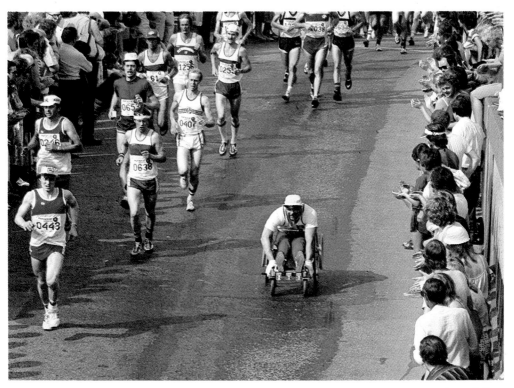

Sports for the handicapped are an integral part of sport in general. *Photo: Collsiöö Pressens bild.*

are playing wheel-chair basketball in particular, the wheel-chairs come into close contact with each other and rapid evasive manoeuvres are necessary. The athlete's fingers can then be jammed both in and between the wheel-chairs. Such injuries are characterized by swelling and tenderness, and abrasions may be present. The swelling should be treated as soon as possible by applying ice and then bandaging.

Injuries caused by wheel-chairs are difficult to prevent, but certain changes in their construction, such as protective frames fitted at the same height as the handle and situated on the same level regardless of wheelchair model, might be beneficial. The skin injuries that occur as a result of crushing or jamming injuries can be prevented if the athlete wears gloves or applies non-irritant tape to exposed areas.

Fractures

Impaired mobility or paralysis is inevitably accompanied by some degree of weakening of the skeleton. Furthermore, in such cases the muscles are often so wasted that they provide little protection for the bones. Fractures can therefore occur relatively easily especially when unexpected loads are applied. Such fractures are often extensive with considerable splintering in the fracture area. Minor fractures are sometimes not discovered immediately if the athlete has impaired sensitivity.

Handicapped people who wear support braces should loosen them during sporting activities as otherwise they may act as levers and contribute towards causing fractures.

Guidelines on the treatment of fractures are given on page 20.

Injuries to muscles, tendons and ligaments

As muscles affected by paralysis become atrophied, certain functions are taken over by other muscles which as a result become stronger from increased use. Arm and shoulder muscles, for example, are often remarkably well-developed in people who depend upon wheel-chairs. The risk of overuse of tendons and tendon attachments, however, is increased by the additional demands made upon specific muscle groups. Guidelines on treatment are given on pages 22–40.

Impaired muscular strength often places greater load on ligaments and increases the risk of ligament injury.

Back and shoulder problems

Anyone who is tied to a wheel-chair spends a large part of his time sitting, and back problems with more or less constant aching are common. A corset can often be beneficial but can be trying to wear for any considerable period, especially in summer.

People in wheel-chairs often suffer from shoulder pain as a result of one-sided repetitive movements in the shoulder joint as the arms are used, not only to carry out extensive routine tasks, but also for mobility.

Urinary tract infection

A great number of handicapped people have problems with urinary tract infections because of paralysis, impaired bladder sensation and constant sitting around. The symptoms of a urinary tract infection can be slight, or absent, so regular bacteriological checks on the urine should be made.

General medical complaints

General medical conditions, including heart disease, high blood pressure, asthma, diabetes and haemophilia do not preclude sporting activity, but it should be undertaken with the advice and supervision of a doctor and/or physiotherapist. Sufferers from these disorders have tended to hold back to a certain extent from participating in physical exercise because of a belief that it could be dangerous for them, but it is now known that it can in fact be positively beneficial and it is likely that the numbers who are keen to indulge in sport despite their medical history will increase in the future.

Diabetes

About 9 per cent of the population suffers from diabetes, and of this group about 5 per cent are insulin-dependent (usually young) diabetics. The disease causes a rise in the blood sugar levels because of the body's failure to produce insulin, and treatment is aimed at keeping the blood sugar levels within normal limits by regulating the diet and by treatment with insulin or other drugs. Regular physical activity is part of the overall management and physical fitness has a definite role to play, affecting both glucose tolerance and insulin sensitivity. There are, however, certain risks involved, especially at a competitive level, of which both athletes and coaches must be aware.

There is a risk that the athlete will suffer from *too low a blood sugar level*. The reason can be irregular or skipped meals, increased or irregular physical activity or altered response to drugs. The symptoms are irritability, fatigue, sweating and pallor, a feeling of faintness and hunger followed by anxiety and also trembling and palpitations. A sensation of numbness in the face can be an early sign. Later the affected athlete can become confused, and can slip suddenly or gradually into unconsciousness. As soon as the diabetic athlete notices any symptoms which he associates with a low blood sugar level (and he is likely to know them well), he must immediately discontinue his sporting activity, take some sugar, a sweet drink or some food which includes plenty of carbohydrates and consult a doctor.

There is also a risk that the athlete will suffer from *too high a blood sugar level* as a result of an infection, negligence with medication or diet or unaccustomed inactivity. Symptoms such as sweating with flushes, thirst, vomiting, abdominal pains and later confusion and air hunger start insidiously over a period that can vary from a few hours to a few days. They need urgent medical treatment.

Thirst, the passage of large amounts of urine and fatigue should cause an athlete to consult his doctor before continuing with his sporting activity.

Asthma

Bronchial asthma occurs in 3 per cent of all children of school age. It can be precipitated by a number of factors including allergy to certain substances (for example, pollen, dust and horse hair), infection, exertion and anxiety. Smoking and cool, damp weather tend to have adverse effects. The principal symptoms are shortness of breath, increased breathing rate, wheezing (particularly when breathing out) and cough.

The majority of known asthmatics will have an attack of asthma if they run hard for a sufficient length of time, but for those who have 'exertional asthma' symptoms *only* occur on physical exercise and they are otherwise free from problems.

There is now a wide variety of effective treatments available for the treatment of asthma, and some of these can be taken preventively before exercise begins. With their help, some top-level athletes who suffer from asthma achieve peak performances.

If symptoms do develop during sporting activity, the athlete should of course stop. This is often enough to stop the attack, but if it is not and usual medication also fails to do so, a doctor should be consulted.

When there are no symptoms, physical activity can and should be encouraged. Swimming has been shown to have positive benefits for asthmatics.

Epilepsy

Epilepsy is a symptom of many conditions and manifests itself in convulsions and disturbed consciousness. During a fit, the epileptic can damage his tongue, lips and teeth by his violent chewing motions, and a rolled-up handkerchief or something similar (nothing rigid) should be placed between his teeth. An unconscious epileptic should be treated according to the guidelines given on page 376, and taken to a doctor as soon as possible.

People suffering from epilepsy are exposed to the obvious risk of drowning if they should have an attack when they are in the water, and they should therefore never swim alone.

Complications

The complications that can occur in sports for the handicapped vary according to the individual athlete's underlying illness. Every athlete and his coach should always be well aware of the particular risks involved and of the measures that should be taken if problems arise.

Difficulties in breathing

Those with disorders of the cardiovascular system (heart and blood vessels) and lungs can be affected by difficulties in breathing during physical exercise. Coaches who train athletes with medical handicaps of this type should pay close attention to their breathing and pulse rate. The training programme should be planned according to the ability of the individual, and if breathing difficulties do develop the affected athlete should discontinue his activity. If the problem is not solved by rest, a doctor should be consulted.

Spasmodic twitches

Spasmodic twitches occur particularly in the legs of people paralysed as a result of degeneration of the nervous system. Bending the foot upwards or stretching the knee for about 5 seconds at a time may stop the twitching but the disabled person himself often knows how best to cope with the situation.

Unconsciousness

Unconsciousness can affect an athlete with, for example, epilepsy. Guidelines for treatment are found on page 376. The unconscious person should be taken to hospital for treatment.

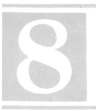

Risks to Children and Adolescents

RISKS OF INJURY TO CHILDREN AND ADOLESCENTS

Regular training of children and adolescents is becoming more common in sport, and competitive sports are indulged in with ever-increasing intensity at ever-decreasing ages. In certain sports, such as figure-skating, swimming and gymnastics, children start regular training when they are five to six years of age, and even in contact sports, such as soccer, training and competition are beginning at earlier ages. In certain sports training for 2–4 hours on 5–6 days a week is not unusual.

Are there any long-term advantages in allowing children to start regular training and competitive activity at such an early age? Children's play has always included running and jumping, which form a natural basis for sporting activity, but the increased demands and increased intensity of regular training can have a negative effect on an adolescent, and a certain caution should be observed. In some sports, swimming and tennis for example, studies have shown that very few winners of junior competitions

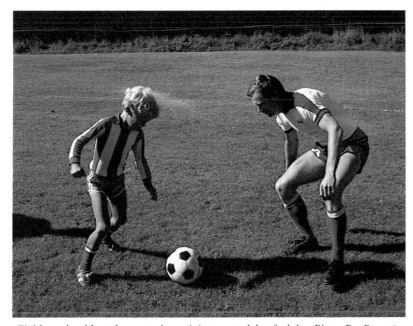

Children should not be treated as miniature models of adults. *Photo: Per Renström.*

become successful seniors — in other words, it is difficult to predict future development. Many young people give up their sporting activities too early because they are no longer enjoying themselves, and children and adolescents should be given the opportunity to try several different sports rather than concentrating exclusively on one.

In principle, sports for children and adolescents should be fun and should not mean painfully hard training. The principles according to which adults train cannot be directly applied to youngsters but must be adapted to their development. The risks of allowing adolescents to train and compete regularly can be looked at from different angles — physiological, psychological and orthopaedic — and the effects of sport on the latter can be divided into three groups:
— effects on the development of the musculo-skeletal system;
— injuries due to accidents (traumatic injuries);
— injuries due to overuse.

Effects on the development of the musculo-skeletal system

The development of the musculo-skeletal system in adolescents is governed by their ability to adapt in response to a changed or recurrent load, for example during training or following injury. Adaptation as a result of prolonged one-sided training can cause permanent changes, exemplified by the tennis player who, at an early age, begins asymmetrical training and loading of his racket arm. This can result in his developing

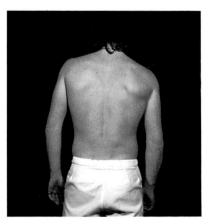 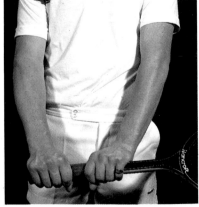

One-sided training in the racket sports, for example, can lead to the athlete developing a 'tennis shoulder'. As the photograph to the left shows this can cause lowering of the shoulder and thus a relative lengthening of the arm. The one-sided training can also lead to an increase in the size of the muscles in the racket arm (the photograph to the right).

a 'tennis shoulder', with an increase in the size of bones and muscles and increased laxity of the joint capsule, ligaments and tendons around the shoulder of the racket arm. This causes dropping of the shoulder and a relative lengthening of the arm. In extreme cases an S-shaped curve (scoliosis) can develop in the thoracic spine.

Another example of the effects of training can be seen in young gymnasts. Long training increases the range of movement in the vertebral column, bringing about permanent changes in vertebral bodies and in the pelvis with increased mobility between the bones that form the pelvic girdle. We do not yet know with certainty what these changes will lead to in the long run, and it is essential that regular training in children and adolescents takes place under medical supervision. At the same time one-sided and repetitive training must be avoided and rules that reward abnormal mobility, for example in marking gymnastic competitions, should be changed.

> The training of children and adolescents should be comprehensive.

Injuries due to trauma (accidents)

Children and adolescents are injured more often than adults, but their injuries are usually less serious. This might be due, amongst other things, to the fact that children are physically smaller than adults, so that less force is involved at the time of an accident. Children's tissues are significantly different from those of adults: their bone structure is more resilient and adaptable, and their muscles, tendons and ligaments are relatively stronger and more elastic. Unlike the situation in adults, the articular cartilages have some blood supply, enabling injuries in those areas to heal to some extent.

The skeleton is the most vulnerable structure in adolescents. Though the bones are adaptable to various stresses, and in this respect superior to those of adults, they are not as adaptable as the cardiovascular system and the muscles. In children and adolescents who participate in regular training, the musculature can develop more rapidly than the skeleton which may be hazardous because of the unusual stress it imposes. Because of the resilience of the tissues, overuse injuries are relatively rare in children and young people, although in recent years their incidence has been increasing noticeably, probably because of more intensive training in younger children.

Injuries to the growth zones (epiphysis)

Growth in length of the skeleton takes place in the growth zones or epiphyseal cartilages. In the femur 70 per cent of the growth occurs in the lower growth zone and 30 per cent in the upper. Corresponding figures for the lower leg are 55 and 45 per cent respectively. The epiphy-

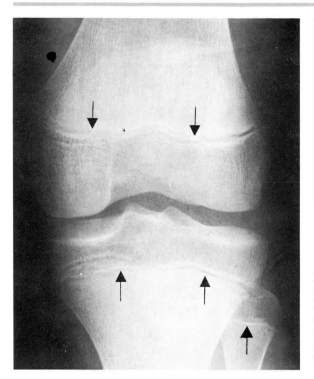

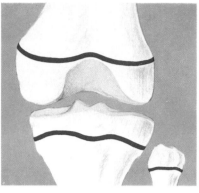

Examples of growth zones. **Left:** an X-ray of a knee joint in which arrows indicate the growth zones of the femur and the tibia. **Above:** a diagram of the corresponding growth zones. The main growth of the lower limbs takes place in these zones.

seal cartilages are weaker than the rest of the skeleton, but, in spite of this, skeletal fractures are commoner than epiphyseal fractures in adolescents. The explanation for this paradox is probably to be found in the types of force that are in action.

The age of the skeleton plays a distinct role in determining the effect of physical training on the epiphyseal cartilages. Hormone factors are also of importance. The epiphyseal cartilages are at their weakest during puberty and towards the end of the growth period when they are beginning to lose their elastic properties.

Epiphyseal cartilages are weaker than normal tendons and ligaments in adolescents, and an impact which would cause a total tear of a major ligament in adults, tends in adolescents to cause an avulsion of the epiphysis. So an impact against the side of the knee joint in children and adolescents may cause an epiphyseal injury while a similar impact in an adult would tear the medial collateral and anterior cruciate ligaments. When tears of major ligaments are suspected in adolescents X-ray examination should be carried out so that the epiphyseal cartilages can be checked and any skeletal injuries discovered.

The epiphyseal cartilages are weaker than the connective tissue joint capsules, so that dislocations of major joints resulting from accidents are less common than injuries to the epiphyseal cartilages in children and adolescents.

In 10 per cent of cases, injuries to the growth zones can cause the normal growth in length to be disturbed. The effects vary. While an injury to an epiphyseal cartilage is healing, the undamaged bone on the opposite side continues to grow. In cases of injury to the growth zone of the lower part of the femur this can mean a difference in length of more than 1 in (2 cm) between the two sides. Sometimes an injury to the epiphysis affects only part of the epiphyseal cartilage. Then only the undamaged part of the cartilage grows during the healing phase, causing the leg to be crooked or angled.

Growth zones can slip in relation to the bone (epiphysiolysis). The injury is not uncommon in the hip joint, in which the femoral head can gradually or suddenly slip from the shaft. Epiphysiolysis should be treated by surgery.

Common fractures

Bone tissue is softer in adolescents than in adults, and the younger the person the less likely it is to break. For this reason, fractures in children show different characteristics. The skeleton also has a better blood supply in children than in adults which reduces the time needed for fractures to heal. Treating fractures in children and adolescents involves principles different from those used in treating adults.

— The fractures heal better and fewer visible signs remain in children and young people than in adults. An X-ray of a fracture taken 18 months after the injury will show perfect healing and no sign of a fracture in an adolescent, while a change in the shape of the bone is often seen in an adult.

— Fractures heal faster in adolescents than in adults, and therefore children and young people do not have to stay in plaster for as long.

— Adolescents sustain different types of fractures to adults. Bones which have not ceased growing are resilient, and can therefore be bent quite vigorously before breaking. An example of this is the 'greenstick' fracture (see page 82).

Avulsion fractures

In adolescents the strength of the tendons, the ligaments and the muscles is greater than that of the bones, while this situation is reversed in adults. This means that children and adolescents usually suffer skeletal injuries as a result of accidents or overuse. The bony attachment of the ligament or muscle is torn away from its origin instead of the muscle or ligament itself tearing. Such avulsion fractures are often located in the growth zones of the flat bones and are most common in the front of the pelvis and also in the ischium where the posterior hamstring muscles have their origins. Avulsion fractures often occur suddenly during hard, rapid loading of the muscles.

When an adolescent has met with an accident that results in injury, and tenderness, swelling and effusion of blood are present in the injured area, an X-ray examination should be carried out. If bone attachments have been torn away and displaced to such an extent that they cannot re-attach to their original site, surgery should be considered in order to reposition the fragments. A displacement of the fragment by only a few millimetres can impair future functioning of the ligaments or muscles if the injury is not treated correctly.

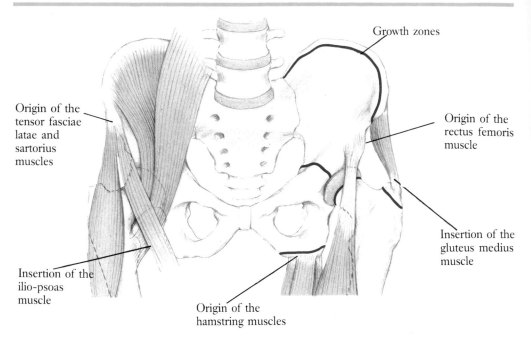

Growth zones

Origin of the
tensor fasciae
latae and
sartorius
muscles

Origin of the
rectus femoris
muscle

Insertion of the
gluteus medius
muscle

Insertion of the
ilio-psoas
muscle

Origin of the
hamstring muscles

Common sites for avulsion fractures.

Sometimes it is not fragments of the bone itself which are torn away but only the periosteum (bone membrane) to which a tendon or a ligament is attached. This can cause a loss of function in the muscle or ligament, but does not show up on an X-ray. For this reason, functional testing of muscles and joint stability is of the utmost importance in order to make the correct diagnosis and choose the correct treatment.

An injury caused by avulsion can be more serious than a straightforward rupture of a muscle or tendon, since it has the same implications as fracture. Injuries due to avulsion should therefore be distinguished from the muscle ruptures that often occur in adults who have been subjected to similar violence. Healing times are longer for avulsion fractures than for ruptures of a muscle and can be anything from 1 to 6 months depending on treatment. It is essential that avulsion fractures are diagnosed at an early stage so that adequate treatment can be started. If these injuries are neglected, the result can be chronic pain and impairment of joint function resulting in instability or impaired mobility.

Adolescents who have tenderness, swelling and effusion of blood in the injured area after an accident should be X-rayed.

Injuries due to overuse

Injuries resulting from overuse in adolescents usually affect the so-called apophyses, that is, those parts of the skeleton which constitute the attachments of tendons, ligaments, muscles or joint capsules.

Inflammation of an apophysis (apophysitis)

In a muscle and tendon unit there are certain high-risk injury areas, such as the attachments of muscles and tendons to bones, the muscle and tendon tissue itself and also the point at which muscle and tendon merge (the muscle-tendon junction). In adults, the muscle or tendon tissue itself is often injured by violence, while the corresponding violence in adolescents causes injuries to the attachments of the muscle or tendon to bone. Studies have shown that physical training increases the strength of tendons and ligaments faster than that of their attachments.

Apophysitis resulting from overuse occurs mainly in specific sports, such as football, long-jump and high-jump, which involve a great deal of jumping and bending the knees, thus exposing the apophyses to great tensile stress and overloading.

The site at which apophysitis most often occurs is that of the attachment of the patellar ligament to the tibia (Osgood-Schlatter's disease; see page 309). Overloading of the apophysis causes inflammation in the attachment of the tendon which manifests itself as pain, tenderness and swelling. An X-ray shows fragmentation of the bone under the attachment of the tendon. Apophysitis also often occurs in the attachment of the Achilles tendon to the calcaneus (apophysitis calcanei; see page 338).

In cases of apophysitis it is essential that the affected athlete rests at an early stage, avoiding the movements that trigger pain, until he feels no more pain and discomfort. The condition can otherwise be of long duration.

The most common cause of apophysitis is one-sided training. Here it is appropriate to give a word of warning against strength training as it is practised by young, growing people. When strength training is carried out with a heavy load, the strength of the muscles develops faster than the strength of the skeleton which can result in apophysitis and also in avulsion fractures. Growing youngsters should therefore practise strength training using only their own body as a load.

Stress fractures

One-sided load on the skeleton can, when intensity and load are too high, lead to stress fractures or fatigue fractures if the adaptive ability of the body is insufficient to cope. Stress fractures can affect children who go in for sporting activity as early as the age of seven years and the frequency of stress fractures in adolescents is increasing. The injury can be caused by frequently repeated movements under normal load, for example long-distance running, or by movements of a lower frequency but with a higher load, for example weight-lifting. The most dangerous combination, however, is a high load and a high frequency. In principle, stress fractures can occur in any bone of the body but are most common in the lower limbs. They occur mainly in the metatarsal bones, and in the tibia, fibula, femur, hip and pelvic bones and vertebral bodies. Stress fractures should always be suspected in people who are subjected to repeated movements or high loads and who complain of pain on exertion. Usually there is no pain or discomfort at rest. Local tenderness and swelling over the painful area are found and a clinical examination usually leads to the diagnosis. If no fracture is discovered on X-ray examination, it should be repeated 3–4 weeks later if the symptoms persist. The diagnosis can then be confirmed. Another diagnostic aid is examination with radioactive isotopes which can confirm the diagnosis at an early stage.

The risk of stress fracture can be reduced primarily by increasing training gradually but also by varied training alternating with regular rest so that the body has time to recover. The surface that athletes use in training can also be of importance, and the construction of the shoes is vital. Anyone running on a hard surface should always wear shoes with good shock-absorbing properties. When there is a change from a hard to a soft surface or vice versa, the intensity of training should be reduced during the transition period.

Cartilage injuries

The collagen tissue of the articular cartilage is better supplied with blood vessels but has poorer tensile strength in adolescents than in adults. Thus children and young people can injure the articular cartilage more easily than adults as a result of sprains and direct blows. A prolonged extreme load on the knee joint, for example in downhill skiing or sailing, can result in injuries to the articular cartilage of the patella. This condition, the patellar femoral pain syndrome (chondromalacia patellae, see page 303), causes pain, arising from the inner surface of the patella or around the patella, which is triggered mainly by running uphill and downhill and by squatting. The articular cartilage of the patella softens and debris gathers. Since the cartilage does not contain any nervous tissue it is not clear why pain is triggered but it may originate from the synovial membrane. The causes of chondromalacia patellae are not known for certain either, but the condition responds to heat therapy and isometric training of the anterior and posterior thigh muscles.

Another cartilage injury that occurs in adolescents is osteochondritis dissecans (see page 301) in which a part of the articular cartilage that has been damaged breaks away and can become free, moving inside the joint where it causes problems.

The diagnosis of these cartilage injuries is made with the help of arthroscopy.

EFFECTS OF PHYSICAL TRAINING ON INTERNAL ORGANS

Good physical fitness is characterized by a high oxygen utilizing capacity. This capacity is influenced by the length and intensity of training. There is also a hereditary factor to consider, and different people have different abilities to achieve good heart and lung function.

Effects on heart and lungs

The lungs have a high reserve capacity and are well able to tolerate hard physical exertion. The heart and blood vessels are more sensitive, but they also possess considerable ability to adapt to increased stress.

A normal heart can *sometimes produce occasional extra beats*. Such extra beats need not cause a break in training and are usually of no significance, but a medical check-up is advisable.

Undiagnosed *congenital heart disease* can cause sudden death during extreme physical activity. *Young people who intend to train regularly should therefore undergo a medical examination* before they begin.

Growing youngsters who train regularly may, even at rest, have a blood pressure which is somewhat higher than normal. If underlying disease has been excluded, there is no reason to discontinue physical fitness training. It is more usual in fact for physical training to bring about a reduction in both blood pressure and pulse rate.

Infection can cause an *inflammation of the heart muscle* (myocarditis), and the risks increase if the body is subjected to physical exertion when an infection is present. An inflammation of the heart muscle usually manifests itself by chest pains, palpitations, fatigue and deterioration of general fitness. Since the symptoms are sometimes slight, the affected athlete does not always consult a doctor but continues his training until the symptoms become worse.

It is essential that a doctor advises when a return to physical activity is safe. At least several months should elapse after the disease shows no further signs of inflammation. For general risk factors with regard to heart and lung function, see also page 128.

Athletes who show signs of an infection, in particular a fever, should avoid all training and competitive activity.

> If relatively easy training causes breathing difficulties, exhaustion or chest pains in an athlete, he must be examined by a doctor.

Effects on kidneys

In athletes who exert themselves, the urine can be coloured red or brown by proteins, red blood cells or waste products appearing in it. During increased load on the body these substances can pass through the kidneys without any significant injury being present. Discoloration may be due to increased decomposition of red blood cells as a result of running on a hard surface, but should, nevertheless, be investigated since the symptom can also be a sign of underlying disease.

Effects on the intestines

The intestines can be upset after strenuous exertion. Nausea, vomiting, abdominal pains and diarrhoea can be present without being signs of any disease. Symptoms that persist for longer periods should, however, be investigated by a doctor since they may be caused by something other than overexertion.

TRAINING

The most decisive stage of an athlete's life from a medical and orthopaedic point of view is probably when he finally decides to concentrate on one particular sport with all that entails in the way of prolonged and planned, intensive training. It would be desirable for the young athlete's physiological qualifications for the sport in question to be analysed, but unfortunately there is as yet no sound medical basis for a reliable judgement.

Regular, targeted training is now starting in younger and younger age groups. Training methods that have been developed for adults are directly applied to children without adapting them either to suit their age or to suit individual variations. With regard to training and competitive activities for adolescents, the trainer and the coach must be aware of the risks that exist for children in the long as well as in the short term. Sport must remain play for children and a means of maintaining physical health for adults. Training activities must therefore be questioned: is it really right to train as hard as athletes do today in order to reach the top level, and are the right training methods being used?

Children are not miniature scale models of adults. They mature at different rates, and puberty can occur any time within a span of about 4–6 years. This physiological inequality in development is often forgotten by coaches and managers.

Physical fitness training Physical fitness training is no more effective for young people between ten and twenty years of age than for any other age group. The anaerobic energy-producing capacity, that is, the ability to produce energy in the absence of oxygen, is lower in ten- to twelve-year-old children than in teenagers. Regardless of age and this capacity, however, young people can benefit from taking part in activities that demand anaerobic energy, and children do not seem to feel tiredness in the same way as adults do.

However, recent findings indicate that adolescents do not lose anything by delaying systematic physical fitness training until they are in their late teens.

Strength training

In growing children the internal organs are able to adapt to great loads while the musculo-skeletal system can easily be damaged. The effects of training in children and young people are seen mainly in the muscles, the cells of which increase in size. This increase in size is directly related to the length and intensity of the training programme. The muscles become stronger when they are trained and lose their strength rapidly when the training ceases.

Children and young people respond to muscular strength training because there is relatively more effect on the musculature than on the skeleton. Under normal circumstances their muscles are not used for strength-requiring activities to the same extent as those of adults, and strength training in growing youngsters therefore has a more obvious effect on their musculature. In adolescence great increases in strength are characteristic of both men and women, but in the early teens the increase in strength is distinctly less than the increase in body size. Athletes in their early teens are therefore not quite as strong as their body size might indicate.

In strength training with a high load, muscular strength develops faster than the strength of the skeleton which can lead to avulsion fractures in which the tendon or attachment of a muscle to a bone is torn away because of the muscle force that is generated.

There are a number of different types of strength training. In isometric training the ability of the muscle to exert power increases but its stamina does not increase as much as in dynamic training. In adolescence the attachments of tendons and muscles in particular are vulnerable, and therefore children and young people should be cautious with so-called isometric work with a load which means that the muscles are working without appreciably changing their length. Light dynamic work, such as running and walking, when the muscles are working by lengthening and shortening, is in most cases sufficient.

Training with heavy weights should be avoided by individuals who are still growing. The load on the vertebral column during weight training, for example, can be so great that the vertebrae are affected. Only the weight of the body should be used as a load in strength training, and only when the skeleton has stopped growing, which in girls happens at about the age of sixteen and in boys seventeen to eighteen years, should systematic strength training with heavy weights start. Before that a growing youngster can perhaps use light weights, but the training intensity should only be stepped up by increasing the number of exercises carried out. *A strength training programme should be specially drawn up according to the growing youngster's age, maturity, body build, physical fitness and sex.*

General mobility training

A considerable part of an adolescent's mobility training consists of basic movements which are carried out more or less automatically, such as moving the body and keeping the balance. This type of movement is hereditary and is controlled by instincts which are passed on genetically and are gradually developed during childhood. Balance, for example, is not fully developed until the age of nine to ten years. Whether physical training can influence development in a positive or negative direction is not known. In most sports there are complex patterns of movement which have to be learned with the aid of the pre-existent instinctive knowledge. When such a pattern has been developed it is difficult to change, so it is important to learn it correctly from the start. The nervous system can incorporate new patterns right into teenage years. It is undesirable to incorporate incorrect information into the nervous system before it is fully developed, as it would subsequently be difficult to alter. Technique training should be carried out during the latter part of the period of growth.

Training in different age groups

7–9 years of age: play, technique and all-round training

Training of children between the ages of seven and nine years should above all be full of variation and fun, that is, the play element should predominate. Light fitness training including different ball games is suitable. All-round training should be the aim. Technique training should be introduced now, as children of this age are very receptive to learning.

10–11 years: general basic training, technique training and all-round training

Training of children between the ages ten and eleven should include technique and co-ordination exercises since this is an excellent time for improving reflexes and mobility technique by training. Play elements are important features in the training, but systematic fitness training and anaerobic training are not meaningful during this period.

12–14 years: general fitness training and learning of technique and tactics

During the age period twelve to fourteen years, which partly coincides with puberty, there are rapid changes in growth and maturity, both physically and mentally. The training must be adjusted to the maturity of the individual youngster. *The body is, both physically and mentally, in a sensitive stage of development, and this must be taken into account.* The play element should be given ample scope. Technique training can also be carried out since the ability to learn continues to be high during this period of growth. Some specialization can begin in the sports for which the young athletes have shown talent. They can be introduced to tactical methods.

15–16 years: preparation for specialized training

In the period fifteen to sixteen years basic physical fitness must be built up, and therefore regular fitness training should become a habit. Anaerobic training can now begin. Comprehensive gymnastics and flexibility training are of great importance during this period, since growth often makes young people stiff and unsupple.

Strength training can start when the muscles and skeleton allow an increased load. Young people at the age of fifteen to sixteen years can start to learn the correct lifting technique, but should only use light weights. *A heavy load should not be used as the skeleton has not yet stopped growing.* The strength training should be intensified by increasing the number of times an element of exercise is carried out, not by increasing the load. *It is important that the athletes spare their backs from overload by using the correct lifting technique!*

During this period, specialization in different sports can be undertaken.

Over 16 years of age: specialized training

Young people who are over sixteen years of age can participate in specialized training which does not differ appreciably from that of adults. Growth in girls tends to be complete by the age of sixteen to eighteen years while the development of boys continues up to the age of eighteen to twenty years.

General comments

When it comes to training and competition for adolescents there has to be an awareness of the risks this entails, both in the short and in the long term. Knowledge of the special characteristics of the musculo-skeletal system in growing youngsters is therefore of great importance. There is a need to question training methods which make such hard, monotonous and regular demands that sport becomes agony rather than the enjoyable pastime it should be. The aim should be to encourage a large number of young people to become active athletes that a vast pool will be available from which top athletes can be produced in the long run. A lasting interest in sports should be founded in adolescence so that in adulthood sport is regarded as a means of maintaining physical health and fitness for the whole of one's life. During the years when adolescents are at their most receptive and find it easy to learn, the stress should be on technical training which can be made interesting and stimulating. Hard physical training and specialization for those who have the ambition to go far, should start at a later stage.

Adolescents have some characteristics which distinguish them from adults. This is especially important to remember when harder and harder training of young children is beginning to be the norm. Age groups create a classification which is purely chronological and tends to ignore the complete physiological picture of a growing youngster. It is quite common for there to be a difference in maturity of more than 5 years between young people in the same age group. Thus, a group of eleven- to twelve-year-old girls or boys, for example, can include youngsters whose biological maturity is on the same level as that of fifteen- to sixteen-year-olds. All training of children and young people must therefore be individual. Coaching courses must be mandatory so that those who train and manage growing young people are well prepared for their task.

In the world of sport there is a widespread opinion that training has a better effect the earlier in life it starts. Scientific studies have still not been able to verify this theory. The question is rather whether too hard and intensive training at an early age can have any adverse effects in later life. Apart from anything else, such training is one reason why many young people give up sport.

— Intensive training of children and young people with the aim of making them into top level athletes should not be carried out without an initial medical examination, and should then be supervised by a doctor.
— Anyone involved in training growing young people should have a sound knowledge of physical development in adolescence.
— Training programmes for children and young people must be drawn up individually. Development, that is, biological maturity, can vary by 4–5 years in youngsters of the same chronological age.
— The training should be adjusted to the individual, not the individual to the training.

9 Training of Different Parts of the Body

After an athlete has been injured there follows a period of rehabilitation. This should be well planned and adapted to be appropriate to the severity of the injury so that healing is not adversely affected. The purpose of rehabilitation after an injury is to achieve:

— no pain;
— full mobility;
— good balance and co-ordination;
— full strength and flexibility.

In this chapter a number of exercises are described which have been compiled in order to help injured athletes to achieve this purpose. Exercises for mobility, strength and stretching, as well as general exercises which are suitable for the various parts of the body, are described. Alternative exercises can be chosen according to experience and the effect the individual athlete believes they have. The exercises that are recommended are also beneficial as preventive measures in order to strengthen parts subjected to wear and strain.

Rehabilitation should only take place in cooperation with a doctor and/ or physiotherapist who can regularly encourage training and evaluate its results.

THE SHOULDER JOINT
Mobility exercises

1. Pendular exercises. Stand leaning forwards supporting your body weight with the hand of your healthy arm on a table or chair. Let the injured arm hang straight down. Swing the injured arm (*a*) forwards and backwards, (*b*) from side to side in front of the body, (*c*) in a

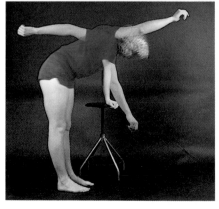 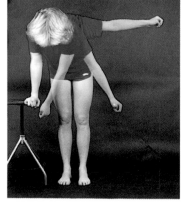

1a, 1b

419

circle, first clockwise, then anti-clockwise. Gradually increase the diameter of the circle.

2. Lie down on your back and hold a stick with both hands. Lift the stick with straight arms, take it back over your head down to the floor and return to the starting position.

2,3

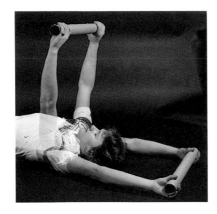 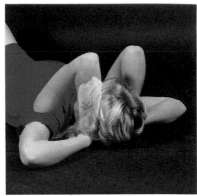

3. Lie down on your back and clasp your hands behind your neck. Lift your elbows forwards and backwards alternately.

4. Stand or sit with your hands on your shoulders. Move your elbows in wide circles.

4,5

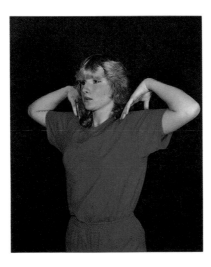 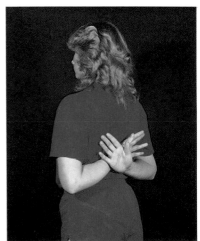

5. Sit on a stool or stand up. Place your hands behind your body. Move your hands as high up your back as possible.

The above exercises should be carried out for short periods several times a day.

Strength exercises

6. Hold your arms straight forwards or out sideways for as long as possible. Increase the intensity of the exercise by holding weights in your hands.

7. Fasten a piece of rubber tubing to wall-bars or a similar support. (*a*) Stand with your back against wall-bars and pull your arms forwards and outwards, forwards and upwards, and forwards and downwards against the resistance of tubing. (*b*) Stand facing the wall-bars and pull your arms backwards and outwards, backwards and upwards, and backwards and downwards against the resistance of tubing.

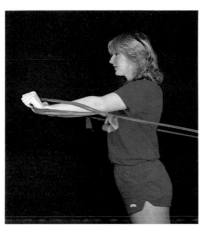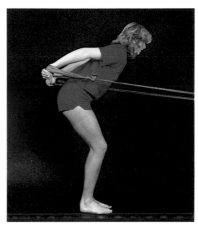

7a, 7b

8. Stand with your side against a door. Fasten a piece of rubber tubing to the door handle. Hold your outer arm close to your body, bend your elbow of your inner arm at a right angle and hold the end of the tubing in your hand. (*a*) Move the forearm inwards 5–10 times. Rest for 30 seconds. Repeat. (*b*) Turn round and repeat the exercise but now move your forearm outwards instead. Change arms and repeat the exercise. Gradually increase the resistance by shortening the length of the tubing.

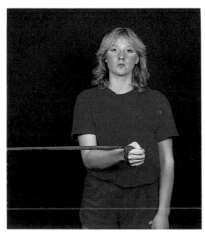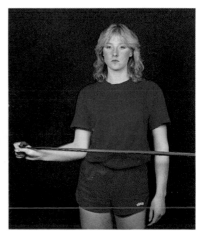

8a, 8b

421

9. Do press-ups, some sitting in an armchair, some lying full length on the floor.

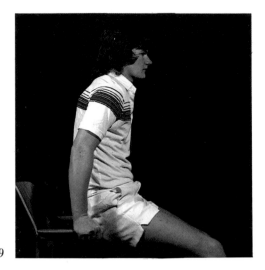

9

10. Weight training. Gradually increase the load of the barbell.

Static stretching exercises (extension training)

Supinators of the arm

11. (*a*) Hold your arms straight out in front of your body and press your hands together, or against a ball, for 4–7 seconds. Relax. (*b*) Hold your arms behind your back, clasp hands or take hold of a door-frame or a friend's hands and stretch with straight arms for 6–8 seconds.

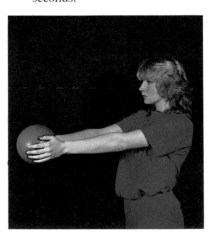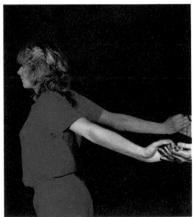

11a, 11b

12. (*a*) 'Tear apart' a towel or a rope behind your back for 4–7 seconds. Let your lower arm relax for 2 seconds. (*b*) Then stretch by pulling the towel or the rope up with your top hand for 6–8 seconds. Change arms and repeat the exercise.

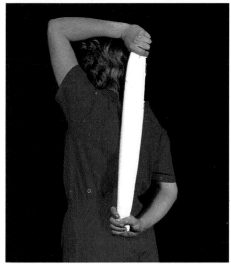

12a

Inward rotators and supinators of the arm

13. (*a*) Hold your elbows bent and press your hands together, or around a ball, for 4–7 seconds. Relax for 2 seconds. (*b*) Put each hand against a door-frame and stretch for 6–8 seconds to the left and right alternately so that the respective arm and shoulder rotate outwards.

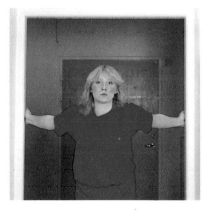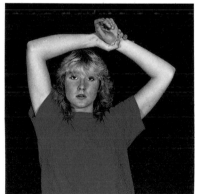

13b, 14a

Adductors and pronators of the arm, extensors of the elbow

14. Hold your hands over your head. (*a*) Pull your right arm to the side and resist with your left hand for 4–7 seconds. Let your right arm relax for 2 seconds. (*b*) Stretch by pulling your right arm behind your head. Hold the arm there for 6–8 seconds. Change arms and repeat the exercise.

General exercises

15. Throw and bounce a light ball with your injured arm.

16. Swim breaststroke and crawl both in water and on land.

THE ELBOW JOINT
Mobility and strength exercises

1. Stand or lie down. Bend and straighten your elbow to its outer limit.

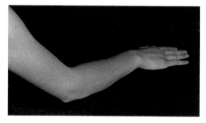

1

2. (*a*) Sit with your forearm flat on a table and the palm of your hand against the table top. (*b*) Turn your forearm so that the back of your hand is resting against the table.

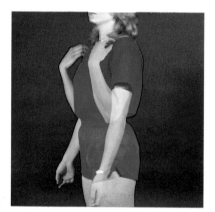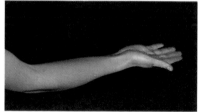

2a, 2b

3. Practise screwing and unscrewing a screw with a screwdriver. Hold your upper arm still close to your body.

4. Hold a dumb-bell in your hand and bend and straighten the elbow joint. Increase the weight of the dumb-bell gradually.

5. Stand up and do press-ups against a wall. Ensure that there is maximum flexion and extension of the elbows.

6. Do press-ups sitting in an arm-chair, lying full length and hanging from a bar.

7. Hold a barbell in your hands. Bend and straighten the elbow joint.

Repeat the above exercises 5–10 times.

Static stretching exercises (extension training)

Flexors and supinators of the arm

8. (*a*) Flex one elbow joint at a right angle. Resist with the other hand for 4–7 seconds and relax for 2 seconds. (*b*) Straighten your arm backwards, take hold of a wall-bar or something similar with your hand and stretch for 6–8 seconds by bending your knees.

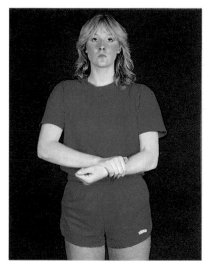 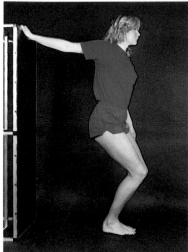

8a, 8b

'Timing'

9. Throw and bounce a light ball.

10. Swim breaststroke and crawl.

11. Practise rowing in a machine or boat.

12. Practise hitting a punchball.

Exercises in cases of 'tennis elbow'

Strength exercises for the wrist:

1. Static training: put your forearm on a table with your hand beyond the edge. (*a*) Bend your wrist down and hold it for 10 seconds. Rest. (*b*) Hold your wrist in a neutral position for 10 seconds. Rest. (*c*) Bend your wrist up and hold it for 10 seconds. Rest.
   The intensity of the exercise can be increased by holding a weight of 1 lb (0.5 kg) in your hand.
   Repeat the above exercises 10–50 times.

2. Dynamic training: exercise 4 under 'Wrist and hand' (see page 427).

Do the following additional exercise: put your forearm on a table with your hand beyond the edge and hold a weight of 2–6 lb (1–3 kg) in your hand. Bend your wrist up and down rapidly 10 times. Rest and repeat the exercise. Gradually increase the weight of the load.

Static stretching exercises Exercise 9 under 'Wrist and hand' (see page 428).

General exercises Exercises 3–4 under 'The elbow joint' (see page 424); exercises 8–9 under 'The shoulder joint' (see page 421–2); exercises 7–9 under 'The back' (see page 431).

WRIST AND HAND
Mobility exercises

1. Clench your fist as hard as possible. Then straighten your fingers and spread them out. If preferred, hold your arms straight out from the body during the exercise.

2. Press your thumb against the base of your little finger. Then move your thumb outwards as far as possible.

3. Put your forearm on a table. The hand, palm downwards, should hang beyond the edge of the table. Bend your hand as far as possible (*a*) down and (*b*) up. Then turn your forearm a quarter of a turn so that your thumb is pointing upwards and bend your hand as far as possible (*c*) down and (*d*) up.

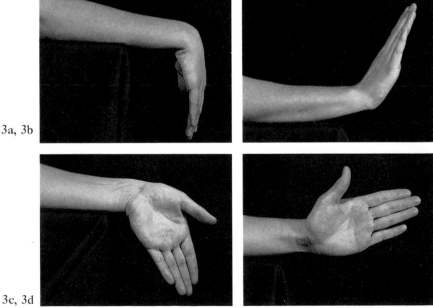

3a, 3b

3c, 3d

Strength exercises

4. Hold your finger-tips together and put an elastic band round them. Spread out the fingers against the resistance of the band.

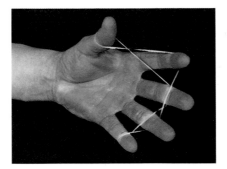

4

5. Squeeze one hand strengthener or a rubber ball repeatedly at a rapid pace.

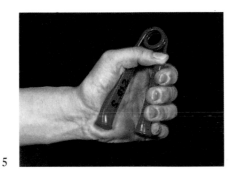

5

6. Hold a dumb-bell in your hand and carry out exercise 3 above (*a–d*).

Static stretching exercises

Flexors of fingers and wrist

7. (*a*) Press the fingers of one hand down against those of the other hand for 4–7 seconds. Relax for 2 seconds. (*b*) Stretch your fingers upwards by pulling them with the other hand for 6–8 seconds.

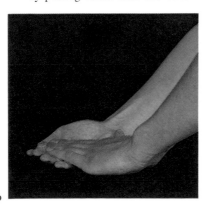 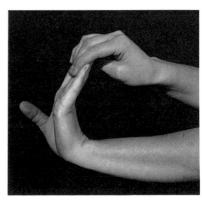

7a, 7b

8. (*a*) Press your hands together in front of your body for 4–7 seconds. Relax for 2 seconds. (*b*) Then stretch by moving your hands downwards, still pressed together, for 6–8 seconds.

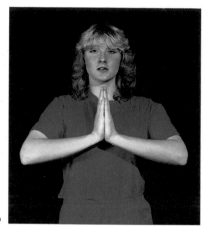
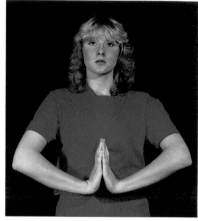

8a, 8b

Extensors of wrist

9. (*a*) Bend your wrist back and resist with the other hand for 4–7 seconds. Relax for 2 seconds. (*b*) Then stretch with a straight, supinated arm and your wrist bent in the other direction for 6–8 seconds.

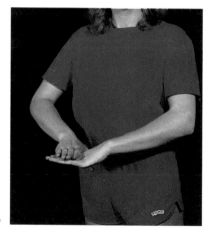
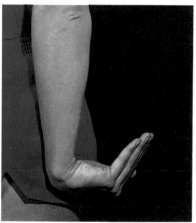

9a, 9b

Repeat the above exercises 3–5 times.

THE BACK
Mobility exercises

1. (*a*) Stand up and bend your back forwards, backwards and sideways and twist to the right and left. (*b*) Lie down on your back with your heels on a chair. Squeeze your buttocks together and lift and lower your pelvis at a rapid pace 10 times. Rest for 5 seconds. (*c*) Repeat exercise *b* once more, but this time keep your pelvis raised and count to 10. Rest for 5 seconds.

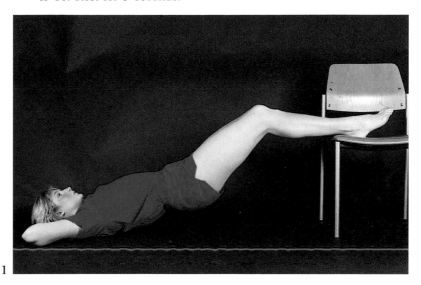

1

2. Lie down on your back with knees bent and feet flat on the floor. Place a ball between your knees, press the knees against the ball, squeeze your buttocks together and lift and lower your pelvis at a rapid pace 10 times. Rest for 5 seconds.

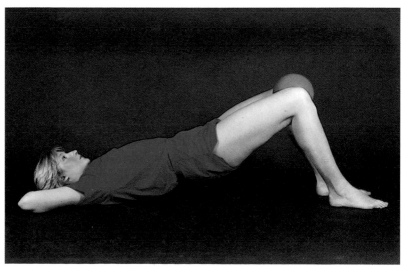

2

3. Sit in a chair with your feet wide apart. Hold your hands on your knees or clasped behind your neck. Turn the upper part of your body alternately left and right 5–10 times. Keep your pelvis and legs still.

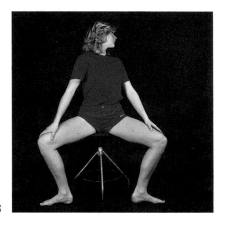

3

4. Practise rowing in a machine or boat.

Practise the above exercises 5–10 times.

Strength exercises

Extensors

5. Lie face down with hands on your lower back. Raise the upper part of your body so that chin and chest are off the floor and hold this position for 5 seconds. Rest for 5–10 seconds. Gradually increase the holding position to 10 seconds.

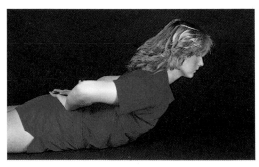 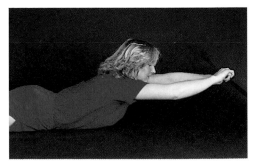

5, 6

6. Lie face down with your arms stretched out in front. Raise the upper part of your body so that chin, arms and chest do not touch the floor and hold the position for 5 seconds. Rest for 5–10 seconds. Gradually increase the holding position to 10 seconds.

Repeat the above exercises 5–10 times.

Straight and oblique abdominal muscles

7. Lie down on your back with knees bent, feet flat on the floor, arms crossed over your chest and hands on your shoulders. Raise your head and the upper part of your body and hold this position for 5–10 seconds. Rest for 5–10 seconds. Repeat the same exercise once more, but this time do rapid 'sit-ups' 5–10 times. Rest.

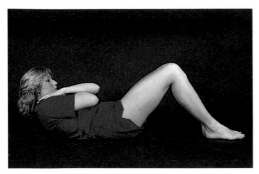 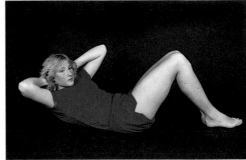

7, 8

8. Lie down on your back with knees bent, feet flat on the floor and hands behind your neck. Raise your head and left shoulder from the floor. Turn diagonally upwards so that your left elbow is turned to the right side, and hold the position for 5–10 seconds. Most of your back should be in contact with the floor. Rest for 5–10 seconds and then repeat the same exercise in the opposite direction.

9. Lie down on your back with knees and hips bent at a right angle. Raise your head and press hands against your knees for 5–10 seconds. Rest for 5–10 seconds.

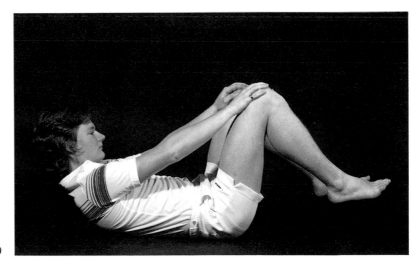

9

Repeat the above exercises 5–10 times.

Static stretching exercises

10. (*a*) Lie down on your back with knees bent; grasp your knees with your hands and 'roll into a ball'. (*b*) If possible, roll over so far that your toes reach the floor when your legs are stretched.

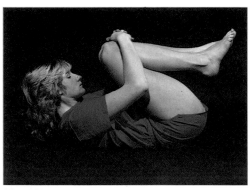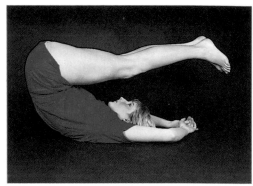

10a, 10b

The back and outside of the hip joint

11. Lie down on your back, bend your right leg and cross it over the left one by turning your hips. Pull up your right leg with your left hand as far as possible. Both your shoulders should remain in contact with the floor. Hold the position in the outer range for 6–8 seconds. Rest for 2 seconds, and then repeat the same movement in the opposite direction.

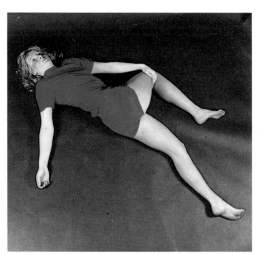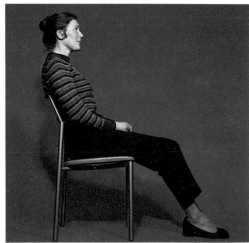

11, 12

12. Good ergonomics, correct lifting technique, good sitting and resting posture, and so on.

THE NECK
Mobility exercises

1. Tilt your head alternately to the left and right.

2. Tilt your head straight forwards.

3. Turn your head alternately to the left and right.

Strength exercises

4. Train the strength of your neck muscles by doing exercises 1–3 above and at the same time resist the movements with your hand.

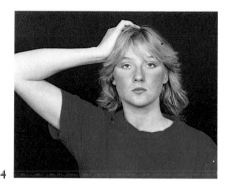

4

Static stretching exercises

The trapezius
muscle

5. Sit on a chair and hold your left hand round the edge of the chair. Tilt your head to the right and at the same time turn it to the left (look at your left shoulder). 'Pull' the edge of the chair up for 4–7 seconds. Relax for 2 seconds, and then stretch by leaning your body to the right. Hold it for 6–8 seconds. Rest and then repeat the exercise, but in the opposite direction.

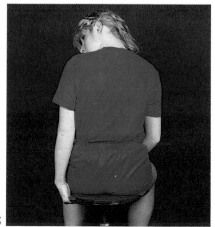

5

THE HIP JOINT
Mobility exercises

Flexors

1. Lie down on your back. Draw up your injured and healthy leg alternately towards your abdomen.

2. Stand up. Draw up your injured leg and healthy leg alternately towards your abdomen.

3. Stand up and place the foot of your injured leg on a table or similar support. Hold your healthy leg straight and shift the weight of your body onto your injured leg so that its knee joint is pressed up towards your abdomen.

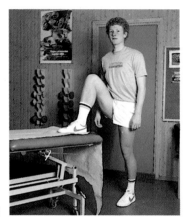

3

Extensors

4. Lie face down with knees straight. Raise your injured and healthy leg alternately.

5. Support the upper part of your body flat on a table. Alternately raise the injured leg and the healthy leg with your knee straight.

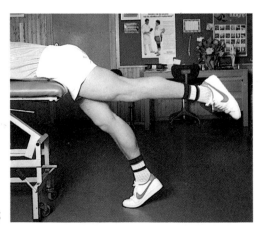

5

Inward and outward rotators

6. Sit on a table with your thighs supported and knees bent. Move your lower legs in turn (*a*) outwards and (*b*) inwards.

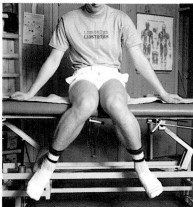 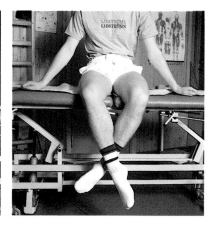

6a, 6b

Repeat the above exercises 5–10 times. For training the adductors and abductors of the hip joint see exercises 19–28 below.

Strength exercises

Flexors

7. (*a*) Lie down on your back. Fasten a weight cuff round the ankle of your injured leg and bend it up towards your abdomen and back again 10–30 times. Change legs. (*b*) Stand up and repeat exercise *a*, but now press your hands against the knee to provide resistance. Bend at the hip.

8. Fasten one end of a piece of rubber tubing to wall-bars or the like and the other end round the thigh of your injured leg. Stand with your back to the wall-bars and move your leg with the knee bent up towards your abdomen so that the tubing is tightened. Change legs.

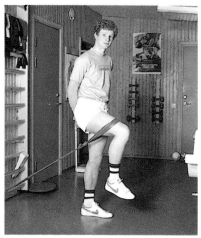

8

Extensors

9. Fasten a weight cuff round the ankle of your injured leg. Support the upper part of your body flat on a table. Raise your injured leg with knee straight and hold the position for 10 seconds. Rest and repeat the exercise at a rapid pace 10–30 times. Change legs.

10. Fasten one end of a piece of rubber tubing to wall-bars or the like and the other end round the ankle of your injured leg. Stand facing the wall-bars. Move your leg straight backwards with knee straight 10–30 times at a rapid pace.

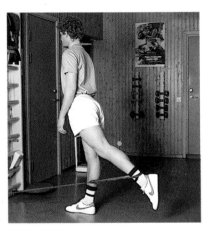

10

Inward and outward rotators

11. Sit on a table with your thighs supported. Fasten a piece of rubber tubing round your ankles. Turn your lower legs outwards against the resistance of the tubing and hold the position for 10 seconds. Rest. Repeat the exercise 5–10 times.

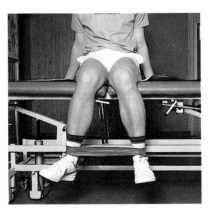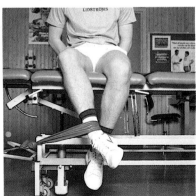

11, 12

12. Sit on a table with your thighs supported. Fasten one end of a piece of rubber tubing to wall-bars or the like and the other end round the ankle of your injured leg. Turn your lower leg inwards against the resistance of the tubing and hold the position for 10 seconds. Rest. Repeat the exercise 5–10 times. Change legs.

436

13. Lie down on your healthy side with knees bent. (*a*) Bend the hip and knee of your injured leg further so that this knee is higher than the knee of your healthy leg and at the same time turn your foot inwards. (*b*) Stretch out your injured leg backwards and at the same time turn your hip and foot outwards. Do the exercise 10–30 times at a rapid pace. Rest and repeat.

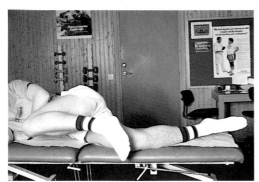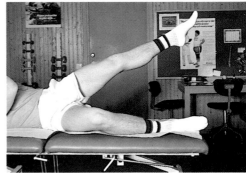

13a, 13b

Static stretching exercises

Flexors

14. Starting position: see picture *14a*. Your hands should be placed on each side of your healthy leg, the knee of which should be straight above your ankle and the foot, which should be pointed straight ahead. Your injured leg should be stretched out backwards with knee resting on the floor. If necessary a cushion can be put under the knee. 'Pull out' the knee of your injured leg for 4–7 seconds without moving it. Rest for 2 seconds. (*b*) Stretch for 6–8 seconds by lifting the knee of the injured leg from the floor, supporting with your toes and lowering your hip so that there is a pull at the front of your thigh.

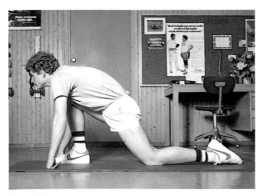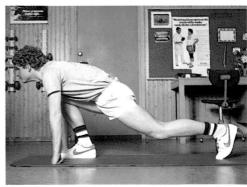

14a, 14b

15. Lie face down on a bed. Bend the knee of your injured leg at a right angle. Ask a friend to lift the thigh of your injured leg up from the bed and press your thigh against the friend's hand for 4–7 seconds. Relax for 2 seconds. Stretch by lifting your injured leg until there is a pull in the groin and hold the position for 6–8 seconds. Rest. The movement should take place in your hip, not in your back.

Extensors

16. Sit on the floor or stand up with straight legs and try gradually to touch your toes with your hands. Bend from your hips, not from your back. The stretching should be felt at the back of your thigh.

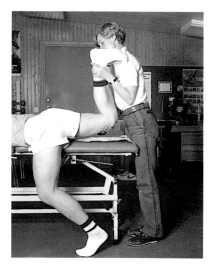

15

17. Lie down on your back on the floor with legs straight. Get assistance from a friend. Put the heel of your injured leg on the friend's shoulder. The friend holds his hands just above the kneecap of your injured leg, keeping the knee joint as straight as possible. Your healthy leg should remain on the floor all the time. (*a*) Press down your injured leg towards the friend's shoulder for 4–7 seconds. Rest for 2 seconds. Stretch for 6–8 seconds with the aid of the friend who raises your injured leg at the same time pressing against your knee to keep it straight. The stretching should be felt at the back of your thigh.

Outward rotators

18. Lie down on your back with healthy leg straight. Grasp the knee of your injured leg with your opposite hand, bend your leg up towards your abdomen, pull your knee towards the healthy hip with your hand and stretch for 6–8 seconds. Rest.

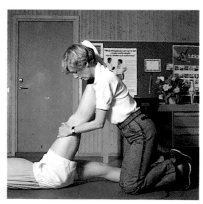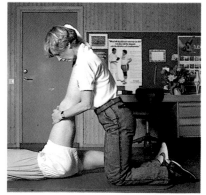

17a, 17b

438

Repeat the above exercises 3–5 times.

Stretch both your left and right leg, but always start by stretching the stiff leg. Compare the stretching of your injured leg with that of the healthy leg to check that there is no overstretching.

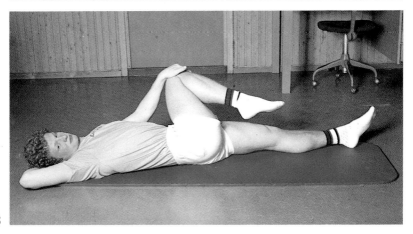

18

THE GROIN
Mobility exercises

The abductors and adductors of the hip joint

1. Lie down on your back. (*a*) Move your injured leg in turn outwards and inwards. (*b*) Move each leg in turn outwards and inwards. (*c*) Raise your injured leg about 4 in (10 cm) from the floor and move it alternately out and in. Change legs.

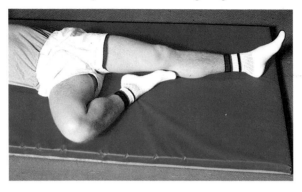

2

2. Lie down on your back. Move the heel of your injured leg up towards the buttocks and at the same time turn knee and hip outwards. Hold the position for 10 seconds. Rest. Repeat the exercise.

Strength exercises

The abductors and adductors of the hip joint

3. Lie down on your back with legs straight and a ball between your knees. Press your legs against the ball for 10 seconds, relax and repeat. Do the same exercise with the ball placed between the feet. Vary the exercises by using balls of different sizes.

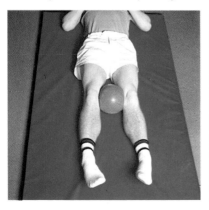 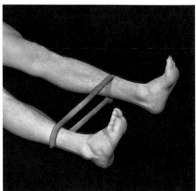

3, 4

4. Lie down on your back and fasten a belt or the like round your lower shins. Press your legs outwards against the belt for 10 seconds, rest and repeat the exercise. Vary the exercise by moving the belt up and down.

5. Sit on the floor leaning back and support yourself with your hands. Ask a friend to sit in the same way opposite and place his feet with the outsides against the insides of your feet. Press your feet inwards for 10 seconds while the friend provides a resistance with his feet. Then place your feet in such a way that the friend's feet have their insides against the outsides of your feet. Press your feet outwards for 10 seconds while the friend provides resistance. Repeat the exercise.

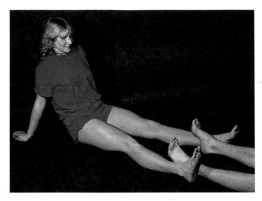

5

6. Fasten one end of a piece of rubber tubing to wall-bars or the like and the other end round the ankle of one leg. (*a*) Stand with the outside of the leg facing the wall-bars and pull the tubing straight out from the wall-bars 10–30 times. (*b*) Stand with the inside of your leg facing the wall-bars and pull the tubing straight out 10–30 times. (*c*) Stand with the inside of your leg facing the wall-bars and pull the tubing diagonally backwards 10–30 times at a rapid pace. Change legs and repeat the exercises.

The value of the exercises can be intensified by gradually increasing the number of repeats and by using a shorter piece of tubing to provide greater resistance.

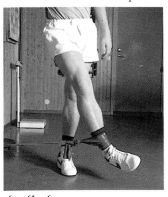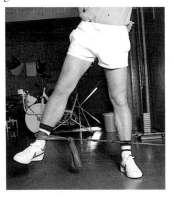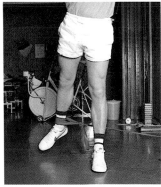

6a, 6b, 6c

Static stretching exercises

The abductors and adductors of the hip joint

7. Sit on the floor with knees bent, the soles of your feet against each other and your elbows on your knees. (*a*) Press knees inwards and resist with elbows for 4–7 seconds. Rest for 2 seconds. (*b*) Stretch by pressing your knees down with your elbows for 6–8 seconds.

441

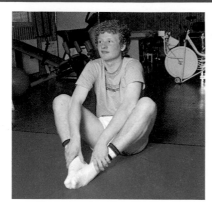
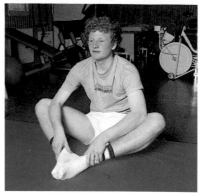

7a, 7b

8. Stand with legs wide apart and body straight. Put the weight of your body on your healthy leg and bend your knee. (*a*) Press the foot of your injured leg against the floor for 4–7 seconds. Relax for 2 seconds. (*b*) Stretch your injured leg for 6–8 seconds by bending your healthy knee further.

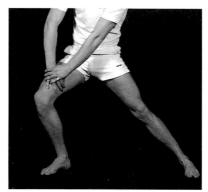
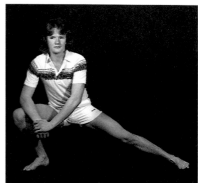

8a, 8b

9. Sit on the floor and bend your healthy leg up under your injured one so that the heel is brought up to your buttocks. Put the foot of your injured leg on the outside of the thigh of your healthy leg. Grasp the outside of the knee of your injured leg with the opposite hand. (*a*) Press the knee of your injured leg against your hand for 4–7 seconds. Relax for 2 seconds. (*b*) Move the knee of your injured leg up towards your body with the aid of the elbow and stretch for 6–8 seconds.

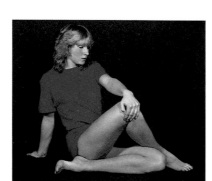
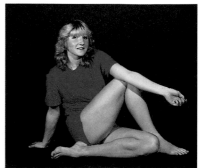

9a, 9b

10. Stand with your injured leg diagonally behind your healthy one. (*a*) Press the foot of your injured leg against the floor for 4–7 seconds. Relax for 2 seconds. (*b*) Stretch the outside of the thigh of your injured leg by bending the knee of your healthy leg.

10a, 10b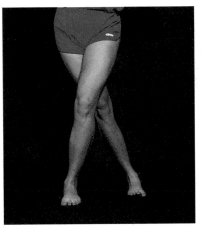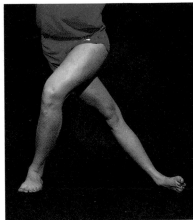

Repeat the above exercises 3–5 times.

General exercises

11. Cycle on an exercise bicycle with gradually increased resistance.

12. Swim breaststroke and crawl in a pool.

Strength exercises

13. Stand with a barbell held on your shoulders. Keep your back straight, bend both knees at an angle of 90° and rise again. Repeat the same exercise with one leg in front of the other. Change legs and do the exercise once more.

Jumping exercises

14. First jump with both feet together, then on one foot at a time.

15. Jump over low hurdles.

16. Play leapfrog.

17. Skip.

18. Hold a barbell on your shoulders, jump and give at the knees when landing.

THE KNEE JOINT
Mobility exercises

Extensors

1. Sit on a flat, firm surface. Put a roll of kitchen-paper or the like under your injured knee. Flex your thigh muscle, bend up your foot and lift your heel from the surface. All the time your knee should be in contact with the roll. Hold your leg in a straightened position for 10 seconds. Rest for 5 seconds. Repeat the exercise.

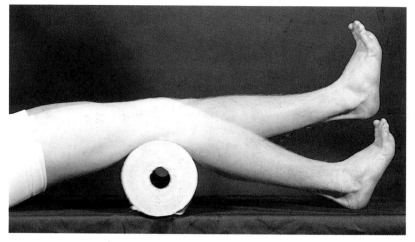

1

2. Repeat exercise 1, this time without putting a roll under your knee.

Flexors

3. Sit on a table with your thighs supported. Bend your injured leg as far as possible. Hold your healthy leg behind the injured one as a support.

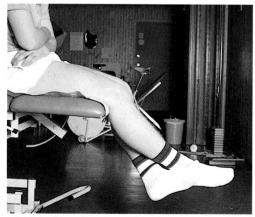

3

4. Lie face down and bend your injured leg as far as possible.

5. Lie down on your back on the floor with the foot of your injured leg up against a wall. Let your foot slide downwards and at the same time bend your knee.

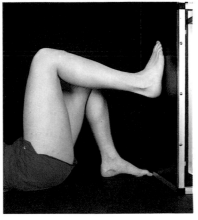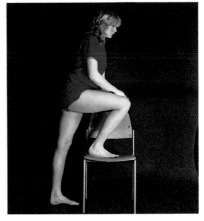

5, 6

6. Stand with the foot of your injured leg on a chair. Slowly stretch forwards so that your knee is bent. Hold the position for 10 seconds. Rest.

The above exercises should be carried out for short periods at a time several times a day.

Strength exercises

Extensors

7. Lie down on your back with legs straight. Bend the foot of the injured leg up, flex your thigh muscle and lift your leg with the knee straight. Hold the position for 10 seconds. Rest for 5 seconds. Repeat 5–10 times.

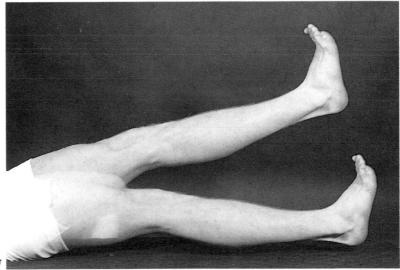

7

8. Lie down on your back. Flex the thigh muscle of your injured leg, straighten your knee and raise and lower your leg with the knee straight 10 times. Rest for 30 seconds. Repeat 10 times.
   The exercise can be intensified by gradually increasing the number of repeats from 10 lifts to 20, 30, 40, and so on.

445

9. Repeat exercise 7 or 8, now with a weight cuff round your ankle. Initially the weight cuff should weigh 4–5 lb (2–3 kg).

10. Sit on a table with your thighs supported. Put the foot of your injured leg on a stool or the like so that your knee is bent at an angle of about 50°. Put the heel of your healthy leg on top of the ankle of your injured leg. Resist with your healthy leg and straighten your injured one against the resistance. Rest for 30 seconds. Repeat the exercise 5 times. Then repeat the whole exercise, now with the knee of your injured leg bent at a different angle, for example, 30°. The exercise should primarily be done with the knee of your injured leg bent at the angle at which the quadriceps femoris is weakest.

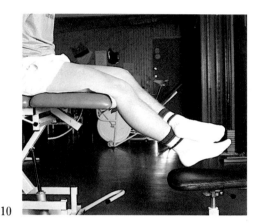

10

11. Sit on a table with your thighs supported. Straighten and bend your injured knee 10 times. Rest and repeat the exercise. Intensify the exercise by fastening a weight cuff around your ankle.

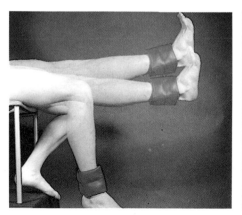 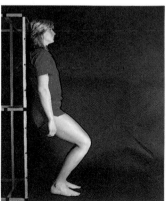

11, 12

12. Stand with your back against a wall. Bend your knees so that your back slides slowly down the wall. Hold the position, knees bent, for 10 seconds. Gradually increase the time for holding the position.

Flexors

13. Sit on the floor with the knee of your injured leg bent and your heel hooked over a step edge, door-sill or the like. Draw your leg backwards so your heel is pressed against the edge and count to 10. Rest for 5 seconds. Repeat the exercise 5–10 times.

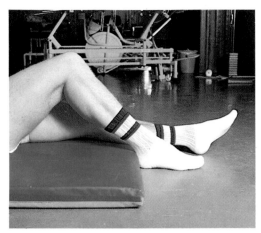 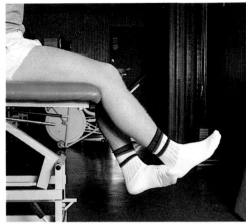

13, 14

14. Sit on a table with your thighs supported. Put your healthy leg behind the injured one, resist with your healthy leg and bend the injured leg against the resistance for 10 seconds. Rest for 5 seconds and repeat the exercise. Exercise your injured leg with knee bent at different angles.

15. Put a piece of rubber tubing round the front legs of a chair. Sit on the chair and press your injured leg backwards against the rubber tubing for 10 seconds. Rest for 5 seconds. Repeat the exercise.

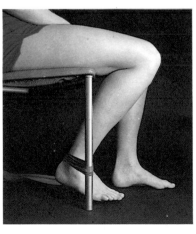 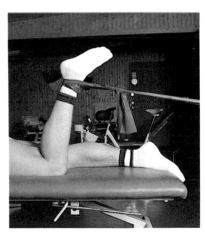

15, 16

16. Fasten one end of a piece of rubber tubing to wall-bars or the like and the other end round the ankle of your injured leg. Lie face down and bend your knee 10 times at a rapid pace against the resistance of the tubing. Rest for 5 seconds. Repeat the exercise. Increase the intensity of the exercise by using a shorter piece of tubing.

17. Repeat exercise 16, now in a sitting position with your thighs supported.

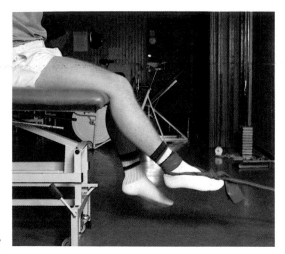

17

Exercise the other muscles of your leg, as well as abdominal and arm muscles.

Load exercises

Flexors and extensors

18. Sit on the edge of a bed or a low table with your injured leg in front of it. Your knee should be bent and your foot pointed straight ahead. Rise to a standing position and sit down again with the aid of your injured leg. The lower the bed or table, the more power will be needed for the exercise.

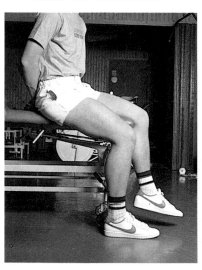 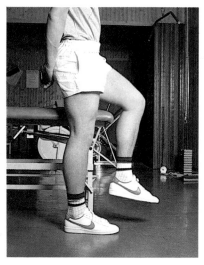

18

19. Kneel on your healthy leg. Rise to a standing position on your injured leg without supporting yourself with your hands. Change legs. Repeat the exercise 10–15 times.

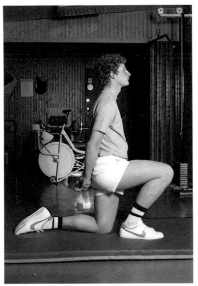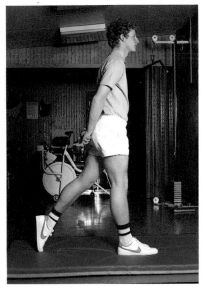

19

20. Stand upright with a light barbell across your shoulders. Bend and straighten your knees.

Combine strength exercises with stretching.

Static stretching exercises

Extensors

21. Lie face down and grasp the ankle of your injured leg with one hand. (*a*) Straighten the leg against the resistance of your hand for 4–7 seconds. Rest for 2 seconds. (*b*) Stretch by drawing the foot as far up as possible for 6–8 seconds. Your thigh should rest against the floor.

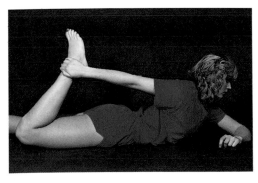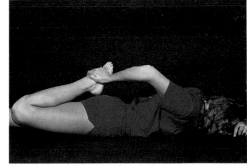

21a, 21b

22. Repeat exercise 21, now in a standing position. Resist your leg with both hands for 4–6 seconds, relax for 2 seconds and stretch for 6–8 seconds. Be careful to hold your hip straight or extended backwards.

Flexors

23. Lie down on your back in a door-way with buttocks as close to the door frame as possible. Put your injured leg against the door frame and let your healthy leg stick out through the door opening. Press the

449

heel of your injured leg against the door frame for 4–6 seconds. Relax for 2 seconds. Stretch by bending your foot up and straightening your knee to its maximum for 6–8 seconds.

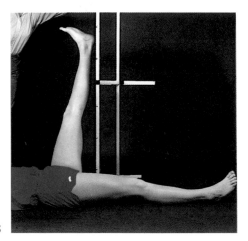

23

24. Put your injured leg on a table. Both legs should be straight, the foot of your healthy leg should be pointed straight ahead and your back should be straight. (*a*) Press your heel against the surface of the table for 4–7 seconds. Relax. (*b*) Stretch for 6–8 seconds by bending up the foot of your injured leg, straightening your knee and bending forwards from the hips with a straight back. For further stretching, the knee of your healthy leg can be bent.

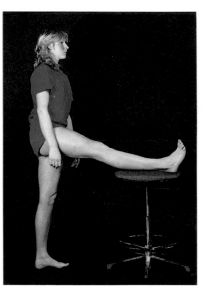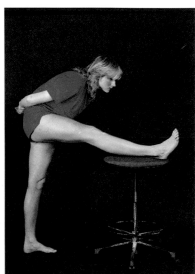

24a, 24b

Repeat the above exercises 3–6 times.

Always start the stretching in the outer range of the muscle. Do the exercises with the injured and the healthy leg alternately.

Chondromalacia patellae

The following exercises are recommended for patients with chondromalacia patellae.

Strength exercises

Exercises 7–10 on page 445 and 13–14 on page 447. When doing exercises 10, 13 and 14, start exercising with the knee joint angled at 30°. The more acutely bent the knee joint, the greater the load on the kneecap. Therefore increase the bending gradually and always train below the pain threshold.

Static stretching exercises

Exercises 3, 5 and 6 on page 440 for stretching the abductors of the leg.

The following general strength exercises (1–4) for the adjacent musculature, (the adductors of the leg (1), the abductors of the leg (2), the extensors of the hip (3) and the straight and oblique muscles of the abdomen (4). For balance and co-ordination exercises see page 460.

1. Lie down on your back with knees bent and feet on the floor. Put a ball between your knees and press them against the ball. Squeeze your buttocks together and raise and lower your pelvis at a rapid pace 10 times. Rest. Repeat the exercise.

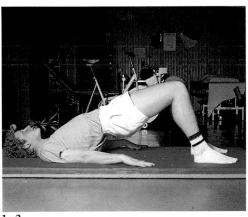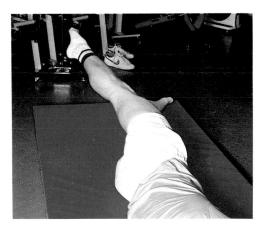

1, 2

2. Lie down on one side with legs straight. Lift your upper leg diagonally backwards and hold the position for 10 seconds. Rest. Repeat the exercise. Then lift and lower your leg at a rapid pace 10 times. Rest. Repeat the exercise. Change legs. The intensity of the exercises can be increased by fastening a weight cuff around your ankle.

3. (*a*) Lie face down with the upper part of your body on a table and your legs over the edge. Lift one leg straight up and hold the position for 10 seconds. Rest. Repeat the exercise. Then lift and lower your leg at a rapid pace 10 times. Rest. Repeat. Change legs. The intensity

of the exercises can be increased by fastening a weight cuff around your ankle.

(*b*) Do the above exercises standing and with a piece of rubber tubing to provide resistance.

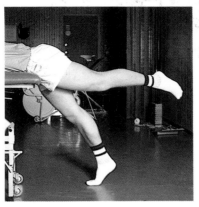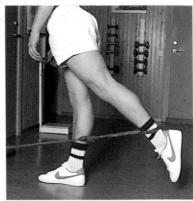

3a, 3b

4. *Abdominal exercises*: see exercises 7–9 on page 431.

Repeat the above exercises 20–50 times twice a day.

Pool exercises

— Swim with moderate leg kicks.
— Walk on the bottom of the pool at a gradually increasing speed.
— Rise from a squatting to a standing position if the pain allows it.

— The whole programme does not have to be done in one go.
— Do the various exercises in turn.
— All the exercises should be done below the pain threshold.

REHABILITATION AFTER SURGERY

Meniscus injuries

About 24 hours after surgery on a meniscus injury, exercises 1–2 on page 444 can be performed. One to two weeks after surgery the patient can add exercises 3–4 on page 444 and also the co-ordination and balance exercises 1–11 on page 460. When there are no signs of pain and swelling in the knee joint, the injured athlete can start doing the strength exercises 7–17 on page 445.

Injuries to the lateral ligaments of the knee

After surgery on injuries to the lateral ligaments of the knee joint, the following exercises are recommended:

Mobility exercises

Exercises 1–6 on page 444.

Strength exercises	Exercises 7–17 on page 445. Gradually increase the intensity of the exercises.
Load exercises	Exercises 18–20 on page 448.
Balance and co-ordination exercises	Exercises 1–11 on page 460.
	When necessary combine the above exercises with the static stretching exercises 21–24 on page 449.

Injuries to the cruciate ligaments

After surgery on injuries to the cruciate ligaments, rehabilitation should take place in consultation with a physiotherapist. When training at home and also when the patient does not have access to a physiotherapist, the following programme can be used.

Exercises 3–5 on page 444 and 13–17 on page 447. Gradually increase the intensity of the exercises. Also exercise the other muscles of the leg and the muscles of the abdomen and the arms.

Exercises 1 and 3–6 on page 460 are recommended for balance and co-ordination.

When the mobility of the knee joint has increased so much that the knee joint can be bent at an angle of about 110° the patient can start cycling on an exercise bicycle. The resistance should be slight at first and be increased gradually.

Twelve weeks after surgery training can be intensified along the following lines:

Mobility exercises	Exercises 1–2 on page 444.
Strength exercises	Exercises 7–12 on page 445.
Static stretching exercises	Exercises 21–24 on page 449.
Pool exercises	— Swim with moderate leg kicks. — Walk on the bottom of the pool at a gradually increasing speed. — Rise from a squatting to a standing position if the pain allows it.
Balance and co-ordination exercises	Exercises 1–7 on page 460. About 4–6 months after surgery, the exercises 8–11 can also be performed.
Track training	This can be started 4–8 months after surgery, but only when a doctor or physiotherapist gives the go-ahead.

453

THE ANKLE JOINT
Mobility exercises

1. Lie down on your back. Bend your foot up and at the same time straighten your toes. Then point your foot while bending your toes.

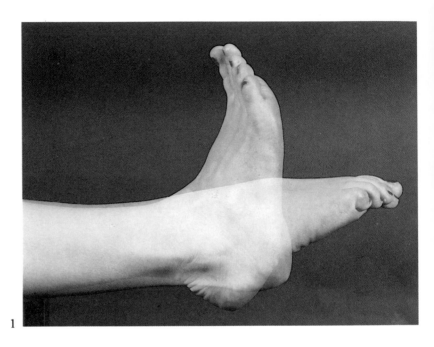

1

2. Sit on a chair with the soles of your feet on the floor. (*a*) Put your feet as far forwards as possible. (*b*) Pull your feet in under the chair and press your heels against the floor.

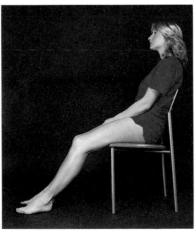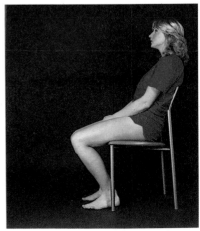

2a, 2b

3. Sit on a chair or lie down on your back. (*a*) Turn the soles of your feet in against each other. (*b*) Turn the soles of your feet away from each other.

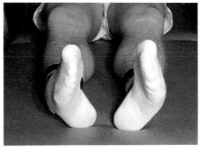 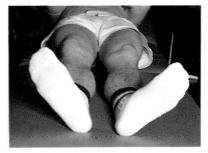

3a, 3b

4. Sit on a chair and roll a golf ball under your foot, both backwards and forwards and from side to side.

5. **Exercises for the toe flexors**: sit on a chair and use your toes to crumple up a towel and smooth it out again. Pick up marbles with your toes.

Strength exercises

6. Support your back against a chair or a wall with your hands. Go up on your toes and down on your heels repeatedly. Intensify the exercise by doing it standing on one leg. When this can be done without pain or swelling the exercise is carried out without support.

7. Walk alternately on your heels and on your toes.

8. When the injury has healed, walk alternately on the outsides and the insides of your feet.

9. Stand with the front part of your feet on a telephone directory. (*a*) Rise up on your toes. (*b*) Lower your heels slowly towards the floor.

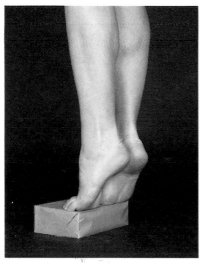 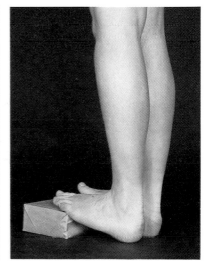

9a, 9b

10. Stand with your injured foot on a step and your healthy foot on the floor. Climb up so that the weight of your body is a load on your injured foot and then step down again. Do the exercise both turned sideways to the staircase and facing it. Intensify the exercise first by doing it on tiptoe, then by taking two steps at a time.

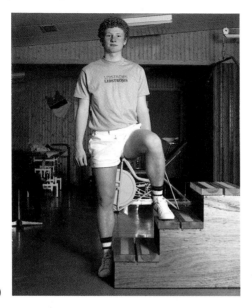

10

11. Sit on a table with your thighs supported. Attach a weight to your foot. Bend your foot up and then lower it slowly.

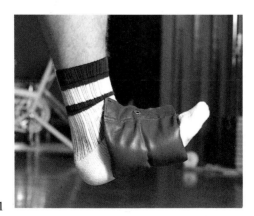

11

The above exercises should be done 5–10 times.

Balance and co-ordination exercises (see page 460) should be started at an early stage of rehabilitation and should be part of the training for at least 6 months after the injury occurred.

Static stretching exercises

The back of the lower leg (the calf muscles)

12. Support your body with your hands at chest height against a wall. Put one leg behind the other. Your feet should be pointing straight ahead and your heels should be in contact with the floor throughout the entire exercise. Bend your front knee and straighten the back one slightly. Press your back foot against the floor for 4–7 seconds. Relax for 2 seconds. Stretch for 6–8 seconds by moving the hips forwards and straightening the back leg so that there is a pull in your calf.

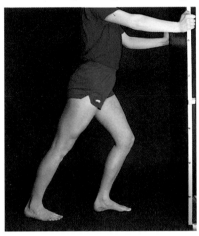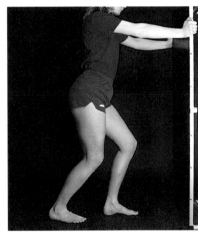

12, 13

13. Stand in the same starting position as for exercise 12, but reverse legs. Press the heel of your back foot against the floor for 4–7 seconds. Relax for 2 seconds. Stretch by pressing the knee of your back leg downwards and forwards for 6–8 seconds. Do not lift your heel from the floor.

Injuries to the arch aponeurosis

14. Kneel with toes bent up. Stretch for 6–8 seconds by leaning your body backwards.

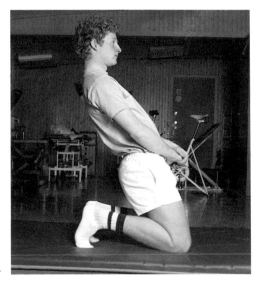

14

The muscles in the front of the lower leg and the foot

15. Starting position: see picture. The back should be straight, the toes and the feet should be pointing straight ahead and straight backwards respectively. Hold the hand just below the knee of the leg, the foot of which is pointing backwards, and lift up. Stretch for 6–8 seconds by pulling the leg up and leaning the body backwards.

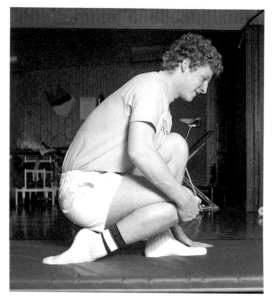

15

During static stretching exercises, the following points should be remembered:

— do warm-up exercises for 5–10 minutes before the stretching is started;
— stretch below the pain threshold;
— muscles cannot all be stretched to an equal extent;
— Not all muscles need to be stretched;
— over-mobility increases the risk of injury;
— start stretching in the outer range of the muscle;
— stretch slowly and gently and do not swing;
— do the exercises regularly.

Rehabilitation after surgery on injured ligaments in the ankle joint

In cases of rehabilitation after surgery on a ligament injury in the ankle joint, the following exercises are recommended when the plaster has been removed after 5–6 weeks:

Mobility exercises

Exercises 1–2 and 4–5 on page 454.

Strength exercises

Exercises 6–7 and 9–11 on page 455.

Anyone who has access to a swimming-pool can use the pool to improve the mobility of the ankle joint by doing the exercises in the water. Strength exercises can also be carried out in a pool, for example with a weight cuff around the injured foot.

Balance and co-ordination exercises Exercises 1–11 on page 460.

Track training See page 462.

Rehabilitation after injuries to the Achilles tendon

In cases of a non-surgical treatment of an injury to the Achilles tendon, the patient should use shoes with ½–1 in (1.2–2 cm) high heels.

The following exercises are recommended:

Mobility exercises Exercises 1–5 on page 454.

Strength exercises These can be started with exercises 6–13 on page 455 after pain and swelling have abated and a doctor or physiotherapist has given the go-ahead.

Rehabilitation in cases of pain in the lower leg

In cases of periostitis, active rest is recommended; all painful movements should be avoided but the muscle groups that are not painful should be exercised. When the problems have disappeared, the whole training programme for the ankle joint can be used. Track training should be started only when a doctor or physiotherapist has given the go-ahead.

BALANCE AND CO-ORDINATION EXERCISES

1. Sit on a chair and 'play' with a ball that is rolled from foot to foot. Use balls of different sizes.

2. Stand on one leg and close your eyes. Change legs.

3. Stand on your healthy leg and 'draw' letters or figures with your injured leg. Your foot should not be in contact with the floor.

4. Stand up and support your body with your hand against a wall. Put the foot of your injured leg on a ball. Move your foot forwards, backwards and sideways without lifting it from the ball. Keep your back straight. Use balls of different sizes. Intensify the exercise by doing it without any support.

4

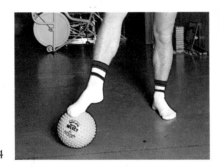
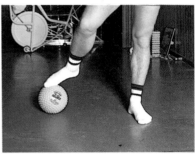

5. Balance on a narrow board or – if possible – outdoors on a fallen tree or something similar.

6. Stand on a balancing board (or on a board that has been put on the rounded side of a hub cap) with both feet and try to keep the board horizontal. 'Rock' the board in different directions by angling your feet.

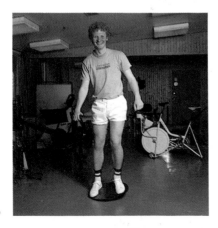

6

7. Do exercises on a trampoline. (*a*) Walk alternately on tiptoe and on your heels. (*b*) Walk alternately on the outsides and the insides of your feet. (*c*) Bounce cautiously up and down. Increase the intensity of the exercise by jumping higher and higher. Jump alternately on your healthy and injured leg.

8. Jump on the spot. Start with low jumps and gradually jump higher and higher.

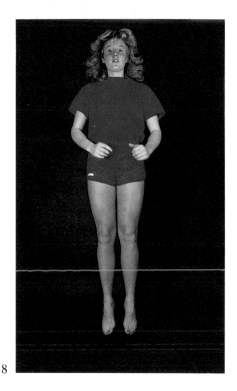

8

9. Skip.

10. Hop on one leg. Hop alternately on your healthy and injured leg.

11. Jump across low hurdles.

Before an injured athlete resumes his specialized sport, his training should be adjusted to suit its requirements, but there should be plenty of time for rest in the programme. After having regained full strength and mobility, an injured soccer player, for example, should train on his own with a football before returning to playing with the team. He should practise dribbling backwards, forwards, sideways and diagonally. In addition, he should practise jumping on the spot and skipping, leg-kicks with jump-ups, side-jumps with the weight of the body on the arms, starting and stopping. Finally he can return to practising with a ball with his team.

Track training

Before an injured athlete resumes track training, he should consult a doctor or physiotherapist in order to get the go-ahead. Alternatives to track training are swimming (crawl) and cycling.

In the preliminary stages of track training, it is appropriate to use interval training. Start, for instance, by alternately walking 100 m and jogging 100 m and repeat this 10 times. Gradually increase to 20 times and then change to alternately jogging 100 m and running 100 m at half speed 10 times. Gradually increase to 20 times and finally intensify the track training by alternately running 100 m at half speed and running 100 m at full speed.

The following points should be remembered when track training:
— the load is high on muscles, ligaments and joints;
— start the training on a soft surface;
— do not run on very hilly ground;
— do not run at full speed at the beginning;
— increased speed means increased load.

Bibliography

Adams, R et al *Games, Sports and Exercises for the Physically Handicapped* (Lea & Febiger, Philadelphia 1972)

Astrand P O & Rodahl K *Textbook of Work Physiology* (McGraw-Hill, New York 1970)

Cantu R C *Clinical Sports Medicine* (The Collamore Press, Lexington, Massachusetts, Toronto 1984)

Cantu R C *Sports medicine in primary care* (The Collamore Press, Lexington, Massachusetts, Toronto 1982)

Cantu R, Gillespie W *Sports Medicine, Sports Science, Bridging the Gap* (The Collamore Press. Lexington, Massachusetts, Toronto 1982)

Cerny, H V *The Complete Book of Athletic and Taping Techniques* (Prentice-Hall, Englewood Cliffs, New Jersey 1972)

Clinics in Sports Medicine *Olympic Sports Medicine* (Saunders, Philadelphia 1982)

Clinics in Sports Medicine *Injuries to Dancers* (Saunders, Philadelphia 1983)

Clinics in Sports Medicine *The Athletic Woman* (Saunders, Philadelphia 1984)

Clinics in Sports Medicine *Nutritional Aspects of Exercise* (Saunders, Philadelphia 1984)

Clinics in Sports Medicine *Profiling* (Saunders, Philadelphia 1984)

Clinics in Sports Medicine *Pediatric and Adolescent Sports Medicine* (Saunders, Philadelphia 1982)

Clinics in Sports Medicine *Skiing Injuries* (Saunders, Philadelphia July 1982)

Clinics in Sports Medicine *Ankle and Foot problems in the Athelte* (Saunders, Philadelphia March 1982)

Cohen I, Beaton G, Mitchell, D *The South African Textbook of Sports Medicine* (Sports Medicine Clinic, Johannesburg 1979)

Cyriax, J *Textbook of Orthopaedic Medicine* (London 1974)

Dandy D J *Arthroscopy of the knee, A diagnostic color atlas* (Lea & Febiger, Philadelphia 1984)

Davies, D J *Rehabilitation of the surgical knee* (CyPress, New York 1984)

Dolan, J & Holladay, L *Treatment and Prevention of Athletic Injuries*

Ehricht, H G *Die Wirbelsäule in der Sportmedizin* (The spine in sports medicine) (J A Barth, Leipzig 1978)

Eriksson, B et al 'Idrottsmedicin' (Sports medicine) *Lakartidningen* (1975) 5

Franke, K *Traumatologie des Sports* (The traumatology of sport) (Georg Thieme Verlag, Stuttgart 1980)

Frankel, V H & Burnstein, A H *Orthopaedic Biomechanics* (Lea & Febiger, Philadelphia 1974)

Frederick E C *Sports shoes and playing surfaces. Biomechanical properties* (Human Kinetics Publishers Inc, Champaign, Illinois 1984)

Gray, M *Football Injuries* (Offox Press, Oxford 1980)

Harris, H & Varney, M *The Treatment of Football Injuries* (Macdonald and Jane's, London 1977)

Heipertz, W *Sportmedizin* (Sports medicine) (George Thieme Verlag, Stuttgart 1976)

Heiss, F *Unfallverhutung und Nothilfe beim Sport* (Accident prevention and first aid in sport) (Verlag Karl Hofmann, Schorndorf 1977)

Helfet A J *Disorders of the knee* (2nd edn) (1982)

Jackson, W D & Pescar C S *The Young Athlete's Health Handbook* (Everest House, New York 1981)

Krejci, V & Koch, P *Musckelverletsungen und Tendopathien der Sportler* (Muscle injuries and tendon complaints in sportsmen) (George Thieme Verlag, Stuggart 1976)

Kulund, D N *The injured athlete* (Lippincott, Philadelphia, Toronto 1982)

Ljungquist, R 'Subcutaneous partial rupture of the Achilles tendon'. *Acta orthop Scand* Copenhagen (1968)

Mangi, R J P & Dayton, O W *The Runner's Complete Medical Guide* (Summit Books, New York 1979)

Marshall J L *The sports doctor's fitness book for women* (Delacorte Press, New York 1981)

Matsen, A F *Compartmental Syndromes* (Grune & Stratton, New York 1980)

Mirkin, G & Hoffman, M *Sportmedicin* (Sports Medicine) (Liber Laromedel, Malmo 1981)

Mirkin, G & Hoffman M *The Sports Medicine Book* (Little, Brown and Company, Boston 1978)

Morehouse, L E & Rasch, P J *Sports Medicine for Trainers* (W B Saunders, Philadelphia 1963)

Muckle, D S *Sports Injuries* (Oriel Press, Newcastle 1971)

Muckle D S *Injuries in Sport* (John Wright & Sons Ltd, Bristol 1978)

McRae R *Clinical orthopaedic examination* (1976)

Mubarak S J & Jargens A R *Compartment syndromes and Volkmann's Contracture* (1981)

O'Donoughue *Injuries to athletes* (Saunders, New York 1980)

Orthopedic Clinics of North America *Injuries in Sport: Recent Developments* (W B Saunders, Philadelphia July 1977) *Ski Trauma and Skiing Safety* (W B Saunders, Philadelphia January 1976)

Peterson, L, Renström, P et al. 'Idrottsmedicin' (Sports Medicine) *Lakartidningen* (1980) *41*

Pforringer, W, Rosemeyer, B & Bar, H W, *Sporttraumatologie – Sportartentypische Schaden und Verletzungen* (Sports traumatology – injuries and traumas typical of different sports (Beiersdorf Medical Bibliothek, Erlangen 1981)

Rapporter i idrottsfysiologi (Reports on sports physiology) – (training at high altitudes, Alpine skiing, motocross, energy demands for running, speed skating, regular physical exercise, soccer, badminton, land and ice hockey, orienteering, cross-country skiing, canoeing, walking, sailing, Alpine sports, team handball, trekking) Trygg-Hansa, Stockholm

Read, M & Wade, P *Sports Injuries – A Unique Guide to Self-Diagnosis and Rehabilitation*   (Breslich & Foss, London   1984)

Schwerdtner, H M & Fohler, N *Sportverletzungen* (Sports injuries) (Verlag Dr. Med, D Straube, Erlangen   1976)

Smillie I S *Diseases of the Knee Joint* (Churchill Livingstone, Edinburgh   1979)

Smillie I S *Injuries of the Knee Joint* (Churchill Livingstone, Edinburgh   1979)

Southmayd, W & Hoffman, M, *Sports Health. The Complete Book of Athletic Injuries* (Quick Fox, New York & London   1981)

Southmayd W., Hoffman M *Sports Health*. The complete book of athletic injuries   (Quick Fox, New York, London   1981)

Sperryn P N *Sport and Medicine* (Butterworths, London   1983)

Subotnick, S I *The Running Foot Doctor* (World Publications, Mountain View, California   1977)

Subotnick, S I *Cures for common running injuries* (Collier Books, Macmillan Publishing Company, New York   1984)

Vinger, F P & Hoerner, F E *Sports Injuries. The Unthwarted Epidemic* (P S G, Thittleton, Massachusetts   1981)

Weisenfeld, F M & Burr, B *The Runner's Repair Manual* (St Martin's Press, New York   1980)

Williams, J G P *A Colour Atlas of Injury in Sport* (Wolfe Medical Publications Ltd, London   1980)

Williams, J G P & Sperryn, P N *Sports Medicine* (Arnold, London   1976)

Yablon I et al. *Ankle Injuries* (1983)

Glossary

abduction – to move or pull away a leg, arm, etc., from the midline of the body.

abductor – any muscle that moves a part of the body away from the midline.

Achilles tendon – the tendon of the gastrocnemius and soleus muscles, attached to the calcaneus.

acromioclavicular ligament – the ligament attached to the acromion and clavicle.

acromion – an oblong process at the top of the spine of the scapula, part of which articulates with the clavicle to form the acromioclavicular joint.

acute – of rapid onset (cf: chronic).

adduct – to move a part of the body towards the midline of the body.

adductor magnus muscle – the large muscle that moves the leg towards the midline of the body.

adrenaline – a hormone produced by the medulla of the supradrenal glands and secreted into the blood. Prepares the body for 'fright, flight or fight'.

agonist – a muscle whose active contraction causes movement of part of the body (cf. antagonist).

amenorrhoea – the absence or stopping of the menstrual periods.

anaemia – a reduced quantity of haemoglobin in the blood, causing excessive tiredness, breathlessness, pallor and poor resistance to infection.

anaerobic energy – energy generated in the absence of oxygen.

ankle joint mortice – the point at which the tibia and fibula are held together by the syndesmosis in the ankle joint.

antagonist – a muscle whose action opposes the agonist; muscles relax to allow agonists to contract.

anterior talofibular ligament – the external lateral ligament between the talus and the fibula.

apophysis – a projection from a bone, or any other part of the body (e.g. the brain).

apophysitis calcanei – inflammation of the Achilles tendon attachment to the calcaneus in adolescents.

aponeurosis – a thin but strong fibrous sheet of tissue that replaces tendon in flat, sheetlike muscles.

arthritis – an inflammation of one or more joints, characterized by swelling, warmth, redness of the overlying skin, pain and restriction of motion.

arthrography – an X-ray technique for examining joints, using a contrast medium.

arthroscopy – the examination of a joint with the aid of an instrument (arthroscope) inserted into it to inspect contents before biopsy or operation.

aspiration – the withdrawal of fluid from body by means of suction.

athlete's foot – a fungal infection of the skin between the toes, a type of ringworm.

atrophy – the wasting away of a normally developed organ or tissue due to degeneration of cells.

autotraction – the traction with one's own muscle strength (or body weight).

avulsion fracture – tearing off of an attachment to a bone.

benign – describing a tumour that does not invade or destroy the tissue in which it originates or spread to distant sites in body (cf. malignant).

biceps – a muscle with two heads.

biceps brachii – the biceps muscle of the upper arm extending from shoulder joint to elbow.

biceps femoris muscle – the muscle situated at the back of the thigh, with two heads.

biofeedback – the giving of immediate information to a subject about body processes (e.g. heart) which are usually unconscious/involuntary.

biomechanics – the mechanical functioning of the human body.

bone marrow – the tissue contained within the internal cavities of bone.

bunion – a swelling of the joint between the big toe and the first metatarsal bone.

bursa – a small sac of fibrous tissue that is lined with a synovial membrane and filled with fluid (synovia).

bursa iliopectinea – the bursa in front of the hip joint.

bursa semimembranosa-gastrocnemia – the bursa in the hollow of the knee (Baker's cyst).

bursitis – an inflammation of a bursa resulting from injury, infection or rheumatoid synovitis.

bursography – an X-ray of a bursa using a contrast medium.

calcaneofibular ligament – the external lateral ligament between the calcaneus and the fibula.

calcaneomedialis nerve – the nerve on the inner side of the calcaneus (medial calcaneal branch of the tibial nerve).

calcaneus – the heel bone.

callus – a mass of blood and granulation tissue (containing bone-forming cells) that forms around a bone end following a fracture.

capitate – head-shaped – having a rounded extremity.

capitellum – (capitulum humen) the round prominence at elbow end of the humerus that articulates with the radius.

carpal tunnel – the space between carpal bones of the wrist and the connective tissue (retinaculum) over the flexor tendons; contains flexor tendons and median nerve.

cartilage – a dense connective tissue composed of a matrix produced by specialist cells called chondroblasts.

cerclage – a steel wire put in a loop around, e.g., a bone during surgery.

cervical brachialgia – a pain from the cervical back region which spreads to the arm.

cervical rhizopathy – a pain from the cervical back region; the pain radiates out into the arm along the area of the nerve.

chondromalacia patellae – the deterioration and softening of the articular cartilage of the patella.

chronic – of long duration involving very slow changes.

clavicle – the collar bone.

claw-foot – a foot with a high instep.

coagulation – blood clotting; process by which a colloidal liquid changes to a jellylike mass.

coccygeal vertebrae – the 4 rudimentary bones at lowest end of backbone; the vestigial human tail.

collagen – a relatively inelastic protein with high tensile strength that is the principle constituent of white fibrous connective tissue (as occurs in tendons).

compound fracture – a fracture in which the skin overlying the bone is lacerated or punctured.

compression – pressing together.

compression rupture – a rupture caused by impact.

concentric contraction – a

467

muscle contraction during simultaneous shortening of the muscle.

condyle – the rounded articular surface at the end of a bone.

conjunctiva – the delicate mucous membrane covering the front of the eye and lining the inside of the eyelids.

contraction – the shortening of a muscle in response to a motor nerve impulse; generates tension in muscle, usually causing movement.

contraindication – any factor in a patient's condition that makes it unwise to pursue a certain line of treatment.

contrast X-ray – an X-ray examination with a contrast medium.

contusions – (bruise) an area of skin discoloration caused by the escape of blood from ruptured underlying vessels following injury.

co-ordination – moving in harmony; the proper functioning of organs in relation to each other to produce the desired effect.

coraco-acromial ligament – the ligament between the beaklike coracoid process and the acromion process of the scapula.

coraco-clavicular ligament – the ligament between the coracoid process and the clavicle.

coracoid process – a beaklike process that curves upwards and forwards from the top of the scapula, over the shoulder joint.

core temperature – the inner temperature of the body.

cornea – the transparent anterior part of the fibrous coat of the eyeball.

costa – a rib.

costoclavicular ligament – a ligament between a rib and the clavicle.

coxa plana – the flattened hip joint ball (osteochondritis of the hip).

coxitis – an inflamation of the hip joint.

crepitus – a crackling sound or grating feeling produced by bone rubbing on bone or roughened cartilage.

cuneiform bones – the 3 bones in the ankle which articulate with the navicular bone.

cutaneous femoris lateralis nerve – the cutaneous nerve on the outer side of the thigh.

cyst – an abnormal sac or closed cavity lined with epithelium and filled with liquid or semisolid matter.

degeneration – the deterioration and loss of specialized function in the cells of a tissue or organ.

deltoid muscle – a thick triangular muscle that covers the shoulder joint and is responsible for raising the arm away from the side of the body.

detached retina – the separation of the retina from the layer of the eyeball to which it is attached.

diabetes – any disorder of metabolism causing excessive thirst and production of large volumes of urine. Used alone, the term most commonly refers to diabetes mellitus.

diabetes mellitus – a disorder of carbohydrate metabolism in which sugars in the body are not oxidized to produce energy due to lack of the pancreatic hormone, insulin.

digitorum longus muscle – the long muscle of a finger.

disc – a rounded flattened structure, such as an intervertebral disc or optic disc.

distal – situated away from the origin or point of attachment or from the median line of the body.

distension rupture – a rupture caused by overstretching.

dorsal – relating to or situated at or close to the back of the body or posterior part of an organ.

dorsiflexion – backward flexion of the foot or hand or their digits i.e. bending towards the upper surface.

dorsum – 1) the back, 2) the upper or posterior surface of a part of the body e.g. the hand.

drawer test – a test used to decide if there is instability in a joint.

dynamic muscle work – muscle work which varies the distance between the origin and attachment of a muscle either by shortening (concentric) or lengthening (eccentric) the muscle.

ectopic bone formation – the misplacement of a bone, due either to a congenital defect or an injury.

endorphin – one of a group of chemical compounds, including encephalins, that occurs naturally in the brain and has pain-relieving properties similar to those of the opiates.

enzyme – a protein that, in small amounts, speeds up the rate of a biological reaction without itself being used up in the reaction (i.e. acts as a catalyst).

epicondyle – the protuberance above a condyle at the end of an articulating bone.

epicondylitis – the inflammation of a muscle or tendon attachment to a protuberance of bone.

epiphyseal cartilage – the growth cartilage at the end of a long bone.

epiphysiolysis – the separation or loosening of an epiphysis from the shaft of the bone.

epiphysis – the end of a long bone, initially separated by cartilage from the shaft of the bone.

erythrocyte – (red blood cell) a blood cell containing the pigment, haemoglobin, the principal function of which is to transport oxygen.

eversion – a turning outward.

exostosis – a benign cartilaginous outgrowth from a bone.

extensor – any muscle that causes the straightening of a limb or other part.

extensor carpi radialis brevis – the short extensor of the radial side of the wrist.

extensor communis digitorum – the common extensor on the radial side of the wrist.

extensor proprius hallucia – the extensor of the big toe.

external fixation – a structure fitted to the outside of the body.

extraoral – outside the mouth cavity.

extrinsic – external; originating outside any particular structure or organism.

facet – a small flat surface on a bone, especially a surface of articulation.

faradic current – a rapidly alternating electric current used to stimulate nerve and muscle activity.

fascia – the connective tissue forming membranous layers of variable thickness in all regions of the body.

fasciculus – a bundle, e.g. of nerve or muscle fibres.

femoral head – the head of the femur.

femoral hernia – a protusion at the top of the femur.

femoralis anteriores cutanei nerve – the nerve that runs at the front of the groin and thigh.

femur – the thigh bone.

fibrocartilage – a tough kind of cartilage in which there are dense bundles of fibres in the matrix.

fibula – the long thin external bone of the lower leg.

flexibility training – a training technique (both active and passive) to improve joint mobility, strength, co-ordination and proprioception.

flexion – the bending of a joint so that the bones forming it are brought towards each other.

fossa – a depression or hollow.

fracture – the breakage of a bone, that may be transverse, oblique, spiral or comminuted.

fusion – (in surgery) the joining together of two structures.

ganglion – any structure containing a collection of nerve cell bodies and often a number of synapses.

gastrocnemius – a muscle that forms the greater part of the calf of the leg; it flexes the knee and foot so that the toes point downwards.

gel – a colloidal suspension that has set to form a jelly.

genitofemoral nerve – cutaneous (skin) nerve that supplies the genitalia and the thigh.

genu valgum – the abnormal in-curving of the legs, resulting in excessive separation of the feet when the knees are in contact.

glenoid cavity – the socket of the shoulder joint.

glenoid labrum – the fibrocartilaginous rim attached to the margin of the glenoid cavity.

glucose – a simple sugar containing six carbon atoms.

gluteus – one of three paired muscles of the buttocks responsible for movements of the thigh: gluteus maximus, gluteus medius and gluteus minimus.

glycogen – a carbohydrate consisting of branched chains of glucose units; the principle form in which carbohydrate is stored in the body.

gracilis muscle – the muscle that runs internally along the femur from the body of the pubis to the upper part of the tibia.

granulation – the growth of small rounded outgrowths, made up of small blood vessels and connective tissue, on the healing surface of a wound or an ulcer.

haematoma – an accumulation of blood within the tissues that clots to form a solid swelling.

haemobursa – an accumulation of blood within the bursa.

haemoglobin – a substance contained within red blood cells, responsible for their colour, and binding and carrying oxygen.

haemorrhage – (bleeding) the escape of blood from a ruptured blood vessel, externally or internally.

haemosiderin – a substance composed of a protein shell containing iron salts which may be present inside certain cells, being one form of iron storage in the body.

hallux – the big toe.

hallux rigidus – the loss of movement in the big toe, causing pain on walking.

hallux valgus – the fixed displacement of the big toe towards the other toes.

hamate bone – the hook-shaped bone of the wrist.

hammer toe – a deformity of the toe, most often the second toe, caused by fixed flexion of the first joint.

hamstring – any of the tendons at the back of the knee. They attach the hamstring muscles (the biceps femoris, semitendinosus and semimembranosus) to their insertions in the tibia and fibula.

head – the rounded portion of a bone which fits into a groove of another bone to form a joint (e.g the head of humerus or femur).

hernia – the protrusion of an organ or tissue out of the body cavity in which it normally lies.

heterotopic bone formation –

formation of a bone in a displaced position.

humerus – the bone of the upper arm.

hydrocele – the accumulation of watery liquid in a sac, usually the sac around the testes.

hydrops – an excessive accumulation of fluid in the body tissues.

hyperextension – an excessive and forceful extension of a limb beyond the normal limits, usually as part of an orthopaedic procedure to correct deformity.

hyperflexion – the forcible bending of a limb to a degree greater than normal.

hypertrophy – an increase in the size of a tissue or organ brought about by the enlargement of its cells rather than by cell multiplication.

illio–inguinal nerve – a cutaneous nerve that supplies the groin area.

ilio–psoas muscle – the composite muscle that bends the hip joint.

ilio–tibial band – the tendon that connects the ilium to the tibia.

ilium – the haunch bone: a wide bone forming the upper part of each side of the hip bone.

immobilization – the procedure of making a normally movable part of the body, such as a joint, immovable.

indication – a strong reason for believing that a particular course of action is desirable.

infraspinatus muscle – a muscle which extends from the spine of the scapula to the greater tuberosity of the humerus.

inguinal hernia – the protusion of a sac of peritoneum, containing fat or part of the bowel, through a weak part of the abdominal wall.

insufficiency – the inability of an organ or part of the body

to carry out its normal function.

internal fixation – the surgical procedure used to stabilize a fracture with the aid of a splint or pin.

intermuscular – between muscles, or among muscles.

interosseal membrane – a membrane placed or occurring between bones which serves to connect them.

interphalangeal joint – the joint between two phalanges.

intervertebral disc – the flexible plate of fibrocartilage that connects any two adjacent vertebrae in the backbone.

intra–articular – with a joint or inside the cavity of a joint.

intramuscular – occurring within the contents of a muscle.

intraoral – occurring inside the mouth cavity.

iritis – the inflammation of the iris.

isokinetic training – a form of muscle training performed at a constant speed and against an adjustable resistance.

isometric training – a form of muscle training used to increase the strength and cross-sectional area of the muscle after injury.

isotonic training – a form of muscle training performed at a constant level of muscular tension, under varying speeds.

'itis – suffix denoting inflammation of an organ, tissue, etc.

joint – the point at which two or more bones are connected.

kinetics – a branch of science which deals with motion produced in bodies by the forces acting upon them.

kyphosis – an excessive outward curvature of the spine, causing hunching of the back.

larynx – the organ responsible for the production of vocal sounds, also serving as an air passage conveying air from the pharynx to the lungs.

lateral – situated relating at or to the side of an organ or organism.

lateral condyle of the femur – the protuberance on the outer side of the lower end of the femur.

lateral malleolus – the protuberance on the outer side of the ankle (the 'outer ankle')

latissimus dorsi – the broad flat triangular muscle of the back and lower chest.

laxity – atrophy, looseness.

ligament – a tough band of white fibrous connective tissue that links two bones together at a joint.

ligamentum patellae – the ligament of the kneecap (the patellar tendon).

limbus – a cartilaginous border which surrounds the edge of the socket of the hip joint.

loose body – a fragment of bone or cartilage that freely moves within a joint.

lumbago – lower backache, of any cause or description.

lumbar – relating to the loin.

lunate bone – a bone of the wrist.

luxation – see dislocation.

lymph – the fluid present within the vessels of the lymphatic system, consisting of the fluid that bathes the tissues, derived from the blood and drained by the lymphatic vessels.

malacia – abnormal softening of a part, organ or tissue, such as bone.

malleolus – either of the two protuberances on each side of the tarsus.

maxilla – either of the pair of bones forming the upper jaw.

medial – relating to or situated in the central region of an organ, tissue or the body.

medial tibioperiostitis – an inflammation of the bone membrane on the inside edge of the tibia.

median nerve – one of the main nerves of the forearm and hand.

membrane – a thin layer of tissue surrounding the whole or part of an organ or tissue lining a cavity or separating adjacent structures or cavities.

meniscus – a crescent-shaped structure such as the fibrocartilaginous disc that divides the cavity of a synovial joint.

metabolism – the sum of all the chemical and physical changes which take place within the body and enable its growth and function.

metatarsal bones – the bones of the foot that connect the tarsus to the phalanges.

monocentric hinge – a hinge with one plane of pivot.

morbus – disease.

Morton's metatarsalgia – a pain in the region of the heads of the metatarsal bones.

mucous membrane – the moist membrane lining many tubular structures and cavities in the body.

muscle belly – the bulging central portion of a muscle.

muscle–tendon junction – the point at which a muscle merges into a tendon.

musculo–skeletal – relating to or composed of muscles and bones.

myelography – a specialized method of X-ray examination of the spinal canal with the injection of a contrast medium.

myositis – any group of muscle diseases in which inflammation and degenerative changes occur.

navicular bone – the boat-shaped bone of the tarsus.

necrosis – the death of some or all of the cells in an organ or tissue caused by injury, disease or lack of blood supply.

neuritis – a disease of the peripheral nerves showing the pathological changes of inflammation.

neuroma – a benign tumour growing from the fibrous coverings of a peripheral nerve.

neuromuscular – relating to or composed of nerves and muscles.

nodule – a small swelling or aggregation of cells.

obturator nerve – the nerve that passes through the large opening (obturator foramen) in the hip bone.

oedema – an excessive accumulation of fluid in the body tissues popularly known as dropsy.

olecranon process – the large process of the ulna that projects behind the elbow joint.

orthopaedics – the science or practice of correcting deformities caused by disease or damage to the bones and joints of the skeleton.

orthosis – the procedure of adjusting or otherwise correcting deformity e.g. in the foot.

osteitis pubis – an inflammation of the pubic bone.

oesteoarthritis – a disease of joint cartilage (associated with secondary changes in the underlying bone) which may ultimately cause pain and impair function of the affected joint.

osteochondritis – an inflammation of a bone associated with pain.

osteochondritis dissecans – the release of a small fragment (or fragments) of bone and cartilage into a joint (frequently the knee) with resultant pain, swelling and limitation of movement.

osteomyelitis – an inflammation of the bone marrow due to infection.

osteophyte – a projection of bone shaped like a rose thorn that occurs at sites of cartilage degeneration or destruction.

pain threshold – the level at which the sensation of pain becomes apparent.

palmar – relating to the palm of the hand.

palpation – the process of examining a part of the body by careful feeling with the hands and fingertips.

patella – the lens-shaped bone that forms the kneecap.

patello–femoral joint – the joint between the patella and the femur.

pectineus muscle – a small adductor in the groin.

pectoralis major – a large fan-shaped muscle (the pectoral muscle) that works over the shoulder joint, drawing the arm forwards across the chest and rotating it medially.

pelvospondylitis ossificans – ossifying inflammation of the pelvic portion of the spine.

periosteum – a layer of dense connective tissue that covers the surface of a bone, except at the articular surfaces.

periostitis – an inflammation of the periosteum surrounding a knee.

peripheral nervous system – all parts of the nervous system lying outside the central nervous system (brain and spinal cord)

peritendinitis – an inflammation of a tendon sheath.

peritoneum – the serous membrane of the abdominal cavity.

peroneal tendons – the tendons of the muscles that arise from the fibula.

peroneus brevis muscle – the short muscle of the leg that arises from the fibula.

peroneus longus muscle – the long muscle of the leg that arises from the fibula.

pes cavus – (claw-foot) an excessively arched foot, giving an unnaturally high instep.

phalanx – (phalanges) the bones of the fingers and toes.

plantar – relating to the sole of the foot.

plantar aponeurosis – the arch sheet in the sole of the foot.

plantar fasciitis – an inflammation of the origin of the arch sheet.

plantaris lateralis nerve (the external plantar nerve) – the nerve on the outer side of the sole of the foot.

plantaris medialis nerve (the internal plantar nerve) – the nerve on the inner side of the sole of the foot.

plasma – (blood plasma) the straw-coloured fluid in which the blood cells are suspended.

pneumothorax – air in the pleural cavity causing collapse of the lungs.

polycentric hinge – a hinge which can move in all directions.

popliteal – relating to the space behind the knee joint.

popliteus muscle – a flat triangular muscle stretching from the lateral condyle of the femur to the upper part of the posterior surface of the tibia.

process – (in anatomy) a thin prominence or protuberance of bone.

prognosis – the assessment of the future course and outcome of a patient's disease.

pronation – the act of turning the hand or foot so that the palm or sole faces downwards.

prophylaxis – any means to prevent disease, such as immunization.

proprioception – the ability to apprehend positional changes of parts of the body or degrees of muscular activity without the aid of sight.

prostrate gland – a male accessory sex gland that opens into the urethra just below the bladder and vas deferens.

prostatis – an inflammation of the prostate gland.

prosthesis – any artificial device that is attached to the body as an aid.

proximal – situated close to the origin or point of attachment or close to the median line of the body.

pseudoarthrosis – a false joint formed around a displaced bone end after dislocation.

psoas muscle – a muscle in the groin that acts jointly with the iliacus muscle to flex the hip joint.

quadriceps extensor muscle – the great muscle in the front of the thigh which possesses four heads.

radial – relating to or associated with the radius.

radial nerve – the nerve on the radial (outer) side of the arm.

radiography – the technique of examining the body by directing X-rays through it to produce images on photographic plates or fluorescent screens.

radius – the outer and shorter bone of the forearm, which particularly revolves around the ulna.

rectus abdominus muscle – the long straight muscle that extends bilaterally along the entire length of the abdomen.

rectus femoris muscle – the straight muscle in front of the thigh (part of the quadriceps).

rehabilitation – the treatment of an ill, injured or disabled patient by massage, electrotherapy and graduated exercises to restore normal health and functions, or to prevent the disability from getting worse.

residual condition – a problem that remains after injury or illness.

resilient arches – the arches of the foot that will resume their original form after pronation or supination.

retinaculum – a thickened band of tissue that serves to hold various tissues in place.

rheumatoid arthritis – a form of arthritis that is the second most common rheumatic disease.

rhizopathy – see cervical rhizopathy.

rotator – a muscle that brings about rotation of a part of the body.

rotator cuff – the area of mergence of the tendons of the subscapularis, supraspinatus, infraspinatus and teres minor muscles.

Ruben's bubble – a rubber bubble used to support breathing.

rupture – the bursting apart or opening of an organ or tissue; tear.

sacral vertebrae – the five vertebrae that are fused together to form the sacrum.

sacro–iliac joint – the joint between the sacrum and the ilium.

sacrum – a curved triangular element of the backbone.

sartorius – the narrow ribbon-like muscle at the front of the thigh, arising from the anterior superior spine of the ilium and extending to the tibia, just below the knee.

scapula – the shoulder blade; a triangular bone, a pair of which form the back part of the shoulder girdle.

sciatica – the pain felt down the back and outer side of the thigh, leg and foot.

sciatic nerve – the major nerve of the leg and the nerve with the largest diameter.

sclerosis – a hardening of tissues, usually due to scarring after inflammation.

scoliosis – a lateral deviation of the backbone caused by congential or acquired abnormalities of the vertebrae, muscle and nerves.

semimembranosus muscle – so called from its membranous tendon of origin; part of the muscles at the back of the thigh.

semitendinosus muscle – remarkable for the great length of its tendon; part of the muscles at the back of the thigh.

separation – dislocation

serratus anterior muscle – one of several muscles arising from or inserted by a series of processes that resemble the teeth of a saw; a chest muscle.

sesamoid bone – an oval nodule of bone that lies within a tendon and slides over another bony surface e.g. patella.

sheath – the layer of connective tissue that envelopes structures such as nerves, arteries, tendons and muscles.

simple fracture (closed fracture) – fracture with no break in the underlying skin.

slipped disc – 'herniated disc'. Protrusion of the inner pulpy material of an intervertebral disc through the fibrous outer coat causing pressure on adjoining nerve roots etc.

soft tissues – muscles, tendons, ligaments, joint capsules, nerves, etc.

soleus – the broad flat muscle of the calf of the leg, beneath the gastrocnemius muscle.

sphincter – a specialized ring of muscle that surrounds an orifice.

spinal stenosis – the narrowing of the spinal canal.

spinous process – the sharp process of a vertebra.

splint – a rigid support to maintain a part of the body in a set position (usually temporary).

spondylolisthesis – a forward shift of one vertebra upon another due to a defect of the joints that normally bind them together.

spondylolysis – a split in a vertebral arch.

spondylosis – the degeneration of the intervertebral discus in the cervical, thoracic or lumbar regions of the backbone.

spongy bone – bone marrow.

static exercise – a type of muscle training without movement.

stellate fracture – a star-shaped fracture of the knee cap caused by a direct blow.

stenosis – the abnormal narrowing of a passage or opening e.g. blood vessel.

sterno–clavicular ligaments – the ligaments between the sternum and the clavicle.

sternum – the breastbone.

strength training – a type of training used to increase the strength and diameter of a muscle by exercising with weights.

subacute – describing a disease that progresses more rapidly than a chronic condition but does not become acute.

subluxation – the partial dislocation of a joint so that the bone ends are misaligned but still in contact.

subscapularis muscle – muscle that extends from the deep surface of the scapula to the lesser tuberosity of the humerus and turns the arm inwards at the shoulder joint.

subungual exostosis – a bone outgrowth beneath a nail.

supination – the act of turning the hand or foot inward so that the palm or sole is uppermost.

supinator muscle – the muscle that turns the forearm inwards in relation to the elbow.

supine – lying on the back or with the face upwards; palm of hand face upwards.

supraspinatus muscle – the muscle situated above the spine of the scapula; turns outward at the shoulder joint and lifts the arm outwards at

an angle of 80–120° to the body.

suture – (in surgery) the closure of a wound or incision with material such as silk or catgut to facilitate the healing process.

syndesmosis – an immovable joint in which the bones are separated by connective tissue e.g. the articulation between the bases of the tibia and fibula.

syndrome – a combination of signs and/or symptoms that form a distinct clinical picture indicative of a particular disorder.

synovia – (synovial fluid) the thick colourless lubricating fluid that surrounds a joint or bursa and fills a tendon sheath; secreted by the synovial membrane.

talus – (astragalus) the ankle bone that forms part of the tarsus.

tarsus – the seven bones of the ankle and proximal part of the foot.

tendinitis – an inflammation of a tendon, often after excessive overuse.

tendon – a tough whitish cord consisting of numerous parallel bundles of collagen fibres that serves to attach a muscle to a bone.

tennis elbow – a painful inflammation of the tendon at the outer border of the elbow, caused by overuse of the forearm muscles.

tenoperiostitis – an inflammation of a tendon attachment to a muscle.

tenosynovitis – an inflammation of the tendon sheath.

tenovaginitis – an inflammatory thickening of the fibrous sheath containing one of more tendons.

tensor – any muscle that causes stretching or tensing of a part of the body.

tensor fasciae latae muscle
(tensor fasciae femoris) – the
tensor muscle of the thigh
fascia; extends from the crest
of the hip to the outer side of
the femur.

thoracic vertebrae – the twelve
bones of the backbone to
which the ribs are attached.

tibia – the shin bone; the inner
and larger bone of the lower
leg.

tibialis anterior muscle – the
muscle at the back of the tibia
that turns the foot inwards and
flexes the toes backwards.

tibialis posterior muscle – the
muscle at the back of the tibia
that extends the toes and
inverts the foot.

tomography – the technique of
using X-rays or ultrasound
waves to produce an image of
a structure at a particular depth
within the body, bringing them
into sharp focus while
deliberately blurring structures
at other depths.

tonus – (tone) the normal state
of partial contraction of a
resting muscle maintained by
reflex activity.

torque – a force producing
rotation.

torsion – twisting.

torticollis – an irresistible
turning movement of the head
that becomes more persistent
so that eventually the head is
held continually to one side.

tourniquet – a device to press
upon an artery and prevent
flow of blood through it.

transcutaneous – through the
skin.

transverse – situated at right
angles to the long axis of the
body or an organ.

trapezius dorsi muscle –
extends from the cervical and
thoracic back region to the
clavicle and scapula.

trauma – a physical wound or
injury e.g. fracture or blow.

triceps – a muscle with three
heads or origins, particularly
the triceps brachii which is
situated on the back of the
upper arm and contracts to
extend the forearm.

trochanter major – (the great
trochanter) a protuberance at
the upper part of the femur
below its neck.

tuberculum majus – (the great
tuberosity) the major tendon
attachment in the articular
head of the humerus.

tuberculum minus – (the lesser
tuberosity) the minor tendon
attachment of the patellar
tendon to the fibula.

tuberosity – a large rounded
protuberance on a bone.

ulna – the inner and longer bone
of the forearm.

ulnar nerve – one of the major
nerves in the arm.

valgus – describing any
deformity that displaces the
hand or foot away from the
midline.

varus – describing any deformity
that displaces the hand or foot
towards the midline.

vertebra – one of thirty-three
bones of which the backbone
is composed.

viscosity – semi-liquidity;
stickiness.

wart – (verruca) a small (often
hard) benign growth in the
skin.

zygomatic bone – either of a
pair of bones that form the
prominent part of the cheeks
and contribute to the orbits.

Index